AF615750

INDIVIDUAL ONSITE WASTEWATER SYSTEMS

Proceedings of the Sixth National Conference 1979

Sponsored by
National Sanitation Foundation

Edited by

NINA I. McCLELLAND

President
National Sanitation Foundation
Ann Arbor, Michigan

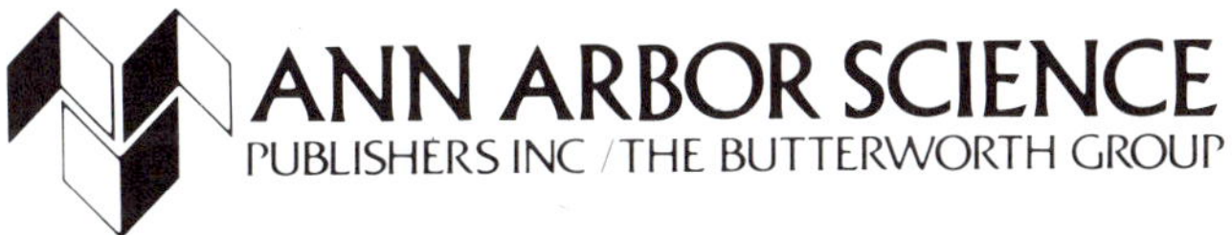

230 Collingwood, P.O. Box 1425, Ann Arbor, Michigan 48106

Library of Congress Catalog Card No. 76-50983
ISBN 0-250-40345-5

Manufactured in the United States of America

PREFACE

The theme of the Sixth National Conference on Individual Onsite Wastewater Systems was "Learning from Experience." Speakers and topics were selected to assure that the audience would be exposed not only to theory, but to actual experiences with onsite alternatives.

This series of conferences, held annually since 1974, has provided a forum for communication between professionals and users concerned with effective utilization of onsite wastewater systems. The kinds of problems for which onsite treatment and disposal should appropriately be considered, selection criteria, management strategies and techniques for rejuvenating failed systems are described in the current publication. Proceedings of each of the preceding conferences are available.

A seventh national conference, cosponsored by the National Sanitation Foundation and the U.S. Environmental Protection Agency, is planned for September 1980.

Nina I. McClelland

Nina I. McClelland is President of the National Sanitation Foundation, Ann Arbor, Michigan, where she oversees the management of research, education and service in environmental quality; and standards development, evaluation and listing services for products and equipment related to health and environment.

Before becoming President, Dr. McClelland was, in turn, Vice President, Technical Services, Director of the NSF Water Research Program and Director of Technical Services. She has been Chemist-Bacteriologist and Chief Chemist in charge of wastewater treatment and industrial waste control for the City of Toledo, Ohio, and holds a Class A Certificate for the Operation of Wastewater Treatment Plants in the state of Ohio.

Dr. McClelland is a nonresident lecturer in the School of Public Health at the University of Michigan. She formerly taught Sanitary Chemistry at the University of Toledo School of Engineering.

She received her BS and MS Degrees from the University of Toledo, and her MPH and PhD Degrees from the University of Michigan. She has written 34 papers on water and wastewater treatment that have been published in technical journals or presented at scientific conferences. She is also a co-author of the Ann Arbor Science eight-volume work, *Applied Chemistry of Wastewater Treatment*, a programmed learning text for wastewater treatment operators, along with K. H. Mancy of the University of Michigan and F. G. Pohland, Georgia Institute of Technology.

A member of numerous professional organizations, she is especially active in the American Chemical Society, the American Public Health Association, the American Water Works Association and the Water Pollution Control Federation. Dr. McClelland was one of the first technical consultants for Ann Arbor Science Publishers, Inc., and is a member of its Editorial Advisory Board.

IN MEMORIAM

It is noted, with a sense of great loss and deep regret, that Paul G. Moe and his associate Raul Zaltzman were fatally injured in an auto accident on February 27, 1980. Paul served with effectiveness as a member of the planning committee for the Sixth National Conference and also as a conference participant. The knowledge and experience as well as the personal and professional cooperation contributed by these colleagues will be missed by all who were associated with them.

Editor

CONTENTS

1

KEYNOTE ADDRESS

The Honorable Jennings Randolph
Senator of West Virginia
United States Senate
Public Works Committee
Washington, D.C. 20510

We all face periods of transition in our national, personal and professional lives. A time of change can often be an uncertain departure from the familiar. I believe that in the sanitation field, and in environmental issues in general, we are in the midst of such a period.

Our national environmental policies and our concern for the environment have undergone great change in the past 25 years. It was in 1956 that the U.S. Congress passed the legislation that first resulted in the federal government upgrading sanitation facilities. That original effort was modest by today's standards, only a $50 million program operated by the Department of the Interior. It was a relatively small beginning, but the beginning of a great transition in our commitment to protecting the fragile environment on which we all depend.

The establishment of the U.S. Environmental Protection Agency (EPA) in 1970 was another step toward reversing the decades of neglect that had fouled so many of our rivers and lakes. The Federal Water Pollution Control Act of 1972 (FWPCA) has served us well in our efforts toward a cleaner and healthier environment. That law has enabled EPA to make more than 12,000 grants to states, cities and towns totaling more than $18 billion. This Act also has allowed EPA to grant funds for up to 75% of eligible project costs. The federal program for the construction of municipal sanitation facilities became the largest single public works program in the nation.

We are now in the process of implementing a program proposed by the

President that will provide more than $40 billion over a 10-year period. The Clean Water Act of 1977 is a component of that effort. In the fiscal year just ended, $4.2 billion were provided under the Act.

The Clean Water Act continued our ongoing commitment and expanded these efforts. This expansion marked another program transition—recognition of the ability of alternative and innovative approaches to solve many sanitation problems, particularly in our rural areas. This latest transition clearly has an effect on many of you attending this conference. You are the pioneers who realized the need for this new dimension in our national program long before we did in Washington. While many of you have pioneered this step, others feel the uncertainty and hesitancy of this approach. New regulations, new policies and unfamiliar procedures have had an effect.

I will not discuss in detail the particular provisions that have brought about this transitional period. I am sure you are acquainted with the provisions of the Act that make available substantial sums of federal money for alternatives to conventional collection and treatment systems.

The Act's impact to date can be seen now with the benefit of more than a full year of operation. The alternative and innovative amendments became effective on October 1, 1978, almost 13 months ago. As with any transitional period, everything has not proceeded as smoothly or rapidly as those of us concerned with rural problems may have hoped. After one year the review is mixed. Perhaps some of you are disappointed that the program has not moved more rapidly. I share that concern. Earlier this month, Chris Beck, who has been nominated to be Assistant EPA Administrator for water, appeared before the Public Works Committee, of which I am chairman. I emphasized the importance we place on the alternative systems program. It must be fully and vigorously implemented, and I intend to see that it is. Tables I and II indicate the status of the alternatives and innovative programs.

Under provisions of the Clean Water Act, a set aside of 2% of each state's allocation was provided to allow extra funding for projects that used alternatives or innovative processes. This allowed EPA to award up to an 85% grant to qualified projects, rather than the usual 75%.

On a national basis, a total of $84 million was available in fiscal year 1979. This included $21 million for innovative projects and $63 million for projects using alternative processes. As of September 30, EPA has awarded only $7.4 million for 28 innovative projects, about one-third of the available funds. In the alternative category, $33.9 million has been awarded to 134 projects. This constitutes slightly better than a 54% utilization.

If these figures seem low, we must keep in mind that this has been a transitional year and that the program will take time to reach its full potential. We should also remember that the states have another 11 months in

Table I. The 4% Set Aside Alternatives for Rural Areas as of September 30, 1979[a]

Amount Available ($ millions)	State	Number of Projects	Amount Used ($ millions)	Amount Used (%)
1.2	Maine	2	0.1	8
6.8	Michigan	1	2.1	31
0.9	Nebraska	10	0.8	89
0.8	North Dakota	3	0.1	13
0.8	Wyoming	1	0.4	50
0.8	Alaska	2	0.4	50
0.8	Idaho	9	2.5	313
2.1	Oregon	1	0.3	14
2.9	Washington	3	2.9	100

[a]FY 1979: $168 million available; $9.8 million used in 33 projects; and $158.2 million unused, or 6%.

Table II. The 2% Set Aside Under Section 202(a)(2) as of September 30, 1979 (utilization by EPA regions)

	Amount Set Aside ($ millions)			Projects Processed			Funds Used ($ millions)			Projects Received for Review			
Regions	1	A	Total	1	A	Total	1	A	Total	1	A	Total	Amount Used (%)
1	1.4	4.2	5.6	1	6	7	1.4	1.7	3.1	2	6	8	55
2	3.2	9.6	12.8	6	7	13	0.8	2.2	3.0	4	14	18	23
3	2.5	7.4	9.8	1	3	4	0.3	1.8	2.1	1	3	4	21
4	2.9	8.8	11.7	2	7	9	1.4	10.0	11.4	5	22	27	97
5	4.6	13.9	18.5	7	21	28	2.2	1.4	3.6	4	17	21	19
6	1.6	4.8	6.4	6	35	41	0.3	1.1	1.4	1	2	3	22
7	1.1	3.2	4.4	5	20	25	0.1	0.7	0.8	17	88	105	18
8	0.7	2.1	2.8	0	10	10	0	4.2	4.2	0	12	12	15
9	2.1	6.4	8.5	0	21	21	0	6.4	6.4	9	103	112	75
10	0.8	2.5	3.3	1	10	11	0.7	4.7	5.4	4	8	12	164

which to finance projects out of the first year's allocation. However, there must not be unnecessary delays, and initiating a new program cannot be an excuse for inaction. The Congress believed that new technologies must be developed and used. Innovation must be encouraged, and we will not permit this effort to be given secondary status.

Under another section of the Act, which I sponsored in the Senate, another set aside of 4% is provided for those states with a rural population of 25% or more. These funds are to be used for alternatives to conventional systems in rural areas. The initial year of this program appears to be less successful than we had hoped. Of the $85.9 million available to the rural states, less than $10 million was approved by the end of the fiscal year.

The state of Washington leads the nation in funding projects using alternative technologies. Three projects have been funded in Washington that used all of that state's $2.9 million set aside. Idaho has nine projects totaling $2.5 million using alternative technology. Here in Michigan, two projects have been approved for $2.1 million. Six other states have approved one or more projects, including Maine, Nebraska, North Dakota, Wyoming, Alaska and Oregon.

There are still 25 states with the mandatory 4% set aside that have yet to approve a project using alternative processes. I regret that my home state of West Virginia is among this group. Certainly we have great need in rural West Virginia and elsewhere to help our citizens with the development of basic sanitation services. In fact, it was the West Virginia situation in particular that stimulated my support of efforts to encourage alternative technologies.

The need for the utilization of new processes is obvious in a great many areas; however, acceptance of these techniques is often slow at all levels of government. Earlier this year, the National Association of Home Builders conducted a survey to determine the acceptance of various types of alternatives. The results show us that we have much work ahead.

The highest level of acceptance among all levels of state, county and local governments was package plants and multiple-home septic tank systems. These were each accepted by approximately 32% of a cross section of government jurisdictions. Land application was next with only 17% acceptance. Acceptance of other techniques was even lower.

In the years ahead, the wisdom of the transition to alternative and innovative techniques for meeting rural wastewater problems will become evident. These techniques will bring substantial savings to the taxpayers. As these savings become known, I am confident that more jurisdictions will accept these methods.

The first hints at the substantial savings are now just beginning to be felt. For example, a sanitation system was proposed in Indiana that included 65 miles of collection lines plus treatment facilities. The estimated cost of this system was $23.2 million. However, EPA has concluded that upgraded onsite systems with central management can provide this area with an efficient sanitation system for $8.3 million. This represents a savings on one project of $14.9 million.

The savings can, of course, be counted in more than one way. In the

Indiana project, for example, the savings at the federal level is coupled with savings to the individual homeowner. I am told that to pay for the construction cost of the onsite system will require only one-tenth as much in monthly costs from each homeowner as for the central system.

Most projects will perhaps represent more modest reductions in cost. However, in the hundreds and possibly thousands of projects in which alternative processes can be used, even more modest savings per project can save us tens of millions of dollars.

Because $75 million remains unobligated from the fiscal year 1979 set aside, one might conclude this effort to have failed. We must remember, however, that this money is available for steps 2 and 3 only, that is, for final design and actual construction. The step one feasibility study, which takes considerable time and effort, must be approved before these funds can be awarded. I understand that while only 33 projects were actually approved last year, many are currently proceeding through the feasibility stage.

It is not only the availability of federal funding that makes alternative and innovative technologies appealing. Private business has seen the potential in such systems to solve problems that cannot be addressed by conventional means.

Later in this conference, you will hear about recent product innovations from several manufacturers. This constant development of new products is a vital function of our free enterprise system. Many of you are pioneers in this field and have come a long way in the development and use of alternative and innovative processes, largely on your own initiative in a field that is still very young. Bear in mind, however, that you have support including my own. I wish you success here and I pledge my continued support.

2

PRACTICE, POLICY, EXPERIENCE: WHERE ARE WE?

R. M. Brown
President, National Sanitation Foundation
Ann Arbor, Michigan 48105

As we begin this Sixth National Conference, I wish to help you understand as precisely as possible what the major thrust of this particular conference has been designed to be. Also, we would ask that at the close of the conference you be prepared to express your best judgment about where we are with the development and utilization of onsite systems and their related technology. The issues interrelate in both instances, and the manner in which you respond to them will, in large measure, reflect your appraisal of current progress with onsite system technology.

Since the First National Conference in 1974, much has happened in the utilization of onsite systems. In just five years we have progressed from the general belief that if septic tanks followed by subsurface disposal were not acceptable, land should not—and could not—be developed, to a beginning acceptance of total reuse technology. It is also recognized that alternatives may be cost-effective for clusters of homes and small community applications. This is progress that could not have been anticipated prior to these conferences.

To identify current practices and regulatory policies, we queried 50 state agencies asking for information we could share with you during this Sixth Onsite Conference. From the 42 states that responded to the questionnaires, we learned that it is usually a dual state and local responsibility to determine the acceptability of onsite wastewater systems. Further, we learned that nearly all of the respondents are using alternatives exclusive of septic tank–soil absorption systems, including home aerobic plants, recycle systems, composting toilets, elevated sand mounds, evapotranspiration and pressure sewers. Eighteen states indicated that they permit surface discharge of effluent from onsite systems. Recycle fluid can be used for flushing, lawn watering and, in some locations, for laundry. Many states have revised their codes as a direct result of implementation of the U.S. Environmental Protection Agency's (EPA) regulations relating to the Clean Water Act Amendments of 1977, which were introduced by Senator Jennings Randolph, our distinguished keynote speaker (see Appendixes A and B).

This year's conference planning committee assembled a series of presentations of real life experience with onsite systems, including programs and their successful resolution; selection criteria; online systems that are innovative applications or technologies; operation, maintenance and management programs; and correction of failed systems.

Since the early 1970s we have known that our energy resources were becoming increasingly scarce; but changes required to cope with the problem have been met with doubt and reluctance. Now we are becoming aware that our western states can soon anticipate a water shortage that may rival our current energy crisis in severity. There is a need now to implement the changes necessary to help minimize problems in the potentially water-short areas. The alternative systems and their appropriate applications can play a key role; however, there are recognized responsibilities with all parties. They must be selected, installed, maintained and managed properly, or they will fail.

To date, some of our experiences can be termed "successful," some not. Nevertheless the circumstances should not be judged only by a pass or fail, success or failure, but in terms of "why" or underlying factors that contributed to the favorable or unfavorable result. If a baker has two cakes in the oven and one falls while the other does not, it is just as important for him to know what he did right to produce the cake that did *not* fall as to know what he did wrong with the cake that failed. In other words, it is just as important to know what is necessary to achieve a favorable result as what contributes to an unfavorable one.

Cases will be presented that relate various experiences. Listen to learn "what went right" or "what went wrong." If those answers are not apparent, inquiries about them should be made. Opinion or appraisal of the particular circumstances may vary depending on whether they are from a manufacturer, a regulatory person, a developer/home builder, a consultant or homeowner. Ultimate evaluation and decision stems from a weighing and reconciliation of even diverging views when group objectives are defined and understood.

Some other questions that should be present during these presentations are: (1) What has worked and what hasn't? Equipment? Policies? Why?

(2) Have we refined and improved our judgment processes? (3) Are we making real progress or merely trading off? (4) How is society benefiting from our efforts? and (5) Will lifestyle adaptations be necessary to achieve even greater progress?

At this point in the development and utilization of onsite systems, we should be able to assess collectively our current experience and progress in a way that will help us to chart a future course. Therefore, it is expected that you will actively contribute to an appraisal and evaluation process that will be made available to you. During the Conference you will be asked to complete an opinion and judgment survey form to help us to determine further, in group judgment, where we are, what is right or wrong, and what we need to address in the immediate future to achieve the most effective application of onsite system technology. The response obtained (see Appendix C) not only will provide us with important information, but may well start shaping the program for the Seventh National Conference in 1980.

It is our hope that this Sixth National Conference challenges you both in expectation and obligation. May your expectations be met in what the conference contributes in knowledge and inspiration. Your obligation can be met in part through your expression of judgment as to how effectively we are serving society with onsite system technology.

APPENDIX A: THE ONSITE WASTEWATER POLICY QUESTIONNAIRE

The Onsite Wastewater Policy Questionnaire was mailed to the states' agency(ies) with oversight responsibility for onsite wastewater systems with the following instruction:

> "We would like to compile information about current state and local policies with respect to onsite alternatives . . . . Would you complete the enclosed questionnaire and return it to us *at your earliest opportunity*? Would you also enclose for our file . . . a copy of your current state code, regulations, and/or policies relating to onsite wastewater systems? Would you also identify who in one of the local agencies within your state could provide us with a copy of local codes, regulations, and/or policies . . . ?"

The codes, regulations and/or policies, as well as the names of local contacts for many of the respondent states, are on file at the National Sanitation Foundation.

ONSITE WASTEWATER POLICY QUESTIONNAIRE

STATE ______________________

1. Who in your state has authority to permit the installation of onsite wastewater treatment systems? (please check)

   ☐ state

   ☐ local agency

   ☐ other

   If other, please explain: ______________________

   ____

   ____

   ____

2. If local agencies have jurisdiction, is there a minimum state requirement they must follow?

   ☐ yes

   ☐ no

3. Are onsite alternatives currently being used in your state?

   ☐ yes

   ☐ no

   If yes, are installations ☐ permanent or ☐ experimental?

4. If there are alternative systems currently being used, are they (*check each* space applicable)

☐ septic tanks	☐ elevated sand mounds
☐ home aerobic plants	☐ evapotranspiration (ET)
☐ blackwater recycle devices	☐ evapotranspiration-infiltration (ETI)
☐ greywater recycle devices	☐ pressure sewers
☐ integrated black-greywater devices	☐ vacuum sewers
☐ composting toilets	☐ grinder pumps
☐ tile fields	☐ wastewater incinerators

   ☐ other innovative alternatives (please describe):

   ____

   ____

   ____

   ____

Onsite Wastewater Policy Questionnaire (continued)

5. What specific criteria do you use for determining size of tile fields?

____

____

____

If home aerobic plants are being used with tile field disposal, do you permit a reduction in field size?

☐ yes

☐ no

If yes, how much? ____________________________

____

____

Do you permit surface discharge?

☐ yes

☐ no

If yes, do you require effluent ☐ filtration
☐ disinfection?

Do you use NSF Standard 40?

☐ yes

☐ no

If yes, is testing (by any agency/laboratory) to assure conformance required?

☐ yes

☐ no

Is your use of Standard 40 by ☐ law
☐ code
☐ regulation
☐ policy?

Is NSF listing required?

☐ yes

☐ no

If the plant has been tested and listed by NSF, do you *require* additional local testing of the plant?

☐ yes

☐ no

If either of the last two questions were answered "yes", please identify what you consider to be unanswered by the NSF program: __________

____

____

Onsite Wastewater Policy Questionnaire (continued)

6. If recycle systems are utilized, how can recycle fluid be used?

☐ flushing only	☐ shower
☐ lawn watering	☐ drinking
☐ laundry	☐ other

If other, please explain: ______________________________

____

____

____

7. Has the Clean Water Act of 1977 prompted you to revise your code, regulations, or policies relating to use of onsite alternative systems other than septic tank/subsurface disposal installations?

☐ yes

☐ no

8. Have you or any member of your staff attended any of the NSF National Conferences on Individual Onsite Wastewater Systems?

☐ yes

☐ no

Is there any specific topic you would like to see included in future programs?

☐ yes

☐ no

If so, identify: ______________________________

____

____

____

Is there someone in your state who should be considered as a speaker for a future program?

☐ yes

☐ no

Name ______________________________

Address ______________________________

Telephone (if known) ______________________________

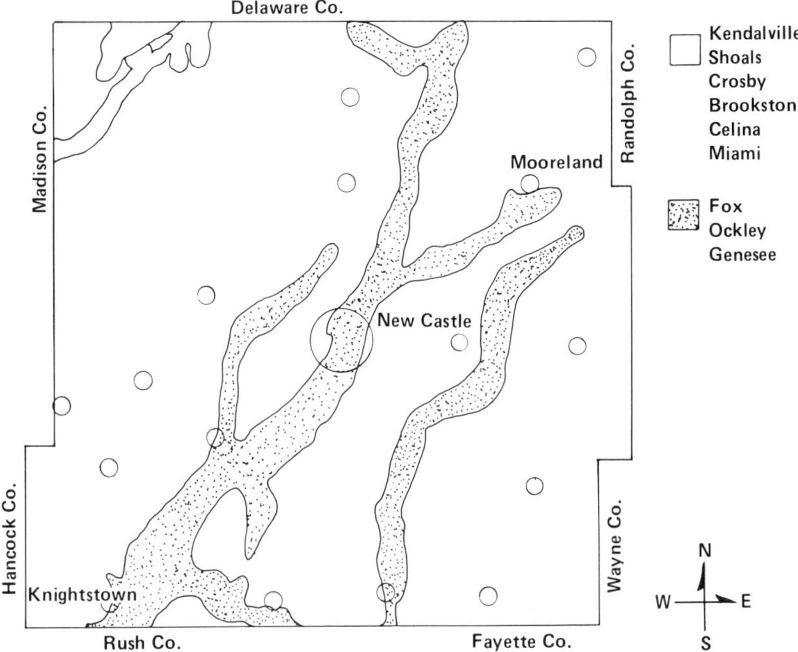

Figure 3. Major soil groups in Henry County.

suitable for septic tanks and absorption fields; other sections represent soils that are unsuitable because of very slow permeability rates, ponding, and an underlying "glacial till," which is present throughout most of the county. This glacial till, which is about 36 inches deep, is like cement, and is where we were placing the onsite systems. The county seat is New Castle; the dots represent outlying communities. While most of the outlying communities are built in soils that are unsuitable for septic tanks and tile fields, the county seat is built in soils that are. Unsuitable soil (Kendalville, Shoals, Crosby, Brookston, Celina and Miami) makes up 78% of the soils within the county. Sand and gravel soils, which, with modifications, are relatively suitable, are in Fox, Ockley and Genesee.

FORMATION OF A TECHNICAL COMMITTEE

One year ago the county's Department of Health developed a technical committee comprised of the president of the Home Builders Association,

Onsite Wastewater Policy Questionnaire (continued)

What is the area of his/her special knowledge and/or experience? Explain:

____

____

____

____

____

9. Do you or your staff have specific needs with which NSF could be of further service?

☐ yes

☐ no

If yes, please identify: ______________________________

____

____

____

10. Will you make available to us a copy of your state

☐ code

☐ regulations

☐ policy?

Please check:

☐ enclosed

☐ will follow

11. To obtain a copy of a *local* code, regulations, and/or policy, contact:

NAME ______________________________

TITLE ______________________________

ADDRESS ______________________________

TELEPHONE (If known) ______________________________

Questionnaire completed by:
(please type or print)

Name ______________________________

Title ______________________________

State of ______________________________

APPENDIX B

STATE ONSITE WASTEWATER POLICIES

	ALABAMA	ALASKA	ARIZONA	ARKANSAS	CALIFORNIA	COLORADO	CONNECTICUT	DELAWARE	FLORIDA	GEORGIA	HAWAII	IDAHO	ILLINOIS	INDIANA	IOWA	KANSAS	KENTUCKY	LOUISIANA	MAINE	MARYLAND	MASSACHUSETTS	MICHIGAN	MINNESOTA	MISSISSIPPI
1. Permitting Authority:																								
State	✓	✓	✓	✓			✓	✓	✓		✓	✓	✓			✓	✓	✓	✓			✓	✓	✓
Local	✓	✓	✓		✓	✓	✓		✓	✓		✓	✓	✓	✓	✓	✓		✓	✓		✓	✓	✓
Other								✓																
2. Minimum State Rules?	✓	✓	✓	✓	✓	✓	✓	✓	✓	✓	✓	✓	✓	✓	✓		✓		✓	✓				✓
3. Alternatives used,										(2)														
Conventionally	✓	✓	✓	✓	✓	✓			✓		✓	✓	✓	✓		✓	✓	✓	✓	✓		✓	✓	✓
Experimentally	✓	✓	✓	✓	✓	✓	✓		✓			✓	✓	✓	✓	✓				✓				
4. Alternatives:																								
Septic Tanks	✓	✓	✓	✓	✓	✓	✓	✓	✓	✓	✓	✓	✓	✓	✓	✓	✓	✓	✓	✓		✓	✓	✓
Home Aerobic Plants	✓	✓	✓	✓	✓	✓		✓	✓		✓	✓	✓	✓		✓	✓	✓	✓	✓		✓	✓	✓
Blackwater Recycle Devices													✓						✓			✓		
Greywater Recycle Devices		✓			✓	✓																		
Integrated Black-Greywater Devices						✓													✓			✓		✓
Composting Toilets	✓	✓	✓		✓	✓	✓		✓			✓		✓	✓		✓		✓	✓		✓	✓	✓
Tile Fields	✓	✓	✓	✓	✓	✓	✓	✓	✓	✓	✓		✓	✓	✓	✓	✓	✓	✓	✓		✓	✓	✓
Elevated Sand Mounds	✓			✓	✓				✓			✓	✓	✓	✓	✓				✓		✓	✓	✓
ET			✓		✓	✓						✓		✓		✓				✓		✓		
ET-I			✓	✓	✓							✓	✓	✓		✓				✓				
Pressure Sewers	✓	✓			✓	✓			✓			✓	✓	✓			✓					✓		✓
Vacuum Sewers		✓			✓				✓					✓										
Grinder Pumps	✓	✓							✓				✓			✓	✓			✓			✓	✓
Wastewater Incinerators		✓			✓		✓						✓							✓		✓	✓	
Others							(A)						Recirculating Filters Ash as Media Stabilization Ponds	Stabilization Ponds Pressure Distributed	Double Sand Filters	Stabilization Ponds Sand Filters Seepage Pits		Oxidation Pond Sand Filters	Leaching Chambers			Lagoons Electro-Osmosis Overland Flow	Sewage Osmosis	Lagoons Sand Filter

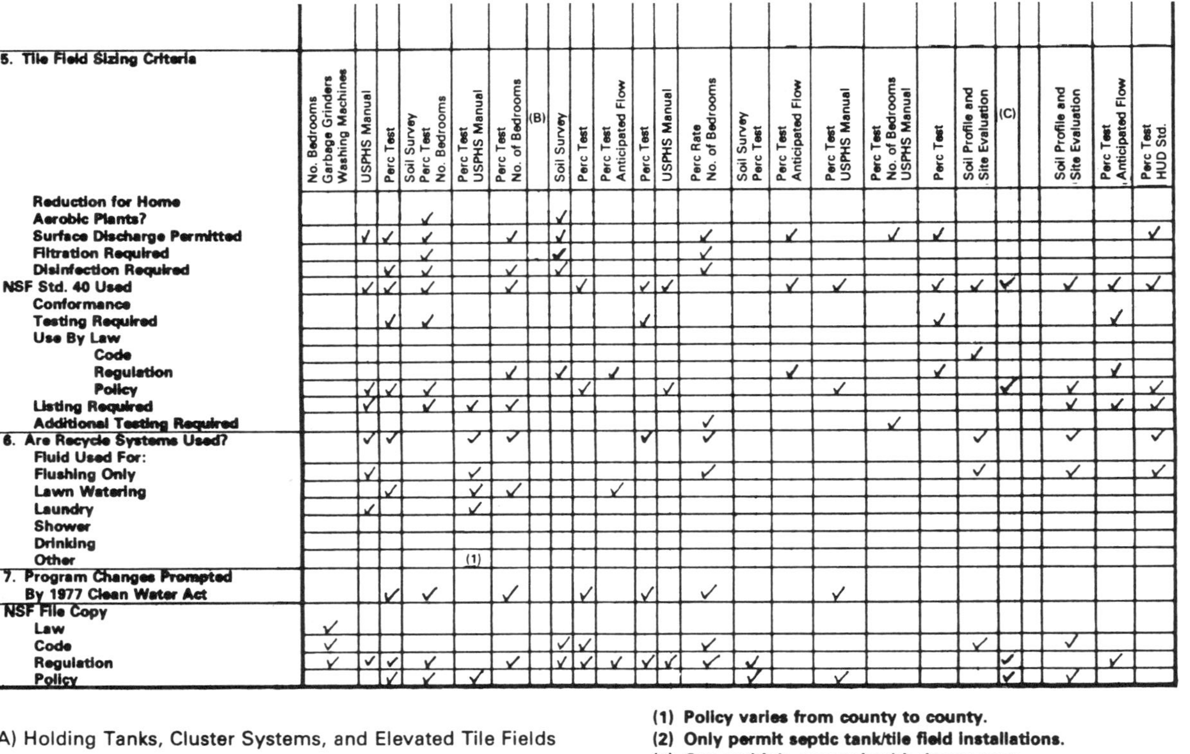

5. Tile Field Sizing Criteria	No. Bedrooms Garbage Grinders Washing Machines	USPHS Manual	Perc Test	Soil Survey Perc Test No. Bedrooms	Perc Test USPHS Manual	Perc Test No. of Bedrooms	(B)	Soil Survey	Perc Test	Perc Test Anticipated Flow	Perc Test	USPHS Manual	Perc Rate No. of Bedrooms	Soil Survey Perc Test	Perc Test Anticipated Flow	Perc Test USPHS Manual	Perc Test No. of Bedrooms USPHS Manual	Perc Test	Soil Profile and Site Evaluation	(C)		Soil Profile and Site Evaluation	Perc Test Anticipated Flow	Perc Test HUD Std.
Reduction for Home Aerobic Plants?				✓				✓																
Surface Discharge Permitted		✓	✓	✓		✓		✓					✓		✓		✓	✓						✓
Filtration Required				✓				✓					✓											
Disinfection Required			✓	✓		✓		✓					✓											
NSF Std. 40 Used		✓	✓	✓		✓			✓		✓	✓			✓	✓		✓	✓	✓		✓	✓	✓
Conformance																								
Testing Required			✓	✓							✓							✓					✓	
Use By Law																								
Code																			✓					
Regulation						✓		✓		✓					✓			✓					✓	
Policy		✓	✓	✓					✓			✓				✓				✓		✓		✓
Listing Required		✓		✓	✓	✓																✓	✓	✓
Additional Testing Required													✓				✓							
6. Are Recycle Systems Used?		✓	✓		✓	✓					✓		✓						✓			✓		✓
Fluid Used For:																								
Flushing Only		✓			✓								✓						✓			✓		✓
Lawn Watering			✓		✓	✓				✓														
Laundry		✓			✓																			
Shower																								
Drinking																								
Other					(1)																			
7. Program Changes Prompted By 1977 Clean Water Act			✓	✓		✓			✓		✓		✓			✓								
NSF File Copy																								
Law	✓																							
Code	✓							✓	✓				✓						✓			✓		
Regulation	✓	✓	✓	✓		✓		✓	✓	✓	✓	✓	✓	✓						✓			✓	
Policy			✓	✓	✓									✓		✓				✓		✓		

(A) Holding Tanks, Cluster Systems, and Elevated Tile Fields

(B) Perc Test
No. Bedrooms

(C) Soil and Site Evaluation
Perc Test

(1) Policy varies from county to county.
(2) Only permit septic tank/tile field installations.
(3) One multiple county health department.
(4) NSF or equivalent required.
(5) Local Health Departments are an extension of the State.
ET - Evapotranspiration
ET-I - Evapotranspiration-Infiltration

	MISSOURI	MONTANA	NEBRASKA	NEVADA	NEW HAMPSHIRE	NEW JERSEY	NEW MEXICO	NEW YORK	NORTH CAROLINA	NORTH DAKOTA	OHIO	OKLAHOMA	OREGON	PENNSYLVANIA	RHODE ISLAND	SOUTH CAROLINA	SOUTH DAKOTA	TENNESSEE	TEXAS	UTAH	VERMONT	VIRGINIA	WASHINGTON	WEST VIRGINIA	WISCONSIN	WYOMING
1. Permitting Authority:																										
State			✓	✓	✓	✓	✓					✓		✓	✓	✓						✓	✓	✓	✓	
Local	✓	✓	✓	✓	✓	✓		✓	✓		✓			✓		✓		✓	✓			(5)	✓	✓		
Other										(3)																✓
2. Minimum State Rules?	✓		✓	✓	✓	✓		✓	✓		✓	✓		✓		✓		✓	✓				✓	✓	✓	✓
3. Alternatives used,																										
Conventionally			✓	✓	✓	✓	✓	✓	✓	✓				✓	✓	✓	✓	✓	✓			✓	✓	✓		✓
Experimentally	✓	✓			✓	✓		✓	✓		✓	✓		✓		✓	✓		✓			✓	✓	✓	✓	
4. Alternatives:																										
Septic Tanks	✓	✓	✓	✓	✓	✓	✓	✓	✓	✓	✓	✓		✓	✓	✓	✓	✓	✓			✓	✓	✓	✓	✓
Home Aerobic Plants	✓	✓		✓	✓	✓	✓	✓	✓		✓			✓			✓	✓	✓			✓	✓	✓	✓	✓
Blackwater Recycle Devices					✓				✓					✓								✓	✓			
Greywater Recycle Devices					✓												✓					✓				
Integrated Black-Greywater Devices					✓																	✓				
Composting Toilets		✓			✓	✓	✓	✓	✓		✓			✓			✓	✓	✓			✓	✓	✓	✓	✓
Tile Fields	✓	✓	✓	✓	✓	✓	✓	✓	✓	✓	✓	✓		✓	✓	✓	✓	✓	✓			✓	✓	✓	✓	✓
Elevated Sand Mounds				✓	✓	✓		✓	✓					✓		✓	✓	✓	✓			✓	✓	✓	✓	✓
ET		✓		✓	✓	✓	✓	✓	✓	✓	✓			✓		✓	✓	✓	✓				✓	✓	✓	✓
ET-I		✓		✓	✓	✓		✓		✓						✓		✓	✓			✓	✓	✓		✓
Pressure Sewers	✓					✓		✓										✓	✓			✓	✓	✓	✓	
Vacuum Sewers																		✓				✓				
Grinder Pumps	✓		✓		✓												✓	✓	✓			✓		✓		
Wastewater Incinerators		✓			✓																	✓	✓			
Others	Lagoons		Lagoons						Low Pressure Systems, Porous Block Systems, V-Ditches, Irrigation			Lagoons		Spray Irrigation, Pressure Dosing	Galleys, Flow Diffusers								(D)	Stabilization Ponds		Pure Cycle

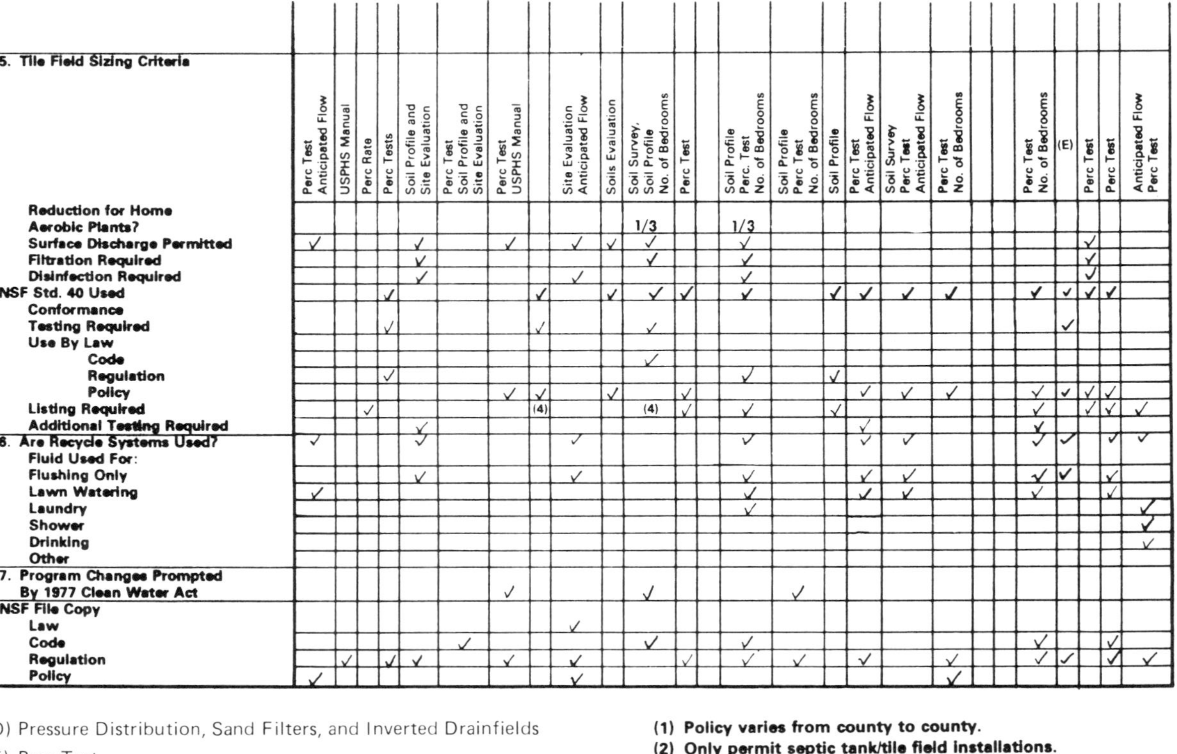

5. Tile Field Sizing Criteria	Perc Test Anticipated Flow	USPHS Manual	Perc Rate	Perc Tests	Soil Profile and Site Evaluation	Perc Test Soil Profile and Site Evaluation	Perc Test USPHS Manual		Site Evaluation Anticipated Flow	Soils Evaluation	Soil Survey, Soil Profile No. of Bedrooms	Perc Test		Soil Profile Perc. Test No. of Bedrooms	Soil Profile Perc Test No. of Bedrooms	Soil Profile	Perc Test Anticipated Flow	Soil Survey Perc Test Anticipated Flow	Perc Test No. of Bedrooms			Perc Test No. of Bedrooms	(E)	Perc Test	Perc Test	Anticipated Flow Perc Test
Reduction for Home																										
Aerobic Plants?											1/3			1/3												
Surface Discharge Permitted	✓				✓		✓		✓	✓	✓			✓										✓		
Filtration Required					✓						✓			✓										✓		
Disinfection Required					✓				✓					✓										✓		
NSF Std. 40 Used				✓				✓		✓	✓	✓		✓		✓	✓	✓	✓			✓	✓	✓	✓	
Conformance																										
Testing Required				✓				✓			✓												✓			
Use By Law																										
Code											✓															
Regulation				✓										✓		✓										
Policy							✓	✓		✓		✓					✓	✓	✓			✓	✓	✓	✓	
Listing Required			✓					(4)			(4)	✓		✓		✓						✓		✓	✓	✓
Additional Testing Required					✓												✓					✓				
6. Are Recycle Systems Used?	✓				✓				✓					✓			✓	✓				✓	✓		✓	✓
Fluid Used For:																										
Flushing Only					✓				✓					✓			✓	✓				✓	✓		✓	
Lawn Watering	✓													✓			✓	✓				✓			✓	
Laundry														✓												✓
Shower																										✓
Drinking																										✓
Other																										
7. Program Changes Prompted By 1977 Clean Water Act							✓				✓				✓											
NSF File Copy																										
Law									✓																	
Code						✓					✓			✓								✓			✓	
Regulation		✓		✓	✓		✓		✓			✓		✓	✓		✓		✓			✓	✓		✓	✓
Policy	✓								✓										✓							

(D) Pressure Distribution, Sand Filters, and Inverted Drainfields

(E) Perc Test
USPHS Manual

(1) Policy varies from county to county.
(2) Only permit septic tank/tile field installations.
(3) One multiple county health department.
(4) NSF or equivlalent required.
(5) Local Health Departments are an extension of the State.
ET - Evapotranspiration
ET-I - Evapotranspiration-Infiltration

APPENDIX C: ONSITE SYSTEMS TECHNOLOGY QUESTIONNAIRE RESPONSE ANALYSIS, BY SECTOR

	Relative Impressions (Value) (+1 to −1)					
	Reg.	Consl.	Ind.	R-D	Other	Total
1. Systems/Technology						
a. Individual Aerobic Treatment Systems	+0.29	−0.40	+1.00	0	+0.33	+0.34
b. Compost Systems	+0.53	+0.87	+0.67	0	+0.33	+0.61
c. Recycle Systems	+0.36	+0.13	0	0	−0.33	+0.28
d. Septic Systems	+1.00	+1.00	+0.17	+0.67	+1.00	+1.00
e. Status-Onsite System Technology	+0.41	+0.53	+0.83	+1.00	0	+0.51
f. Utilization-Onsite System Technology	+0.19	−0.27	−0.50	−0.33	+0.33	+0.03
g. Dependability-Onsite System Tech.	−0.7	+0.07	+0.33	−0.33	−0.67	−0.05
2. Administration and Regulation (Agency)						
a. Knowledgeability-Onsite Technology	+0.94	−0.67	−0.29	−0.75	−0.67	+0.30
b. Responsiveness/Receptiveness to Use	+0.66	−0.67	−0.86	−1.00	−0.33	0
c. Assistance with Problem Situations	+1.00	−0.40	−0.29	−1.00	−1.00	+0.40
d. Reasonableness of Rules	−0.19	−0.93	−0.43	−0.75	−0.67	−0.37
e. Promptness of Decisions	−0.47	−1.00	−1.00	−0.75	−0.67	−1.00

3. Manufacturing, Installing, Service (Ind)						
a. Responsibility/Reliability of Agents	0	+0.33	+1.00	0	0	+0.57
b. Dependability-Equipment & Materials	−0.40	−0.67	+0.29	0	−0.5	−0.21
c. Dependability-Service	−1.00	−0.67	+0.43	−0.50	+0.5	−1.00
d. Immediacy of Service Upon Request	−0.73	−1.00	+0.71	−1.00	+1.0	−0.64
e. Responsiveness to Major System Failure	−0.27	−0.33	+0.43	−0.50	0	−0.21
4. Serving Societal Needs with Onsite Systems						
a. Significant Need Filled	+1.00	+0.72	+0.72	+0.33	+0.50	+1.00
b. Future Service-Benefits Promising	+0.75	+1.00	+1.00	+1.00	+1.00	+1.00
c. Obstacles to Progress Being Addressed	+0.77	+0.44	+0.40	0	+1.00	+0.73
	Order of Priority					
5. Area of Greatest Need of Attention/Import.						
a. Systems/Equipment Design	5	3	1	3	3	5
b. Industry Representations/Services	6	6	6	6	6	6
c. Agency Policies/Procedures	3	1	2	2	1	3
d. Land Development/Use Policies	1	5	3	5	3	2
e. Systems Technology	3	2	4	4	1	4
f. Homeowner/Occupant Responsibility	2	4	5	1	5	1
No. of Respondents.	76	24	11	5	4	120

STATUS AND UTILIZATION OF ONSITE SYSTEMS TECHNOLOGY

Opinion Survey of Participants in Sixth National Conference

With the knowledge and experience you have, please express your views on the following issues by checkmarks.	Regulatory (76)			
	(+) Favorable Impression	(±) No Impression	(–) Unfavorable Impression	
1. Systems and technology	#	#	#	Value
a. Individual aerobic treatment systems	39	14	23	+16
b. Compost systems	44	18	13	+31
c. Recycle systems	39	19	18	+21
d. Septic systems	61	11	3	+58
e. Status of onsite system technology	41	17	17	+24
f. Utilization of onsite system technology	34	19	23	+11
g. Dependability of onsite system technology	21	25	25	-4
2. Administration and regulation (agency)				
a. Knowledgeability of systems and technology	43	17	13	+30
b. Responsiveness and receptiveness to proposed use	37	21	16	+21
c. Assistance with problem situations	44	20	12	+32
d. Reasonableness of rules and regulations	32	19	26	+6
e. Promptness of decision rendering	20	22	35	-15
3. Manufacturing, installing and servicing (industry)				
a. Responsibility and reliability of representatives	19	35	19	0
b. Dependability of equipment and materials	17	35	23	-6
c. Dependability of service rendered	9	42	24	-15
d. Immediacy of service when requested	13	39	24	-11
e. Responsiveness to major system failures	16	39	20	-4

4. **Serving societal needs with onsite systems**				
a. A significant societal need is being served	50	16	10	+40
b. Future service benefits are very promising	43	19	13	+30
c. Obstacles to future progress are being addressed	45	17	14	+31

5. Please identify by priority number (1, 2, 3 only), those items in the following list which require the more immediate attention and improvement (1 = highest priority):	#/pts.	Average Assigned Priority
a. Systems and equipment design—i.e., mechanical/electrical; effluent disposal; sizing criteria, etc.	48/80	1.66
b. Industry representations and services	35/78	2.23
c. Agency policies and procedures	57/106	1.96
d. Land development and use policies	59/94	1.60
e. Systems technology—i.e., state of the art; responsiveness to need; reliability, etc.	57/106	1.96
f. Homeowner/occupant responsibility	53/91	1.72
g. ______	______	

6. What questions should we have asked and did not?

______

______

______

7. Please identify your area of involvement:

Industry (manufacturer, seller, installer, service/repair)	______
Regulatory (federal, state, local/regional)	______
Consultant (engineer, architect, planner, adviser)	______
Research/Development (institutional, private practice, non-industry)	______
Land/Subdivision Developer, Homebuilder	______
Other (specify) ______	______
Have major involvement (25% or more of work time)	______
Years of experience with onsite systems	______

STATUS AND UTILIZATION OF ONSITE SYSTEMS TECHNOLOGY

Opinion Survey of Participants in Sixth National Conference

	Consultants (24)			
With the knowledge and experience you have, please express your views on the following issues by checkmarks.	(+) Favorable Impression	(±) No Impression	(−) Unfavorable Impression	
1. **Systems and technology**	#	#	#	Value
a. Individual aerobic treatment systems	17	4	13	−6
b. Compost systems	16	5	3	+13
c. Recycle systems	8	10	6	+2
d. Septic systems	18	4	3	+15
e. Status of onsite system technology	15	2	7	+8
f. Utilization of onsite system technology	7	5	11	−4
g. Dependability of onsite system technology	7	9	6	+1
2. **Administration and regulation (agency)**				
a. Knowledgeability of systems and technology	3	8	13	−10
b. Responsiveness and receptiveness to proposed use	3	8	13	−10
c. Assistance with problem situations	1	16	7	−6
d. Reasonableness of rules and regulations	0	10	14	−14
e. Promptness of decision rendering	0	9	15	−15
3. **Manufacturing, installing and servicing (industry)**				
a. Responsibility and reliability of representatives	8	8	7	+1
b. Dependability of equipment and materials	6	13	4	−2
c. Dependability of service rendered	4	13	6	−2
d. Immediacy of service when requested	3	13	6	−3
e. Responsiveness to major system failures	5	13	6	−1

4. **Serving societal needs with onsite systems**				
a. A significant societal need is being served	17	3	4	+13
b. Future service benefits are very promising	20	2	2	+18
c. Obstacles to future progress are being addressed	13	6	5	+8

5. Please identify by priority number (1, 2, 3 only), those items in the following list which require the more immediate attention and improvement (1 = highest priority):	#/pts.	Average Assigned Priority
a. Systems and equipment design— i.e., mechanical/electrical; effluent disposal; sizing criteria, etc.	16/37	2.31
b. Industry representations and services	10/23	2.30
c. Agency policies and procedures	17/29	1.71
d. Land development and use policies	8/14	1.75
e. Systems technology— i.e., state of the art; responsiveness to need; reliability, etc.	15/24	1.60
f. Homeowner/occupant responsibility	12/24	2.00
g. ____________	______	

6. What questions should we have asked and did not?

____

____

____

7. Please identify your area of involvement:

Industry (manufacturer, seller, installer, service/repair) ______

Regulatory (federal, state, local/regional) ______

Consultant (engineer, architect, planner, adviser) ______

Research/Development (institutional, private practice, non-industry) ______

Land/Subdivision Developer, Homebuilder ______

Other (specify) ____________ ______

Have major involvement (25% or more of work time) ______

Years of experience with onsite systems ______

STATUS AND UTILIZATION OF ONSITE SYSTEMS TECHNOLOGY

Opinion Survey of Participants in Sixth National Conference

With the knowledge and experience you have, please express your views on the following issues by checkmarks.	Industry (11) (+) Favorable Impression	(±) No Impression	(–) Unfavorable Impression	
1. **Systems and technology**	#	#	#	Value
a. Individual aerobic treatment systems	8	1	2	+6
b. Compost systems	5	5	1	+4
c. Recycle systems	3	5	3	+0
d. Septic systems	5	2	4	+1
e. Status of onsite system technology	7	2	2	+5
f. Utilization of onsite system technology	3	2	6	–3
g. Dependability of onsite system technology	5	3	3	+2
2. **Administration and regulation (agency)**				
a. Knowledgeability of systems and technology	3	2	5	–2
b. Responsiveness and receptiveness to proposed use	1	1	7	–6
c. Assistance with problem situations	1	6	3	–2
d. Reasonableness of rules and regulations	2	3	5	–3
e. Promptness of decision rendering	0	2	7	–7
3. **Manufacturing, installing and servicing (industry)**				
a. Responsibility and reliability of representatives	7	4	0	+7
b. Dependability of equipment and materials	4	2	2	+2
c. Dependability of service rendered	4	5	1	+3
d. Immediacy of service when requested	5	5	0	+5
e. Responsiveness to major system failures	4	5	1	+3

4. **Serving societal needs with onsite systems**				
a. A significant societal need is being served	8	1	1	+7
b. Future service benefits are very promising	10	0	0	+10
c. Obstacles to future progress are being addressed	5	4	1	+4

5. Please identify by priority number (1, 2, 3 only), those items in the following list which require the more immediate attention and improvement (1 = highest priority):	#/pts.	Average Assigned Priority
a. Systems and equipment design– i.e., mechanical/electrical; effluent disposal; sizing criteria, etc.	11/21	1.91
b. Industry representations and services	3/6	2.00
c. Agency policies and procedures	5/6	1.20
d. Land development and use policies	8/16	2.00
e. Systems technology– i.e., state of the art; responsiveness to need; reliability, etc.	5/9	1.80
f. Homeowner/occupant responsibility	4/9	2.25
g. ________________	______	

6. What questions should we have asked and did not?

____

____

____

7. Please identify your area of involvement:

Industry (manufacturer, seller, installer, service/repair)	______
Regulatory (federal, state, local/regional)	______
Consultant (engineer, architect, planner, adviser)	______
Research/Development (institutional, private practice, non-industry)	______
Land/Subdivision Developer, Homebuilder	______
Other (specify) ________________	______
Have major involvement (25% or more of work time)	______
Years of experience with onsite systems	______

STATUS AND UTILIZATION OF ONSITE SYSTEMS TECHNOLOGY

Opinion Survey of Participants in Sixth National Conference

R&D (5)

With the knowledge and experience you have, please express your views on the following issues by checkmarks.	(+) Favorable Impression	(±) No Impression	(–) Unfavorable Impression	
1. Systems and technology	#	#	#	Value
a. Individual aerobic treatment systems	2	1	2	0
b. Compost systems	1	3	1	0
c. Recycle systems	2	1	2	0
d. Septic systems	4	0	1	+2
e. Status of onsite system technology	4	1	0	+3
f. Utilization of onsite system technology	0	2	3	–1
g. Dependability of onsite system technology	1	2	2	–1
2. Administration and regulation (agency)				
a. Knowledgeability of systems and technology	1	0	4	–3
b. Responsiveness and receptiveness to proposed use	0	1	4	–4
c. Assistance with problem situations	0	1	4	–4
d. Reasonableness of rules and regulations	0	2	3	–3
e. Promptness of decision rendering	0	1	4	–3
3. Manufacturing, installing and servicing (industry)				
a. Responsibility and reliability of representatives	1	3	1	0
b. Dependability of equipment and materials	1	3	1	0
c. Dependability of service rendered	1	2	2	–1
d. Immediacy of service when requested	1	1	3	–2
e. Responsiveness to major system failures	1	2	2	–1

4. **Serving societal needs with onsite systems**				
a. A significant societal need is being served	2	2	1	+1
b. Future service benefits are very promising	3	2	0	+3
c. Obstacles to future progress are being addressed	1	3	1	0

5. Please identify by priority number (1, 2, 3 only), those items in the following list which require the more immediate attention and improvement (1 = highest priority):	#/pts.	Average Assigned Priority
a. Systems and equipment design— i.e., mechanical/electrical; effluent disposal; sizing criteria, etc.	3/4	1.33
b. Industry representations and services	3/6	2.00
c. Agency policies and procedures	4/6	1.50
d. Land development and use policies	4/8	2.00
e. Systems technology— i.e., state of the art; responsiveness to need; reliability, etc.	5/12	2.40
f. Homeowner/occupant responsibility	3/3	1.00
g. ______	______	

6. What questions should we have asked and did not?

______

______

______

7. Please identify your area of involvement:

Industry (manufacturer, seller, installer, service/repair)	______
Regulatory (federal, state, local/regional)	______
Consultant (engineer, architect, planner, adviser)	______
Research/Development (institutional, private practice, non-industry)	______
Land/Subdivision Developer, Homebuilder	______
Other (specify) ______	______
Have major involvement (25% or more of work time)	______
Years of experience with onsite systems	______

STATUS AND UTILIZATION OF ONSITE SYSTEMS TECHNOLOGY

Opinion Survey of Participants in Sixth National Conference

Other (4)

With the knowledge and experience you have, please express your views on the following issues by checkmarks.	(+) Favorable Impression	(±) No Impression	(−) Unfavorable Impression	
	#	#	#	Value
1. **Systems and technology**				
a. Individual aerobic treatment systems	2	1	1	+1
b. Compost systems	2	1	1	+1
c. Recycle systems	1	1	2	−1
d. Septic systems	3	1	0	+3
e. Status of onsite system technology	1	2	1	0
f. Utilization of onsite system technology	2	1	1	+1
g. Dependability of onsite system technology	0	2	2	−2
2. **Administration and regulation (agency)**				
a. Knowledgeability of systems and technology	1	0	3	−2
b. Responsiveness and receptiveness to proposed use	1	1	2	−1
c. Assistance with problem situations	0	1	3	−3
d. Reasonableness of rules and regulations	0	2	2	−2
e. Promptness of decision rendering	0	2	2	−2
3. **Manufacturing, installing and servicing (industry)**				
a. Responsibility and reliability of representatives	1	2	1	0
b. Dependability of equipment and materials	0	3	1	−1
c. Dependability of service rendered	1	3	0	+1
d. Immediacy of service when requested	2	2	0	+2
e. Responsiveness to major system failures	0	4	0	0

4. **Serving societal needs with onsite systems**				
a. A significant societal need is being served	2	1	1	+1
b. Future service benefits are very promising	3	1	0	+2
c. Obstacles to future progress are being addressed	2	2	0	+2

5. Please identify by priority number (1, 2, 3 only), those items in the following list which require the more immediate attention and improvement (1 = highest priority):	#/pts.	Average Assigned Priority
a. Systems and equipment design— i.e., mechanical/electrical; effluent disposal; sizing criteria, etc.	3/5	1.67
b. Industry representations and services	2/4	2.00
c. Agency policies and procedures	3/4	1.33
d. Land development and use policies	3/5	1.67
e. Systems technology— i.e., state of the art; responsiveness to need; reliability, etc.	3/4	1.33
f. Homeowner/occupant responsibility	4/9	2.25
g. ______	______	

6. What questions should we have asked and did not?

______

______

______

7. Please identify your area of involvement:

Industry (manufacturer, seller, installer, service/repair) ______
Regulatory (federal, state, local/regional) ______
Consultant (engineer, architect, planner, adviser) ______
Research/Development (institutional, private practice, non-industry) ______
Land/Subdivision Developer, Homebuilder ______
Other (specify) ______ ______
Have major involvement (25% or more of work time) ______
Years of experience with onsite systems ______

3

CASE A–A HENRY COUNTY, INDIANA EXPERIENCE

Lynn Bowers
Health Officer
Henry County Health Department
New Castle, Indiana 42362

INTRODUCTION

The Health Department in Henry County, Indiana (Figure 1) consists of three sanitarians for a county population of 53,000. One of its functions is to hand out onsite permits. A problem came before the Department in which a gentleman who had built a home wished to have his permit issued. The home was located in an area comprising 92 homes, of which 32 had failing septic tanks and/or disposal fields. During the past two or three years the people living there had been complaining vigorously to the Health Department because of its part in granting these permits. A section of a county ordinance, which is designed to handle this kind of problem, is entitled "Article 4, Permit and Inspection for New Construction or Alterations." It states, "BEFORE commencing construction . . . an individual must obtain a septic permit . . ." (Figure 2). However, this man came after he built his home. Typically, what happens is that an individual goes before the Planning Commission and Building Commission and obtains a building permit. He then goes to the Health Department, having already built the structure, to seek the onsite wastewater system permit. These permits were always granted; they have never been denied.

SOIL COMPOSITION IN HENRY COUNTY

A map of major soil groups in the county (Figure 3) demonstrates the problem in Henry County. The colored area represents soils that are relatively

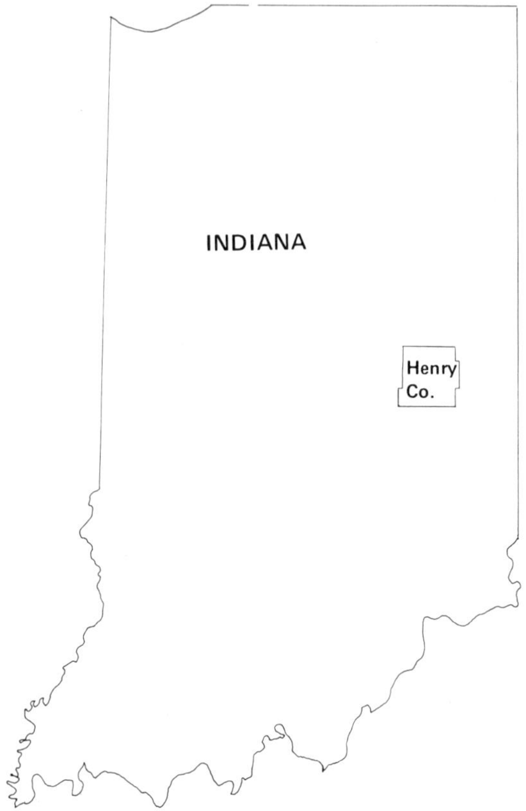

Figure 1. Location of Henry County, Indiana.

ARTICLE IV

Permit and Inspection for New Construction or Alteration

Section 401: Before commencement of construction of any building or private residence where a private sewage disposal system or privy is to be installed or where any alteration or addition of an existing private sewage disposal system is planned, the owner or agent of the owner shall first obtain a written permit signed by the County Health Officer.

Section 902: Passed and adopted by the Commissioners of Henry County, State of Indiana, on this 16th day of June, 1969.

Board of Commissioners of
Henry County

Figure 2. County ordinance.

community commissioners, planning commission members, realtors, bankers and a number of other people interested in this problem. The committee began to look at onsite requests and made it very clear through the local media that anyone planning to build a new home should first present a request for a septic tank and tile field permit to determine whether this type of system could be expected to work. Not everyone has cooperated. After one year, it appears to work relatively poorly, but at least an effort is being made to involve those most concerned.

INVESTIGATING THE PROBLEM

Having discerned the problem in one area, the question arose whether there was a problem elsewhere in the county in terms of pollution only. Figure 4 is a map of a qualitative method which tries to determine and demonstrate pollution in the county.

Recently, sanitarians took 14 water samples from random streams and ditches throughout the county from north to south (depicted by dots on

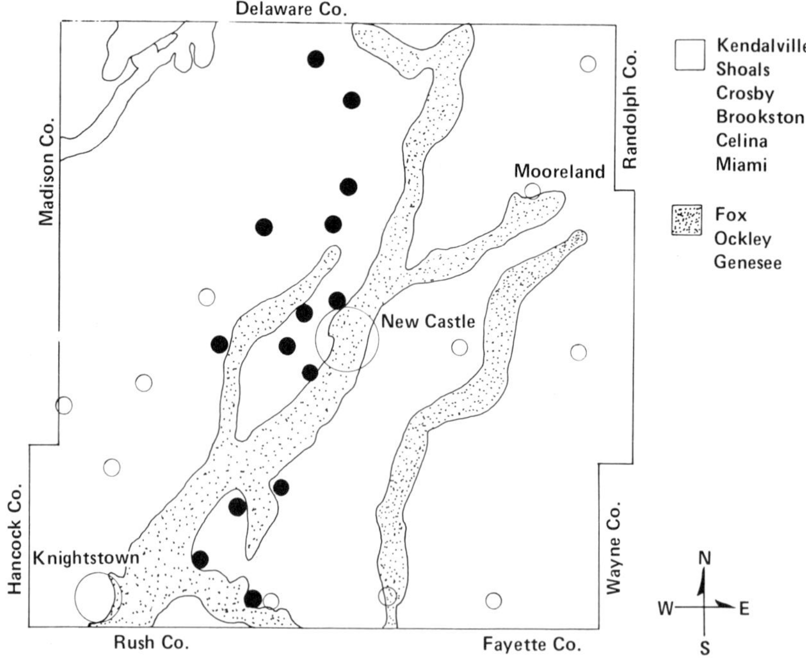

Figure 4. Pollution in Henry County.

the map in Figure 4). These were sampled for fecal coliform counts, which is the parameter used in the state of Indiana as a direct measure of human contamination. Table I demonstrates the incredible counts that were determined.

To go wading in a body of water in the state of Indiana, the water must have less than 200 fecal coliforms per 100 cc; to go swimming and immerse head and face, it must have less than 10; to drink or use it for cooking, it must have none. Not one of these samples showed a zero count; only one had 10 (Number 9). (Number 9, incidentally, happens to be a point downstream from a new sewage disposal plant for the county seat.) The committee felt that a significant pollution problem had indeed been demonstrated. If we have pollution we must then determine if we also have disease.

RESULTS

We looked at the population of the counties surrounding Henry County (Table II). Henry County has a population of 53,000, of which 23,000 live within the county seat of New Castle. There are six other surrounding counties (Madison, Delaware, Hancock, Rush, Wayne and Randolph). Madison, Delaware and Wayne Counties are one and one-half to three times the size of Henry County. Hancock County is about the same size as Henry County, while Rush County is quite a bit smaller. With that in mind, we began to compare diseases that could be contributing to pollution (salmonella, shigella, forms of communicable diarrhea, hepatitis, infectious hepatitis, and certain

Table I. Fecal Coliform Counts in Samples from Streams and Ditches

Samples	Location	Results, No./100 ml
1	¾ mi. west of 75 West on C. R. 200 North	770
2	¼ mi. north of U.S. #36 on 300 West	3,900,000
3	Fall Creek, south edge of M-Town	540
4	¼ mi. west of Prairie Rd. on 800 North	67,000
5	¼ mi. west of Mt. Summit on U.S. 36	2,500,000
6	St. Road #3 at C.R. 200 North	580,000
7	¼ mi. west of N.C. on St. Rd. #38	620,000
8	1½ mi. west of N.C. on St. Rd. #38	160,000
9	1 mi. west of Spiceland Pk. on 200 South	10
10	⅛ mi. west of S. Main St. on Southview Drive	8,200
11	K-town Park, ¼ mi. south of U.S. #40	480
12	⅛ mi. north of U.S. 40 on C.R. 575 West	40
13	¼ mi. east of Dunreith on U.S. #40	310
14	Brook Beezer, Bond St. Spiceland	54,000

Table II. Population Data

County Populations (1974)	
Madison	139,400
Delaware	130,600
Henry	53,200
Hancock	40,300
Rush	20,900
Wayne	79,200
Growth of Henry County	
1900-1950	25,088-45,505 408/yr
1950-1975	45,505-53,934 337/yr
1975-2000 (projection)	53,934-55,201 (1995 peak) 50/yr

central nervous system (CNS) infections, namely, viral meningitis and encephalitis). We obtained data from the State Board of Health because all counties must report disease to them; thus, within the limits of reporting, data in Table III are relatively valid. In terms of infectious hepatitis, compared with all surrounding counties, including much larger ones, Henry County had at least nine cases in the period 1976-1978. We had at least five cases of diarrheas (about half of that of the surrounding counties). In terms of viral meningitis and encephalitis, Henry County leads all others. In fact, 12 cases were reported this fall and summer alone (Figure 5). It would seem that even considering the larger counties, Henry County is not a very healthy place in which to live.

One obviously does not leap from septic tanks that fail to CNS infections; however, if you look at the past record of civilization, one of the greatest

Table III. Selected Diseases in Henry County, October 1976–July 1979

Hepatitis Infections	No.	Diarrheas (Shigella, Salmonella)	No.	CNS Infections (Viral Meningitis/ Encephalitis)	No.
Henry	9	Henry	5	Henry	7
Hancock	1	Hancock	0	Hancock	3
Rush	2	Rush	0	Rush	1
Delaware	3	Delaware	13	Delaware	4
Wayne	8	Wayne	4	Wayne	4
Madison	4	Madison	11	Madison	1

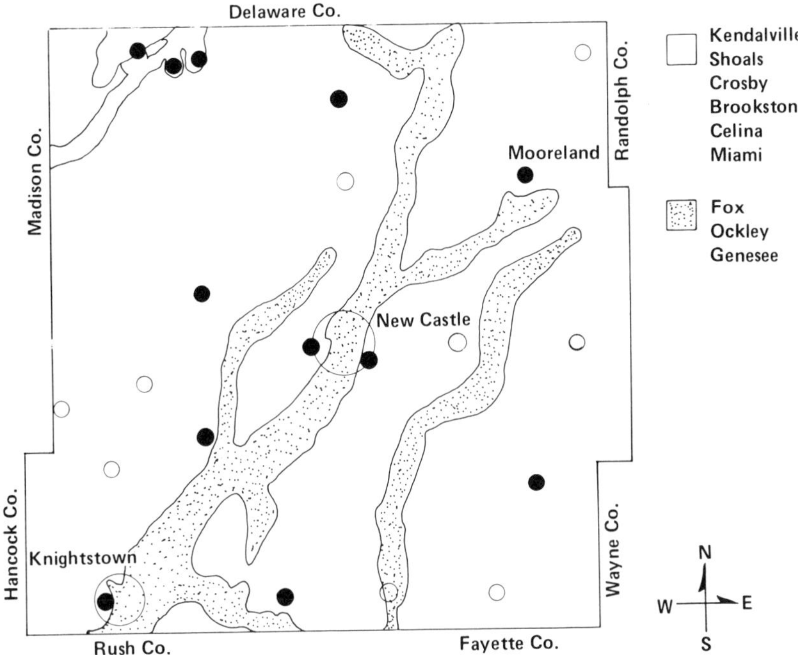

Figure 5. Twelve reported cases of viral meningitis and encephalitis.

contributions mankind has made has been in the form of sanitation. Improved sanitation conditions in western Europe brought the plagues of Europe and dysentery under control. We can learn from history and, if we are going to prevent similar episodes, we must begin by cleaning up our land.

Having established these facts, we then began to determine the impact of our technical committee. Prior to 1978, not a single septic tank permit had ever been denied. In many instances, permits were given after the tanks and fields were already assembled and in place. Our sewer ordinance for Henry County was enacted in 1969. After looking at the criteria and causes for failures, permits began to be denied. Enough evidence was gathered to confirm the existence of a problem in Henry County and it was concluded that perhaps it is unreasonable to continue building with those problems.

CONCLUSIONS

What was the impact? From November 1978 to the present, 322 permits have been requested; 152 were allowed and 170 were denied. Three of these denials involved housing additions of greater than 30-40 homes. In 1977-1978, prior to this, 388 requests were made and not one was denied. Although we do not want to bring the county to a standstill in housing and population growth, our concern is to protect the health and common good. We have had an enormous impact in the county. In 1979 the average cost to build a three-bedroom home in Henry County, Indiana is about $65,000 for land and house. The 129 homes that were denied equals about $11,000,000 worth of construction that has not occurred, mortgage loans not made, jobs not had, real estate not sold and tax revenues not realized. The solutions to these problems will not be simple. Presently, our short-term solutions include utilizing our soil conservation service and obtaining our own soil scientists to help us determine onsite land and soil analyses. In the long term, Henry County will probably have to go toward regional wastewater management districts to obtain sufficient funds and expertise to solve the problem.

4

CASE B–VILLAGE CENTRE: ONSITE WASTE TREATMENT AT A COMMERCIAL COMPLEX

David E. Calhoun, Manager
Marketing, Customer and Technical Services
Thetford Corporation
Ann Arbor, Michigan 48106

Douglas Cobb, President
Commercial Industrial Construction
Village Centre Partnership
Great Falls, Virginia 22066

Jack R. Sutherland, P.E.
Director, Bureau of Wastewater Engineering
Department of Health
Commonwealth of Virginia
Richmond, Virginia 23232

INTRODUCTION

Onsite wastewater systems are traditionally thought of in relation to the requirements of the nonurban single family residence. However, there is another element of American society that also often finds the matter of wastewater disposal troublesome. That element of society is the commercial and industrial community, which supports this nation's growing suburban and semirural population. The economic and environmental burden of wastewater disposal is as great for nonurban commerce and business as it is for the individual nonurban homeowner. All citizens share in both the benefits and penalties of whatever method and means is employed for wastewater disposal, whether that waste originated at the residence, the school, the workplace or the local shopping center.

This case describes the innovative way in which a commercial development benefitted both economically and environmentally by using complementing onsite wastewater systems. The discussion will cover three aspects of the project. Douglas Cobb, developer of Village Centre, will describe the project from his perspective. Then David Calhoun will discuss his involvement as the supplier of the Cycle-Let waste treatment and water recycling system used there. Finally, Jack Sutherland, Director of The Bureau of Wastewater Engineering for the Commonwealth of Virginia, will discuss the state's position in reviewing the wastewater disposal plan.

THE PROJECT

Great Falls, Virginia is a semirural community on the Potomac River, just North of Washington, D.C. Within a five-minute drive of the heart of Great Falls live about 12,000 people, and the population is growing. The residents of Great Falls recognized the need for more consumer services, which meant an opportunity that few developers on the east coast get—the opportunity to create a complete downtown for a community. The Great Falls Citizens Association initially feared that development would mean just another shopping center—the familiar, ugly "strip" of stores behind huge asphalt parking lots that plagues thousands of American neighborhoods.

The Citizens Association wanted a town center to complement the attractive rolling hill, rural setting and the basic good taste of homes throughout the vicinity. As a commitment had been made to constructing a shopping complex that incorporated a whole spectrum of stores, shops, community facilities and services, it was necessary to find a design that the local citizens could accept and be proud of. The model plan was found in the Early American community of Old Sturbridge Village, Massachusetts—colonial buildings around a village green. As the project plans began to take shape in late 1977 and early 1978, the plan was to use a septic tank and soil absorption system for the wastewater from the development because the county did not expect to put a sewer collection system through the area for seven or eight years. The necessary preliminary approvals from the Fairfax County Department of Health were obtained; however, the drainfield was sized at about three acres and would take up almost 25% of the 13-acre site that had been purchased at the intersection of Georgetown Pike and Walker Roads. The drainfield had to be located in such a way that once in place it hindered access to a part of the site scheduled for future development. The real magnitude of the problem can be illustrated by applying some dollar values. The value of ground covered by the three-acre drainfield was about $2.50/ft^2, or $110,000/ac, for a total of $330,000. In searching for an alternative, the Cycle-Let system manufactured by Thetford was investigated. The manufacturer looked at the wastewater disposal requirements to determine if there were a better alternative to the three-acre drainfield.

As a result of working with Thetford, a revised site plan was compiled and submitted to the Fairfax County Department of Public Health and approval was requested for an innovative approach to wastewater disposal from Village Centre. The full cooperation and support of the County Division of Environmental Health and the Bureau of Wastewater Engineering in Richmond was received. They approved the plan and today Village Centre is a reality.

Every building on the 13-acre Village Centre complex is an accurate representation of an Early American architectural style (Figure 1). The nearly 60,000 ft^2 of usable space in the center's 12 multitenant buildings have finished wood plank floors, painted and finished walls, and exposed beam and plank ceilings. Village Centre includes a large community room, commercial stores and shops, restaurants, a bank, the town newspaper, and numerous medical and other professional offices. Soon the community post office will be added to the complex.

The economic and environmental benefits of using the Cycle-Let system at Village Centre are clear. A septic tank and drainfield are still used for some of the wastewater, but the size of the drainfield now is only about one acre. The two-acre portion of valuable land no longer required for a drainfield could now be used to its full potential.

The \$220,000 value of the land saved more than offset the cost of Cycle-Let and the 70 toilets and urinals associated with it. The use of this recycling system substantially reduces the water bills for tenants and virtually eliminates charges for sewer service.

The environmental benefits are just as obvious. Before Cycle-Let, the annual wastewater flow at Village Centre was calculated to be 4.9 million gallons. Now the calculated annual flow to the drainfield is 1.9 million gallons. That means 3 million gallons of sewage annually that will not be going either to a municipal plant or into the soil. The wastewater treatment system at Village Centre was paid for with private capital, not taxpayer dollars, because the environmental and economic benefits were right.

THETFORD CORPORATION

Thetford Corporation first learned of the Village Centre project in the fall of 1978. The first task was to understand the volume and characteristics of the wastewater that could be produced by a complex like Village Centre. Only after volumes and characteristics are known can a wastewater management strategy be developed that will satisfy the test of both economics and environment.

A list of tenants had already been drawn up, waiting for space at Village Centre. By taking this list of tenants and then analyzing the type of business

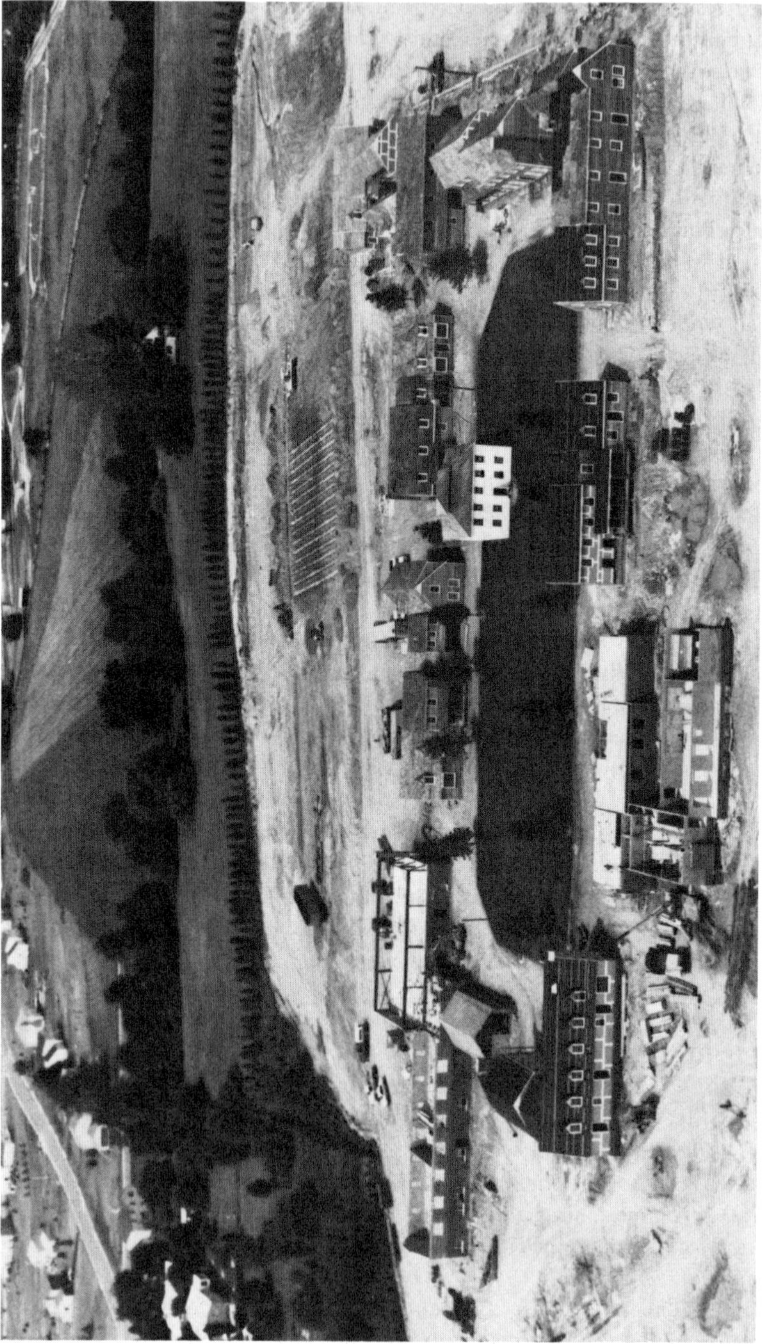

Figure 1. Village Centre, Great Falls, Virginia.

each represented, identifying the number of employees each would have, calculating greywater flows and determining the level of public access to restrooms in each business, it was possible to quantify and qualify the wastewater stream at Village Centre. The total calculated wastewater flow at the site was 13,254 gpd. Of this, 6865 gallons originated at toilets and urinals and 6389 gallons was greywater, originating at hand sinks and food and product preparation centers. The task was to find a solution to what was regarded as a wastewater disposal problem.

The calculated volume of greywater for the site was 6389 gpd; however, by the use of flow-reducing fixtures and appliances, this volume was reduced by 17% to 5354 gpd.

Daily blackwater fixture flushes were calculated at 804. The wastewater management strategy that resulted was that of employing complementing systems, one for greywater and one for blackwater. The Cycle-Let system at the Centre has a design capacity of 1000 fixture flushes per day to allow for the inevitable tenant changes. In addition, the Cycle-Let will process 150 gpd of greywater. The system has a two-day surge or shock load capacity of 2000 fixture flushes per day. The high-quality processed water that is recovered for reuse in flushing fixtures is stored in an 800-gallon tank. This volume of water provides an entire day's supply for flushing at design capacity. The septic tank will receive 5204 gallons of greywater. The septic tank effluent, plus 150 gallons of water processed through Cycle-Let, thus puts 5354 gallons into the soil absorption system.

The following services were provided: blackwater treatment system design and engineering; engineering support for the architects and consulting engineers; system fabrication and assembly; field engineering support for installation; system startup and service personnel training; and one year of field engineering support to the service organization.

Documentation of these data, along with equipment drawings and site drawings, were submitted to Fairfax County with the permit application. The blackwater treatment system consists of a collection system (including Microphor toilets and Spartan urinals), a waste treatment system, an ultrafiltration system and a water polishing system.

The Cycle-Let system occupies 400 ft^2 of floor space in the basement of one of the buildings and is made up of four subsystems. The tasks and functions performed by the system are as follows:

1. The waste treatment module provides rapid biodegradation of waste;
2. The ultrafiltration system provides efficient solids/liquid separation;
3. The water polishing system consists of three elements: activated carbon adsorbers for color and odor removal; ultraviolet light-generated ozone for disinfection of the processed water; and storage and pressurization of the water for return to toilets and urinals for flushing; and
4. The electrical control system provides for microprocessor monitoring and control of the system to ensure the system's failsafe operation.

An overall schematic view of Village Centre shows the total wastewater collection and disposal system (Figure 2).

In addition to equipment costs, there were other cost benefits. The projected operation and maintenance costs for the system are $1200–$1500 to replenish the carbon columns, ultraviolet lamps and pump diaphragms, and $2000 for electrical power costs, for a total of approximately $3500. That is approximately 25% of what the annual sewer rate costs would be if Village Centre were on central sewer service.

Village Centre offered a perfect opportunity to employ an onsite treatment and disposal system. The project has attracted, and will continue to attract, national attention because of the unique character of the complex. All who are interested in innovative and alternative approaches to onsite disposal can feel a measure of accomplishment in this project and the wastewater treatment technology employed here.

THE COMMONWEALTH OF VIRGINIA POSITION

It is the stated policy of the Bureau of Wastewater Engineering in Virginia to encourage the development of any new methods, processes

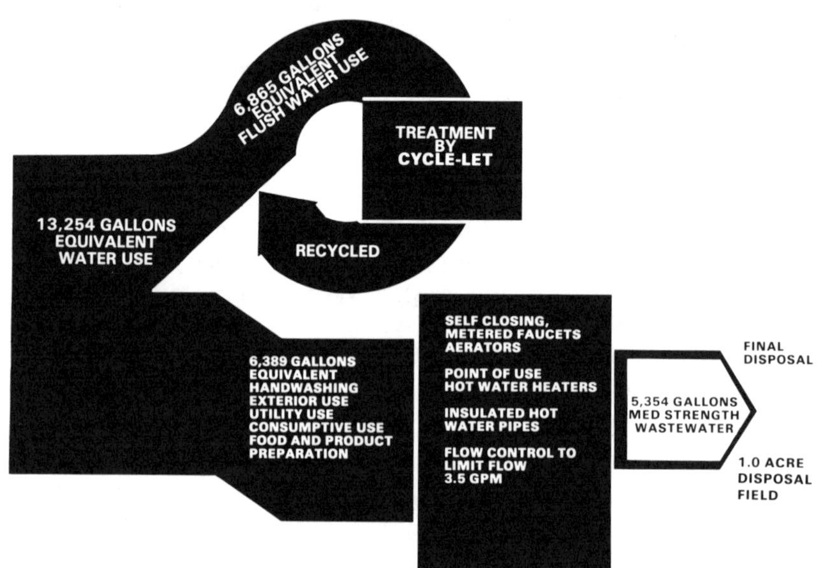

Figure 2. Thetford waste management strategy, Village Centre, Great Falls, Virginia.

or equipment that appear to have application for the treatment and/or disposal of sewage. When the Fairfax County Department of Public Health submitted the Village Centre site and wastewater disposal plan for review, two significant aspects of the proposed wastewater management strategy were recognized immediately. First, this was an innovative combination of complementary wastewater disposal schemes, which appeared to offer both economic benefit to the developer and environmental benefit to the community. The second aspect of the plan was that it appeared to have real potential for use not only at Village Centre, but elsewhere in the state of Virginia as an alternative approach to wastewater disposal needs. The method of treatment and disposal proposed for Village Centre seems to represent the kind of innovation the Bureau is trying to encourage.

However, in confirming both the benefits of the Village Centre approach and the desirability of using such an approach in other applications throughout Virginia, the state would want to have a complete understanding of the design parameters of both the soil absorption system and the Cycle-Let system, and documented evidence of its successful performance.

The Bureau already had more than five years of experience with smaller models of Cycle-Let. The first installation of this system anywhere in the United States was in Prince William County, Virginia, in 1974. Today, this product has been installed in seven different counties in Virginia. The performance of many of those installations has been well documented by an independent Virginia-based wastewater laboratory, the Thetford Corporation and the state of Virginia. After five years of observation, the Bureau was satisfied as to the system's performance for such applications as service stations, individual wholesale and retail outlets, recreational and community center facilities, etc.

Even so, the Village Centre project was on a scale four times larger than any of the earlier Virginia installations. Rather than serving a single building with a predictable resident, this application was serving twelve buildings with a complex array of tenants.

The permit request submitted by Village Centre was well documented with respect to projected volumes and flowrates. Design drawings and details on the Cycle-Let system and the soil absorption field were reviewed. Following review of this information, we recommended that Fairfax County, as part of the permit authorizing the Village Centre wastewater disposal plan, set up a program with the manufacturer and developer to gather operating and performance data on volumes, flows and process bioparameters.

The monitoring program has a twofold purpose. First, it ensures Village Centre, Thetford Corporation and the state of Virginia that the design of this wastewater system is indeed a workable solution for the safe and sanitary disposal of sewage at and from the Village Centre complex. Second, it develops documentation of satisfactory performance that will allow this innovative technology to be applied to other wastewater disposal problems in Virginia. The need for sound and thorough documentation cannot be overstressed in assessing the viability of innovative and alternative technologies for sewage treatment.

The waste treatment system installation is impressive. It is well engineered, and if it performs as well as earlier smaller models, the quiet revolution in sanitary wastewater treatment methods will be well on its way.

CONCLUSIONS

Today, Village Centre is a reality. It demonstrates the innovative employment of onsite disposal systems to satisfy both economic and environmental objectives. It also demonstrates the effectiveness of developers, equipment suppliers and state health departments working together to solve wastewater problems.

REACTION PANEL

T. C. Williams
Chairman of the Board
Williams & Works, Inc.
Grand Rapids, Michigan 49506

Dr. Bower's point seems to be that enforcement is the key to the success of any program and that we should now begin to enforce the laws we have and put more emphasis in our meetings on enforcement of the present rules, regulations and laws.

In connection with the presentation by Mr. Calhoun, I would like to know the estimated annual costs of operation and maintenance. He mentioned the cost of power and carbon (some $35,000 a year), but there must be some labor and related costs involved in the long-term operation and maintenance of the greywater system.

I am also curious to know the cost (and who pays it) of the monitoring program described by Mr. Sutherland. The capital cost of the total system was not given in the presentation—I assume it is something less than $200,000 for the combination of the blackwater and greywater system; however, if it was $200,000, that figure equates to about $33,000,000/mgd. This is not an economic solution in places where public sewers and wastewater treatment facilities are available. It *is* an economic solution when you are farther than $200,000 from the connection to such a system.

To Mr. Cobb, I have a question as to the acceptance by the prospective occupants of the shopping center. I expect there would be little or no question in terms of the prospective occupants, but I wondered if that was any kind of problem to him. It would appear that it shouldn't be and that we can learn a lesson from his method of presentation of this information to his prospective occupants.

Harold D. Baar
Deputy for Environmental Health
Michigan Department of Health
Lansing, Michigan 48909

In response to the Henry County case, it concerns me that land use decisions focus entirely on whether soils are suitable for septic tanks. Certainly the suitability of soils is an important criterion in land use decision, but it shouldn't be *the* decision. So often we consider what comes out of the pipe at the end and how it is disposed of as the most critical factor in deciding how land should be used. We do not take into account the impact in the development of schools, roads, police and fire protection, commercial needs, the needs for drainage, other utilities or the impact on energy costs. While I commend the efforts in Henry County toward code enforcement, I will caution that they should not endeavor to do this by themselves but through education and coordination with other county agencies, in particular the Planning Agency, to address the broader scope of the impacts on land development.

It was mentioned in the presentation that within a year the permits denied accounted for $11,500,000 in lost building construction. As a regulatory agency, those losses are always illuminated for us. What we do not hear, and of equal importance, are the liabilities that go with that kind of construction. What is it going to cost Henry County to correct its past practices and what would it cost to continue as it is now? If the soils are completely unsuitable for onsite sewage disposal, the only permanent correction is an extension of municipal sewers. Those costs are high and rising and are a tremendous price to pay for an absolute lack of planning.

The final point concerning the Henry County case is that sanitarian registration is being attacked by the sunset laws in seven states throughout the United States, including Michigan. Sanitarians are not alone here; engineers and anyone else who is licensed by the state is currently under attack. People are asking, "What is the benefit of having people licensed and certified when a sanitarian, for example, inspects soils which he knows will not work, yet issues the permit?"

The Virginia case presentation left many questions unanswered. Very little was presented about the operation and maintenance. To be truly helpful, we should have the full presentation. I am apprehensive about drainfields of one acre in size and the capability of the soils to absorb the amount of effluent with what will be the effective mounding created by the loading rates. There is also concern about the construction of drainfields that large and equal distribution throughout the field. Many factors will influence that drain system, and the portion of the total wastewater system, whether properly controlled or not, will influence how others perceive that system. There was brief mention that the shopping center includes a medical complex. Was any thought given to how any toxic or hazardous wastes generated by that, or any other, tenant are handled by the Thetford system in its processing and reuse of the wastewater?

Returning to the analogy about whether the cake rises or falls (and we must look for the reason for its rise or fall), even a fallen cake may not be bad eating sometimes. The proof of this case is going to be in the "eating," i.e., the experience two or three years from now. I would hope that through this conference, the literature and other means this will continue to be studied. We can benefit from the *full* picture and make better informed judgments in future.

Allan N. Young, Jr.
President, Cromaglass Corporation
Williamsport, Pennsylvania 17701

Probably we would all agree that we need more control and acceptance of new regulations and methods of handling situations such as those discussed this morning.

Starting with the case of Village Centre in Virginia, I ask, "So, what's new?" Many people in our industry have been working with projects such as this for several years. The question is, "How do we obtain the acceptance of these new methods through regulatory agencies and (perhaps this is the forum through which we must work) organizations such as NSF and these meetings. As with this situation, we have had alternatives recommended in Virginia that were not accepted. It is attributable only to Thetford's persistance that this project was accepted. There are projects in New Hampshire in which large apartment house developments have been built outside the sewered areas, where only 16 apartment units could have been built using standard methods; however, 48 apartments were constructed on the same land using alternative methods and water-saving techniques. *That* is cost-effective. There are other areas in water-scarce islands in the Caribbean where they have been recycling water for several years–complete recycling–for toilet flushing and gardening purposes.

On the situation in Henry County, Dr. Bowers made what I believe to be a very important point. Regulatory agencies, if they had regulations, certainly were not holding to them properly. I have been informed that the direct discharges of sewage to ditches in that area of Indiana is disgraceful. "This is not the way to do it. It is against reasonable sanitary engineering practice." There are projects near Henry County—near the city of Indianapolis—where methods for effluent subsurface disposal are being used properly despite government regulations.

Lowell Welker

Director, Environmental Health
Allen County General Health District
Lima, Ohio

The theme for this session is "Real World Problems and Their Resolution." Resolution might be defined as a statement of opinion or determination and we have heard both.

Certainly there is a place in the entire onsite sewage disposal problem for alternatives and innovations. These case studies have demonstrated good planning for taking care of domestic wastes. This is very important. In fact, it is where management starts in the whole procedure in taking care of domestic wastes.

Unfortunately, in the Henry County case, the systems that were installed in previous years were doomed to fail. This is what we are trying to overcome with modern technology. Many of us feel that one of the best ways to do this is to treat domestic waste immediately after its discharge from the household, instead of putting it into a tank and letting it putrify. I am speaking of the individual aerobic system for homes. I believe they have a place in areas where offlot discharge is not allowed; however, there are many other innovative and alternative ways to handle a treated effluent. I would like to share some ideas that I have encountered. Try to apply these thoughts to yourself and your activity, whatever it might be, with onsite sewage disposal systems—both those that work and those that fail. I have learned that it takes less time to do a thing right than to explain why it was done wrong.

A year ago, Henry County was groping to change some things within the county. Groping is not a dirty word. Einstein was once asked how he worked and he said, "I grope." As was evident in Dr. Bowers' presentation, a fault recognized is half corrected. We note that the number of permits being issued was cut almost in half in one year's time. Henry County has made some big steps in trying to correct a problem and we shouldn't be afraid to take a big step if it is indicated to do so because you can't cross a chasm in two small jumps.

Looking at the Virginia project, this may be classed as an achievement. Just a few years ago, this would have been impossible. We are making progress.

Over the years, I have been rather outspoken and forward in my actions and I have met with a lot of opposition. In most cases, I have learned that when others oppose you, it is often an indication that you are on the right track. What we are experiencing today are really the good old days that we shall long for in a few years. Wisdom is knowing what to do next; skill is knowing how to do it; and virtue is doing it. All progress that we make in the area of onsite sewage disposal is a result of change, but all change is not necessarily progress.

In closing, I want to make this statement: Someone once said that there are three kinds of people in the world; those who make things happen; those who watch things happen; and those who wondered what happened.

Allan J. Coviello
General Manager, Waste Treatment Products Division
Thetford Corporation
Ann Arbor, Michigan 48106

I would like to congratulate Dr. Bowers and Henry County for their courage and behavior, which give the public health professions a good image. Dr. Bowers, by using good problem-solving techniques, came to some major conclusions that could affect the lives of all the people in his county. I am impressed by his attempt to set up a technical committee made up of concerned people throughout the county. It is unfortunate that the committee has not functioned properly. I think the situation we see in Henry County–permits being allowed for onsite systems that should not be installed–is typical across the United States. I have been in 800 counties in this country during the last six years, and it is obvious to me that septic tanks and drainage fields are continuously being installed that should not be installed.

Some of the comments implied that the panacea to this problem is the regional sewer. If Henry County has not started its step one procedures, it is five or ten years away from that goal. If ever I have seen an opportunity for a county to come forward and continue to use its problem-solving and creativity to look at all alternatives and combinations of alternatives and central treatment devices, Henry County is that county. It is an ideal fit and I encourage Dr. Bowers down his path.

5

DECENTRALIZED APPROACHES TO RURAL LAKE WASTEWATER PLANNING–SEVEN CASE STUDIES

Gerald O. Peters, Jr.
Project Manager
WAPORA, Inc.
Chevy Chase, Maryland 20015

Alfred E. Krause
Project Officer
EIS Preparation Section
U.S. Environmental Protection Agency, Region V
Chicago, Illinois 60604

INTRODUCTION

The largest federal public works program now active in the United States is the Construction Grants Program for wastewater treatment under the Clean Water Act (Section 201), as amended. The President has proposed levels of funding for this work of approximately $4.5 billion over each of the next ten years.

Until comparatively recently, the relationship between this cleanup effort and private sewage treatment has been uneasy at best. Applicant facilities plan proposals often looked on the widespread use of individual systems as a priori evidence of water quality problems. Where water quality problems actually existed, often only casual efforts were made to determine any cause and effect relationships between individual systems and the problem.

Another important problem of these earlier days was a strong emphasis on regionalization of wastewater treatment: a regionalized sewer system serving a number of discrete areas was considered preferable to a number of systems with local treatment plants, and both were preferable to continued reliance on individual systems. The whole hierarchy of values was oriented against private systems.

The rising costs of indiscriminate regionalization and an awareness of the limited capabilities of even the massive Section 201 funding were some of the immediate causes of the 1977 amendments to the Clean Water Act. These amendments recognize the great potential role of individual systems and indeed provide for a higher level of federal funding for them. They also recognize the need for continuing public management of such systems, including periodic monitoring and inspection.

Even before the amendments were passed, however, U.S. Environmental Protection Agency (EPA) Region V noticed that there were literally hundreds of municipalities and sewer districts with construction grant projects in an early planning stage distinguished by certain characteristics:

1. Most were in rural areas.
2. Most involved total or partial sewering of rural lakeshores.
3. Most had a substantial seasonal population.
4. Most reaching the planning stage had received only a casual consideration of the real role of private systems in water quality problems, or of the use of such systems in solving them.
5. Most reaching the planning stage were unusually expensive in terms of size and population served.

Table I.

Project	Location	Comments	Lake Area (ac)
Crystal Lake	Benzie County, Michigan	1 large lake 1 small nontributary lake	9,792
Crooked and Pickerel Lakes	Emmett County, Michigan	2 medium lakes	2,400 1,100
Salem Township	Kenosha County, Wisconsin	8 nontributary lakes	43.2- 464
Steuben Lakes	Steuben County, Indiana	11 lakes; 9 tributaries	34 -1,000+
Nettle Lake	Williams County, Ohio	1 small lake	95
Green Lake	Kandiyohi County, Minnesota	1 large lake 2 tributaries	5,406 1,697 945
Otter Tail Lake	Otter Tail County, Minnesota	1 large lake 5 small lakes	14,746 4,000 T

Not only did these projects exhibit a high local cost ($4000 or more per dwelling even after a 75% federal grant), but they also often showed typical environmental problems, such as destruction of wetlands or endangered species habitat. Many of the local costs were so high that they themselves became major impacts on the human environment, causing potential population displacement.

SELECTION OF PROJECTS

In July 1977, EPA Region V selected seven typical projects of this type as the subject for seven individual environmental impact statements (EIS). All involved substantial environmental impacts and all featured a high cost per dwelling served. The seven projects were Crystal and Crooked/Pickerel Lakes in Michigan; Green and Otter Tail Lakes in Minnesota; the eleven Steuben Lakes in Indiana; Nettle Lake in Ohio; and the eight Salem Township Lakes in Wisconsin. Together these projects included 35 different lakes at different stages of shoreline development and lake trophic conditions; their general characteristics are shown in Table I.

As shown in Tables I and II, the seven projects included lake areas ranging from single small lakes to single large lakes to complexes of eight or more

Project Background

Hydrology				
Volume (ac-ft)	Minimum Depth (ft)	Retention (yr)	1977 Population (permanent/seasonal)	Facilities Plan Design Population (permanent/seasonal)
616,896	64	64	2,600/3,200	4,830/5,170
24,173 13,636	10 13	NA	420/420	1,200/800
362- 4,891	5-20	0.6- 5.1	4,400/4,300	7,500/7,500
427-17,610	8-30.3	0.1-10.6	4,800/6-15,000	6,000/8-19,000
NA	NA	NA	110/550	250/1000
113,500 33,600 14,200	21 20 15	3.7 0.5	2,401/4,164	5,146/3,184
339,158 35,000 T	23	2.43 0.3-9.1	1,114/5,174	1,506/6,996

lakes. Proposed project environmental problems ranged from cost impacts to secondary development to interbasin transfer to possible impact on endangered species habitat. Existing lakewater quality ranged from pristine to highly eutrophic, with elevated bacteria levels.

The engineering response of the applicant's consultants ranged from comparatively straightforward to bewilderingly complex; in its original form, one project serving 10,000 people had about 85 miles of interceptor and collector sewers. Almost all lacked any definite determination of project need or water quality impact on the lakes served. Local costs ranged from high to exorbitant; on one project, about 30% of the population served faced local and private costs ranging between $1\frac{1}{2}$ and $2\frac{1}{2}$ times the value of the average single family dwelling. Local reaction ranged from passive acceptance to vigorous support to ferocious controversy.

None of the projects represented a simple failure of engineering competence by the original consultants. All were firms not only of recognized ability, but of known eminence in their fields. This suggested that some of

Table II. Facilities

Project	Proposal	Present Worth Cost[a] ($)	Cost/Existing Total ($)	Cost/Existing Local ($)
Crystal Lake	Sewer around lake + existing plant replacement + combined sewer separation	18,000,000	9,400	2,800[b]
Crooked and Pickerel Lakes	Sewer around lakes + treatment at existing plant in Petoskey	3,900,000	12,600	2,800+[b]
Salem Township	Sewering around 8 lakes + 1.5 mgc actual sludge + 1.6 mile outfall	13,800,000	4,419	
Steuben Lakes	65.2 miles of sewer around 8 lakes + regional STP	23,200,000	5,562	2,229[b]
Nettle Lake	Sewer around lake + aeration lagoon	1,300,000	4,800	2,500[b]
Green Lake	Sewer around lake + lagoons	8,400,000	7,700	4,100
Otter Tail Lake	Sewer around lake + lagoons + land application	11,380,000	4,800	2,170

[a]Capital Costs + 20 years operation and maintenance, less salvage value.
[b]Does not include private costs to homeowner for lateral connection. For Nettle Lake indoor plumbing + construction of bathroom.

the problems posed by these projects might be beyond the grasp of existing technology and that later facilities plans might not show great improvement. There was a definite need to examine new or neglected techniques that might allow adequate response to project needs at a cost bearable to the population served.

EPA Region V therefore instructed WAPORA, Inc., its EIS consultant, to examine innovative, alternative and other conservation-oriented approaches, some for the first time in an EIS or facilities plan. These included:

1. realistic use of flow reduction and water conservation measures;
2. use of land application of wastewater, mound systems, cluster septic tank systems, low-pressure sewers, composting toilets and onsite maintenance and upgrading;
3. use of several of these systems in combination, tailoring service to the needs of individual project subareas; and
4. evaluation of administrative and management approaches to the use of such systems.

Plan Proposals

Dwelling Annual ($)	Environmental Issues
292[b]	High local cost; seasonal population displacement; actual water quality impact; EIS request by state and applicant.
NA	High local cost; seasonal population displacement; secondary impact; interbasin transfer.
370–525	High local costs; seasonal population displacement; actual water quality impact; discharge to chain of lakes in nearby Illinois.
260[b]	High local costs; seasonal population displacement; actual water quality impact; secondary impact, especially on wetlands and endangered species habitat.
200[b]	Extremely high local cost (1½ times value of average dwelling) for 33% of population served by privies; retired population displacement; impact on archaeological site; secondary impact on endangered species habitat.
234 permanent 180 seasonal	High local costs; displacement of seasonal and retired population; secondary impact on wetlands; local controversy.
302 permanent 302 seasonal[b]	High local costs, actual water quality impact; displacement of seasonal and retired population; secondary impact.

population served by privies, private costs include lateral connection + installation of

All new alternatives were to be evaluated for their impacts on the natural and human environment, consistent with the National Environmental Policy Act (NEPA). A special issue-oriented format was adopted to make the statements particularly comprehensible.

Completion of the seven individual impact statements is to be followed by an overall generic EIS on problems of rural lake sewering. This statement is to use the seven projects and their thirty-five lakes as case studies to develop specific recommendations for future project planning. These recommendations will include methods of documenting project need and water quality impact, alternative approaches specifically requiring consideration in particular cases, and many other elements. The generic statement will also attempt a general case survey of the dynamics of rural lakeshore development. Eventually, this will lead to preparation of a *Rural Lakes Sewer Project Handbook*, summarizing these recommendations, to be distributed to grant applicants, consulting engineers and government bodies at all levels.

Five of the seven draft EIS's have been published. The remaining two were to be published by December 1979. Work on the EIS's has produced valuable insights into the process of planning rural wastewater facilities and their effects on water resources, environmentally sensitive areas and the human environment. The EIS's and studies undertaken in support of their development should become models for evaluation of alternative technologies in rural areas. Of particular interest are the use of both conventional and innovative methods for documenting public health and water quality problems caused by existing onsite septic tank–sewage absorption systems.

DEVELOPMENT OF ALTERNATIVES

The facilities plans for which the EIS's were prepared all recommended sewering of lakeshore properties and centralized treatment. To compare alternative technologies and management approaches with the Facilities Plans recommendations, a variety of wastewater management plans were developed for each community. Development of these alternative plans generally followed five steps:

- Analysis of Available Data
- Screening of Alternative Technologies
- Preliminary Alternative Design
- Economic Analysis
- Revision of Alternatives

Data presented in the facilities plans and acquired from other local and state sources were reviewed for use in the EIS's to describe the existing natural and manmade environments and to provide the basis for the design and evaluation of alternatives. The data on condition and effects of existing onsite systems were generally insufficient to justify total area sewering and centralized treatment. In all study areas, the available data failed to document significant public health problems, groundwater contamination or other water quality problems, despite the age and frequently improper siting, design and maintenance of onsite systems. Soils suitable for subsurface disposal of septic tank effluent were found in all or parts of the study areas on or near presently developed sites.

A number of alternative technologies were incorporated into the wastewater management plans developed for the EIS's. A list of these technologies is presented in Table III according to their function. Many other potentially viable technologies were not incorporated, either because they involved discharge of excessive nutrients to area lakes (e.g., small lagoons, package plants) or because insufficient site information was available to justify their cost (e.g., aerobic treatment, evapotranspiration systems).

For those plans that avoided central sewers, the lack of detailed, site-specific data resulted in the use of conservatively high estimates for the

Table III. Alternative Technologies Incorporated in Wastewater Management Plans

Function	Technology
Flow and Waste Load Reduction	– Low-flow toilets – Pressure toilets – Composting toilets – Low-flow shower heads – Air-assisted showers – Faucet flow restrictors – Phosphorus ban
Collection	– Pressure sewers – Vacuum sewers – Holding tanks – Blackwater/greywater separation
Wastewater Treatment	– Septic tanks – Slow-rate land application – Marsh/pond system
Effluent Disposal	– Onsite subsurface disposal unit – Hydrogen peroxide treatment of subsurface disposal units – Multifamily, offsite subsurface disposal units – Elevated sand mounds – Rapid infiltration – Wetlands discharge – Dosed subsurface disposal units
Sludge Disposal	– Land application – Composting

rehabilitation, replacement and abandonment of onsite systems. An example of the assumptions made for one study area is presented in Table IV. These estimates were later revised downward for several study areas after field data collection.

To generate costs that could be equitably compared on a present worth basis, all alternatives for a community were based on one population projection. This effort at uniformity was later determined to have sacrificed reality. For nonsewered alternatives in lake communities near urban employment centers, growth is likely to be limited by the amount of land that can be developed with onsite systems. Developable land would not be a restriction with centralized collection and treatment.

Economic analysis of the preliminary alternatives included 20-year present worth and estimation of 1980 average user charges. While many interesting cost relationships were recognized, the most significant and conclusive finding had to do with conventional onsite systems. Even with the high assumptions for renovation and replacement, high housing densities (some approaching four houses per acre), and allowances for holding tanks or offsite cluster

Table IV. Assumed Levels of Replacement, Rehabilitation, Abandonment, and New Construction of Decentralized Facilities: Crystal Lake, Michigan, Preliminary Draft EIS, Alternative 3

Existing Systems–1980

- 59% of existing onsite soil absorption units would be abandoned. Septic tank effluent pumps would transport wastewaters to new multifamily filter fields.
- Most of the remaining systems would be replaced or rehabilitated according to the following figures:

	Pre-1964[a] Systems (%)	Systems Installed 1964-1980 (%)
Replace septic tank	75	25
Replace soil absorption unit with drainfield	50	25
Replace soil adsorption unit with mound	25	10
Install holding tank	2	0
Hydrogen peroxide renovation of drainfield	10	10

Future Systems–1980-2000

- Future housing would be accommodated with a mix of system designs:

Conventional septic tank/drainfield	56%
Septic tank/dosed drainfield	19%
Septic tank/mound	20%
Cluster system	5%
Hydrogen peroxide renovation	2%

[a]1964 was the first year that local health codes for onsite systems were in effect.

systems, the present worth for continued use of onsite systems was substantially less expensive than any method of centralized collection and treatment. An even greater savings in 1980 average user charges resulted from higher federal funding of capital costs for alternative technologies and from deferment of sewerage costs for new housing.

Because of the substantial economic advantages and unresolved concern over the actual condition and water quality impacts of "continued use," major field data collection efforts were initiated in August 1978. The techniques used and pertinent results are summarized in this chapter. More detailed discussions of the innovative data collection techniques are presented in Chapters 37 and 38.

In five study areas, the new data plus modeling of lake eutrophication potential indicated that most existing onsite systems were not causing public health or water quality problems. Because of the poor design and/or maintenance of those systems causing problems, rehabilitation or replacement and publicly supervised maintenance of existing systems with provision for holding tanks or cluster system for the worst cases was judged to be a reliable approach to wastewater management in those five study areas. New alternatives were described and costed that maximize the continued use of onsite systems but that still assume conservatively high estimates for renovation and replacement. Table V presents a brief description and cost data for the alternatives recommended by EPA in the draft EIS's.

FIELD EVALUATIONS OF ONSITE SYSTEMS PERFORMANCE

Present EPA guidance on the eligibility of new collector sewers for federal fundings (Program Guidance Memorandum 78-9) requires that alternatives to conventional sewers be evaluated. Where an alternative is feasible and cost-effective, sewers will not be eligible. The cost analysis performed for the Seven Lakes EIS indicates that renovation and replacement of onsite systems is cost-effective for these communities, even at high levels of construction and at moderately high housing densities. The feasibility of renovation and replacement was addressed through collection of new data on the extent of problems related to existing onsite systems and analysis of factors that caused the problems.

The first source of information on the type, extent and causes of onsite failures should be the local officials responsible for community sanitation and local contractors who install and repair onsite systems. These individuals can provide the most valuable, readily available information on onsite systems short of conducting field investigations. In some cases, the information provided by review of file data and interviews may be adequate for making

Table V. EPA Recommendations and Economic Statistics for the Seven Lakes Study Areas

Project	EPA Draft EIS Recommendations	Present Worth ($ million)	Average 1980 User Charge ($/yr/household)	Percent Savings[a]	
				Present Worth	User Charge
Crystal Lake Area Sewage Disposal Authority, Benzie County, Michigan	Sewer or cluster 1/6 of lake + replace existing plant + onsite upgrading + cluster systems as necessary.	7.5	60	59	86
Green Lake Sanitary Sewer and Water District, Kandiyohi County, Minnesota	Renovate and replace existing onsite systems. Upgrade two existing STP's or replace with rapid or slow-rate land application.	5.1 5.4 4.5	130[b] 120 130	39 36 46	19 25 19
Salem Utility District #2, Kenosha County, Wisconsin	Minor reduction in Service Area by using cluster systems and existing systems. Conventional collection and land application for most of area.	13.5	280	13	15

Steuben Lake Study Area, Steuben County, Indiana	Onsite upgrading + cluster systems.	8.3	50	64	89
Otter Tail Facility Planning Area, Otter Tail County, Minnesota	Centralized sewerage for one small area; cluster systems + onsite systems renovation and replacement.	7.1	165	31	53
Springvale-Bear Creek Sewage Disposal Authority, Emmet County, Michigan	Onsite upgrading + cluster systems.	1.2	90	67	86
Nettle Lake Study Area, Williams County, Ohio	Decision has not been made.	NA	NA	NA	NA

[a]Compared with EIS estimation of costs for centralized collection and treatment proposed in Facilities Plan.
[b]Three options for treatment and disposal remaining for analysis by the applicant.

appropriate conclusions on whether to continue using onsite systems. However, such information may be insufficient for facilities planning for the following reasons:

1. Not all problems are reported to officials because of the costs of appropriate repairs or because homeowners or their neighbors do not recognize the problem, as in the case of groundwater contamination.
2. Health departments rarely monitor the operation and effects of onsite systems. They normally address existing problems on a complaint basis only. Typically, neither the funds nor the authority to monitor existing systems are available to the local official.

Table VI. Field Methods Utilized in Investigating the Impacts of Onsite

			Problems
Method	Surface Ponding of Septic Tank[a] Effluent	Household Backup	Aquifer Contamination
Sanitary Survey	Locate	Locate and quantify frequency of occurrence	
Well Sampling (total and fecal coliform and NO_3)			Quantify contamination
Aerial Photography	Locate		
Septic Leachate			Device can be used on well-water sample
Shallow Groundwater Flow Monitoring			
Shallow Groundwater Sampling			
Surface Water Sampling			

[a]May include other systems such as cesspools, etc.

3. Contractors are reticent to provide specific information on unresolved problems because of uncertainties about actions that might be taken against their customers.

When official and contractor information is not sufficient to evaluate the cost-effectiveness and feasibility of "continued use" for all or parts of a community, several conventional and innovative field data collection methods are available. The methods used in preparation of the Seven Lakes EIS's are presented in Table VI. For each method, the types of problems are listed that they can detect or quantify. Costs to use these methods shown in the table are based on the following assumptions:

Wastewater Management Systems on Water Quality and Public Health

Covered				
Discharge of Septic Tank[a] Effluent to Surface Water				
Direct	Via Groundwater	Nearshore Plant Growth	Other Information	Cost (based on hypothetical lake situation discussed in text) (%)
Locate		Locate and identify	Occupancy Water use System design Public attitudes Public education	10,800
			Background concentrations for lake nutrient budgets	3,000
Possible by use of thermal scanning device		Locate	Land use Wildlife habitat Topography Housing counts Lake morphology	3,000
Locate only	Locate only			11,800
	Identify source		Groundwater flow data for lake nutrient budgets	5,000
	Quantify contamination			3,100
Quantify contamination	Quantify contamination			3,100

- development located primarily near lakeshores;
- 600 homes;
- total shoreline of 9 miles;
- sanitary surveys conducted for 25–40% of residences;
- surface and shallow groundwater samples taken for nutrient and bacteriological analysis at 30 sites in the vicinity of effluent plumes entering the lake;
- shallow groundwater and surface water sampling in conjunction with the shoreline septic leachate survey; and
- wellwater sampling in conjunction with a sanitary survey.

This hypothetical lake situation is presented so that an economic comparison can be made of the field evaluation techniques. The cost presented could vary greatly depending on factors such as time of year, lake morphology, resident cooperativeness and the detail of results required.

Sanitary surveys are house-to-house interviews with residents on the usage, design and condition of their existing onsite systems. The survey should include inspection of the lot, well and lakeshore in the company of the resident. In the context of 201 Facilities Planning, there should be three basic goals in performing a sanitary survey:

1. to identify public health problems and potential water quality problems to aid in determining grant eligibility for collector sewers;
2. to provide a basis for identifying feasible water conservation and onsite technologies to be included in cost-effective analysis of alternative approaches for wastewater management; and
3. to evaluate design, usage and site limitations that may be affecting performance of onsite systems.

Because of the cost involved, sanitary surveys should be conducted only when these goals cannot be achieved by other methods. When they are conducted, however, the results will be of most use when the surveyor has a basic knowledge of soils, water quality and design of onsite systems. The sanitary survey form developed by WAPORA, Inc. during the course of several surveys is based on the surveyor having this knowledge. A copy of the form is presented as Appendix A. It covers seven main topics, including:

1. location and description of the property;
2. occupancy, including size of household, duration of occupancy, intended use and planned additions;
3. type of sewage disposal systems;
4. service history of the system;
5. water-using facilities;
6. site characteristics; and
7. sketch of the property, surface drainage facilities and sanitary facilities.

A well inspection form is also included so that wellwater samples and probability of contamination can be evaluated.

For 201 Facilities Planning, a partial survey covering 10–50% of residences may be adequate. The amount of coverage should depend on the uniformity of soils, water resources and system age.

There are several advantages in conducting a sanitary survey that may not be available with other survey methods:

1. It is the only method for obtaining quantitative data on the frequency and causes of sewage backups in the house or plumbing.
2. The interview can be used to determine socioeconomic characteristics and water usage patterns, as valuable planning data are not otherwise available for small communities with no metered water supply.
3. Insight may be gained into problems that may not have been suspected previously, such as unregulated system installation and maintenance practices.
4. The survey can serve as an effective public participation tool, allowing the interviewer to provide information to the public on the facilities planning and construction grants process, the range of alternatives being examined, preliminary findings, and means by which the public can participate in the decision-making process. In return, the interviewer can determine public opinion relating to the project from those most directly affected by it.

Disadvantages to the sanitary survey include the following:

1. The cost is high.
2. The information provided by the resident may not be complete or reliable. Residents may be unwilling to discuss problems with their systems for fear of expensive repairs. They may not be knowledgeable regarding their systems, particularly if they are renting the property.
3. Unless conducted for all dwellings, the assumption must be made that a partial survey fairly represents the entire community. Costs for "continued use" alternatives depend on the validity of that assumption.
4. Results of the survey may be biased by the time of day, week or year conducted. Permanent residences occupied all day are more likely to be included and are also more likely to have onsite problems because of greater wastewater flows.

Sampling of wellwaters will provide invaluable information on the effects of onsite sewage disposal on groundwater aquifers. Conventional parameters for analysis by health department or commercial laboratories are total coliforms, fecal coliforms and nitrates. Fecal streptococci can also be analyzed, but bacterial counts are normally too low to provide meaningful fecal coliform:fecal strep ratios for evaluating the bacteria's source. Ammonia nitrogen could be a valuable analysis, particularly if local soil conditions do not facilitate oxidation of this pollutant to the nitrate form.

A new, potentially powerful and inexpensive method for detecting short-circuiting of wastewater to wells was applied to several wells in Seven Lakes study areas. Fluorescence analysis for detergent brighteners is highly sensitive to minute concentrations of these organic molecules because of naturally low background concentrations and the inherently low detection limits of the equipment. Whereas bacteria may die off and nitrates may be diluted to concentrations near background, fluorescent organic materials present in nearly all sewage would show whether there exists any direct hydrologic connection between onsite sewage and water supply systems. The technique of fluorescence analysis is discussed in Chapter 37.

To evaluate the effects of onsite sewage disposal on wellwater quality using bacterial indicators and nitrate data, only those wells protected from contamination by surface runoff should be sampled. An inspection of the well for proper surface drainage, grouting of the annular space around the well casing, integrity of well seal and proper well venting should be documented. Otherwise, well data may be used to justify community sewering in situations in which a community water supply or renovation of the wells would be more appropriate.

In addition to providing information on local aquifer contamination, well data might also be useful in estimating nutrient loads to lakes from groundwater recharge. Another possible use is as background reference data for shallow groundwater sampling programs in locations directly affected by effluent plumes.

Aerial imagery of all Seven Lakes study areas was acquired by EPA's Environmental Photographic Interpretation Center (EPIC) for detection of surface malfunctions (ponding). Three types of imagery were acquired, including normal color photographs, color infrared photographs and black and white thermal infrared scans. High-resolution, normal color film was found to be the most successful format for this purpose. More information on this work is provided in Chapter 38.

Advantages of the aerial survey include the following:

1. It is relatively inexpensive.
2. Total coverage of a study area is possible.
3. The survey can be completed quickly and without mobilizing equipment and manpower.
4. The imagery provides current data on land use, wildlife habitat areas, wetlands, housing density and number, waste disposal sites, aquatic plant growth, transportation, topography, lake morphology, etc.

Limitations of the methods are as follows:

1. For greatest benefit, the imagery should be collected during wet seasons before foliage grows.
2. Clear weather is required for the flyover.
3. Direct discharges to streams or lakes, groundwater problems and household backups would not be detected.

4. A small percentage of surface malfunctions may be obscured by heavy foliage directly over the malfunctions.

The septic leachate detector is a newly developed device capable of detecting near ultraviolet fluorescent organics derived from whiteners, surfactants and natural degradation products, which are persistent under the combined conditions of low oxygen and limited microbial activity. Operated continuously while drawn along a lake's shoreline or stream, this device can pinpoint the location of effluent emergence into surface waters. It was also used during field studies to detect effluent in samples taken through ice holes in winter and to trace the shape and relative strength of effluent plumes in groundwaters sampled from test sites. More information on the operation and applications of this equipment is presented in Chapter 37.

Septic leachate surveys allow rapid detection of effluents that may be adversely affecting surface water quality. No other currently available technique can accomplish this effectively. Once located, the effluent plume can be sampled and analyzed by standard laboratory methods to determine the degree of pollution on a highly site-specific basis.

Advantages of the septic leachate survey are as follows:

1. All lakeshore onsite systems that directly or indirectly (via groundwater) discharge to surface waters can be identified in a short time.
2. The equipment can be used in different modes to sample continuously using a submerged pump or to test discrete samples drawn from any source.
3. Waters pumped through the equipment during a continuous shoreline scan can be captured and saved for analysis without resampling at that location.
4. Because of naturally low fluorescence of most surface waters, the very low detection limit of the equipment and the persistence of the fluorescent organics, effluent plumes can be detected even after use of a sewage disposal system is discontinued and in conditions of moderately high mixing or dilution.

The following are the limitations of the detector:

1. The equipment is new, and few trained operators are available who can use it effectively and interpret the data realistically.
2. To date, the data output of the detector can only be expressed in relative terms. Use of the equipment to predict actual proportions of wastewater in samples or to estimate concentrations of other contaminants in samples is not justified.

Another device developed by Dr. Kerfoot is a groundwater flowmeter. This was used in several of the study areas to determine groundwater flow direction and rate along shorelines. In addition to providing new data on groundwater hydrology, the meter, when used in conjunction with the septic leachate detector, can verify the source of effluent plumes detected in surface waters. The meter has shown that significant variations in groundwater flow occur over relatively short distances and that lake level can significantly alter groundwater flow at a given location. The use of this meter could provide a rational method for locating new or replacement subsurface sewage disposal units in situations where distances to wells, lakes or streams are limited.

Sampling and laboratory analysis of groundwaters directly affected by onsite sewage disposal was undertaken in conjunction with the septic leachate surveys and during very detailed monitoring of 17 onsite systems serving lakeside dwellings. During the septic leachate surveys a specially fabricated stainless steel well point was used to sample groundwater at a depth of 18 inches into lake sediments beneath detected effluent plumes. Calculation of nutrient breakthrough to the lake was based on expected nutrient concentrations and conductance of wastewaters, assumed background conductance and concentrations of nutrients, and on the assumption that the center of the surface water effluent plumes coincided with the center of the groundwater effluent plumes. Later, detailed site work showed both that background conductance varies too much to support the calculations, and that locating the center of a groundwater effluent plume is considerably less certain than initially believed. A new method to estimate nutrient breakthrough incorporating the septic leachate detector, groundwater flowmeter and a modified well point sampler is being developed.

RESULTS OF THE FIELD EVALUATIONS

The results of our extensive investigations are summarized in Table VII for the seven study areas.

Because many of the existing onsite systems were constructed prior to enforcement of present sanitary codes and because of shallow depth to groundwater in lakeshore areas, the percentage of systems not conforming to the codes is very high. Small lot sizes, substandard design of septic tanks and soil absorption units, and inadequate separation distances between onsite systems and wells or lakes are typical in these communities. Based on this information and the difficulty of complying strictly with present design codes for conventional onsite sytems, the facilities planners concluded that continued use of onsite systems was not feasible. As previously mentioned, however, documentation of public health and water quality problems was not provided in the facilities plans.

Surface malfunctions—the most obvious type of problem—were relatively infrequent. The highest surface failure rate, 8%, occurred in Salem Utility District #2, an area characterized by moderately to highly impermeable soils. With the exception of this community, for which EPA has not recommended continued use of onsite systems, there were an estimated 45 surface malfunctions in the other six communities. Nearly all were caused by old, poorly maintained onsite systems. An example of what can be done about such problems is provided by the Steuben County Health Department's dye testing and enforcement program undertaken before the EIS was initiated. Out of approximately 125 discharges and surface malfunctions, only four remained in 1978.

A more frequent problem is the backup or sluggish operation of some systems. Of the residents having this problem, a majority claimed that backups occurred on holiday weekends and other times when guests increased the hydraulic loading on the systems. Other systems performed poorly in spring when soils were wet, while a few had a low capacity year round. Many of the residents claiming recurrent backups, and some who have not had this problem, have avoided installing clothes washers and dishwashers or have altered their water use habits. However, few have installed or have even known about effective water conservation devices that are available.

Elevated nitrate concentrations, defined as greater than 4 mg/l NO_3-N, were found in up to 8% of the wells sampled. A total of six wells out of the 437 sampled before and during preparation of the EIS's had nitrate concentrations exceeding the 10 mg/l drinking water standard.

Total coliform counts above 1/100 ml were detected in wellwater samples from three of the four communities in which well surveys were conducted. The highest percentage of positive samples, 29%, was found in the Green Lake study area. While this rate is high, the condition of the sampled wells was not reported, and it is inconclusive whether the contamination was caused by onsite systems.

Plumes of effluent were found to emerge from the groundwater into lakes in all of the study areas except Nettle Lake, where there appears to be little or no groundwater inflow to the lake. However, sampling of lakewater at the point of plume emergence indicates that few are contaminated with indicator bacteria or show nutrient concentrations above background levels. Exceptions to this general finding were bacteria present in plumes resulting from sewage in overland runoff and nutrients in groundwater plumes passing through acidic, organic soils.

Stream source plumes were found entering one or more lakes in each study area. The "streams" ranged in size from major tributaries to the lakes down to small ditches with a limited drainage area of a few acres. Stream source plumes were located during septic leachate surveys. Sources of wastewater included municipal sewage treatment plant effluents, direct discharges, surface runoff and groundwater leachate. In the Steuben Lakes, a large, previously unrecognized source of nutrients was found by using the leachate

Table VII. Investigations Conducted, Nonconformance with Local

Study Area	Investigations Conducted[a]	Number of Lakeshore Residences	D.U. Onsite Systems in Nonconformance with Local Sanitary Codes (%)	Surface Ponding (%)	Recurrent Backups (%)
Crystal Lake Area Sewage Disposal Authority, Benzie County, Michigan	A,B,C[b],D, E,F,G,H	500	54 (B)	3 (B)	20 (B)
Green Lake Sanitary Sewer and Water District, Kandiyohi County, Minnesota	A,B,C,D, E,F,G,H	677	47 (B)	1 (D) 1 (B)	11 (B)
Salem Utility District #2, Kenosha County, Wisconsin	A,D,E,G,H	1,273	No data	8 (D)	NA
Steuben Lakes Study Area, Steuben County, Indiana	A,C,D,E. F,G,H	3,513	90 (A)	<1 (D)	NA
Otter Tail Facility Planning Area, Otter Tail County, Minnesota	A,B,C,D, E,F,G,H	1,440	85 (A + B)	<1 (D) <1 (B)	2 (B)

Codes and Problems Quantified in the Seven Lakes Study Areas

Elevated Well Nitrates (>4 mg/l) (%)	Coliform in Wells (>1 count 100/ml) (%)	Effluent Plumes (%)	Number of Stream Source Plumes	Comments
4[b]	0	18 (90)	~7	Aerial photography was conducted during summer months; foliage may have prevented the detection of some malfunctioning systems. EPIC photography detected "suspected beds of submerged aquatic vegetation" (49) but not ponding of septic effluent.
7[b]	29[b,c]	9 (64)	8	A major undocumented source of phosphorus loading was observed originating from the discharge stream of an unnamed lake in the Study Area. Sampled wells were not checked for casing integrity. Contamination may have resulted from poor installation.
NA	NA	5 (65)	~37	Only two plumes were found to be of groundwater origin; the others represented overland runoff or bog drainage inflows.
0	10	2 (65)	5	Prior to the EIS's, eight dye test programs were conducted by the Steuben County Health Department. Approximately 126 malfunctioning systems along lakeshore areas were located and repaired immediately after discovery.
8	5	16 (235)	5	A nearly one-to-one relationship was noted between plumes and permanent dwelling units in the first septic leachate study, which took place in the winter. The second survey, which took place during Labor Day, located far fewer plumes. These changes were probably due to elevated water level in Otter Tail Lake and changes in groundwater flow from winter to summer. Direct discharges of septic effluent are suspected based on information gathered in sanitary survey.

Table VII,

Study Area	Investigations Conducted[a]	Number of Lakeshore Residences	D.U. Onsite Systems in Nonconformance with Local Sanitary Codes (%)	Surface Ponding (%)	Recurrent Backups (%)
Springvale-Bear Creek Sewage Disposal Authority, Emmet County, Michigan	A,B,D,E	212	78 (B)	4 (D) 8 (B)	9 (B)
Nettle Lake Study Area, Williams County, Ohio	A,B,D,E	284	44 (A + B)	0 (B) 0 (D)	10 (B)

[a]A - Interview with local health department; B - sanitary survey; C - well sampling; itoring; G - shallow groundwater sampling; H - surface water sampling.
[b]Obtained prior to WAPORA study.
[c]Based on MPN.

detector. That source showed a larger phosphorus load than all of the groundwater effluent plumes combined. Because of the possibility that direct discharges of sewage could be the source of stream source plumes, sanitary surveys and leachate detection in tributary areas may be necessary.

Sanitary codes requiring minimum depths to groundwater beneath soil absorption units could have a significant effect on the design and cost of "continued use" alternatives. Yet analysis of lakewaters at the point of plume emergence, even where drainfield or dry wells are actually in the groundwater, indicates that in nearly all cases, water quality standards are not being violated. In most cases, bacteriological and nutrient analyses were not measurably higher than center-lake samples. Detailed investigations of nutrient transport, groundwater flow and aquatic plant growth were conducted for 17 lakeside onsite systems. All systems chosen for investigation represented worst case conditions for depth to groundwater, system age and proximity to lakes. Septic leachate analysis of surface and groundwaters, continued

Elevated Well Nitrates (>4 mg/l) (%)	Coliform in Wells (>1 count 100/ml) (%)	Effluent Plumes (%)	Number of Stream Source Plumes	Comments
NA	NA	24 (51)	2	
NA	NA	0 (0)	1	No substantial groundwater plumes of effluent from nearshore septic units were observed along the shoreline of Nettle Lake. Some variation in background conductance usually occurs as a result of the inflow of different types of groundwater; this was lacking along the shoreline of Nettle Lake, indicating very little groundwater inflow.

D - aerial photography; E - septic leachate scan; F - shallow groundwater flow mon-

shallow groundwater sampling onlot and beneath the lake, sanitary survey interviews with the resident, nutrient analysis of wellwaters, groundwater flowmetering, nutrient analysis of soils and lake sediments, and quantification of nearshore plant growth were conducted for each site. Because earlier survey results had shown that bacterial contamination of lakes through groundwater effluent plumes was not a problem, bacteriological analysis was not included.

Interpretation of groundwater, plant and soil chemistry data from these detailed site evaluations has not been completed at this time. Quantification of nearshore plant growth and correlation with the location of effluent plume emergence showed that some stimulation of attached algae growth occurs where there is suitable substrate for attachment. The amount of growth was relatively small and was seen as a problem by the residents only in a highly oligotrophic lake where it is the only aquatic plant growth to be found.

CONCLUSIONS

Extensive field data collection has shown that the actual public health and water quality problems caused by onsite systems in these lakeshore communities are not as extensive as nonconformance with sanitary codes might indicate. The natural assimilative capacity of soil/groundwater/surface water systems in these hardwater, glacial lakes and lakeshores is greater than they had previously been considered to have.

Caution is advised against the use of these findings in other communities where similar field investigations have not been undertaken, especially in areas with neutral or acid groundwater, high groundwater inflow rates or organic soils. Advantage of the natural assimilative capacity of soil/water systems should only be taken where it is evaluated by field investigations.

APPENDIX A

SANITARY SURVEY FOR CONSTRUCTION GRANTS APPLICATION

(Page One)

Resident:	Study Area:
Owner:	Surveyor/Date:
Address of Property:	Weather:
Lot Location:	Approximate Lot Dimensions:
Tax Map Designation:	____ feet by ____ feet

Preliminary Resident Interview

Age of Dwelling: __years. Age of sewage disposal system: __years.

Type of Sewage Disposal System:

Maintenance: __years since septic tank pumped. Reason for pumping:
__years since sewage system repairs (Describe below)
Accessibility of septic tank manholes (Describe below)

SANITARY SURVEY FOR CONSTRUCTION GRANTS APPLICATION

(Page Two)

Dwelling Use: Number of Bedrooms: __actual, __potential, __planned
Permanent Residents: __adults, __children
Seasonal Residents: __, length of stay __
Typical Number of Guests: __, length of stay __

If seasonal only, plan to become permanent residents: __
In how many years? __

Water Using Fixtures (Note "w.c." if designed to conserve water):

___Shower Heads	___Dishwasher
___Bathtubs	___Other Kitchen
___Bathroom Lavatories	___Clothes Washing Machine
___Toilets	___Water Softener
___Kitchen Lavatories	___Utility Sink
___Garbage Grinder	___Other Utilities

Plan for Changes:

Problems Recognized by Resident:

Resident Will Allow Follow-Up Engineering Studies: __ Soil Borings
__ Groundwater
__ Well Water Sample

Water Supply

Water Supply Source (check one)
___Public Water Supply
___Community or Shared Well
___On-Lot Well
___Other (Describe)

If public water supply or community well:
___Fixed Billing Rate $ /
___Metered Rate $ /
Average usage for prior year: /

SANITARY SURVEY FOR CONSTRUCTION GRANTS APPLICATION

(Page Three)

If shared or on-lot well: ___Drilled Well
___Bored Well
___Dug Well
___Driven Well

Well Depth (if known): ___ feet total ___ feet to water table

Well Distance: ___ feet to house ___ feet to septic tank
___ feet to soil disposal area
___ feet to surface water

Visual Inspection: Type of Casing
Integrity of Casing
Grouting Apparent?
Vent Type and Condition
Seal Type and Condition

Water Sample Collected: ___ No
___ Yes
(Attach Analysis Report)

Surveyor's Visual Observations of Effluent Disposal Site:

Drainage Facilities and Discharge Location:

Basement Sump

Footing Drains

Roof Drainings

Driveway Runoff

Other

Property and Facility Sketch

ACKNOWLEDGMENTS

The authors wish to recognize the valuable assistance of many individuals who aided in the development of the "Seven Lakes" Environmental Impact Statements. A list of the organizations and key personnel involved is presented in each EIS, available on request from the EIS Preparation Section, Region V, U.S. Environmental Protection Agency.

Preparation of this paper and of the "Seven Lakes" EIS's was funded under Contract No. 68-01-4612 between U.S. Environmental Protection Agency and WAPORA, Inc.

6

AN OVERVIEW OF ALTERNATIVE ONSITE WASTEWATER TECHNOLOGY

Gwendolyn M. Buchholz
Senior Engineer
James M. Montgomery Consulting Engineers, Inc.
Walnut Creek, California 94596

INTRODUCTION

More than 50 million people in the United States live in unsewered communities and rely on onsite systems for wastewater treatment and disposal. Onsite treatment and disposal systems were originally developed to serve homes in rural or recreational communities; however, as the number of people moving from urban areas to unsewered communities increases, so does the use of onsite systems and the potential for system failures. To prevent or eliminate failing systems, rural residential communities have been encouraged to construct central wastewater collection, treatment and disposal facilities, which may result in annual costs of $200–300 per household.

Increasing capital and maintenance costs of central wastewater facilities have prompted federal and state agencies to place increased emphasis on maintaining the use of onsite wastewater systems. The Clean Water Act of 1977 (PL 95-217) provides for construction grants for individual onsite systems under the U.S. Environmental Protection Agency's (EPA) Construction Grants Program. Availability of federal (and, in some cases, state) construction grant funds and increased public support for onsite systems has resulted in the need for an in-depth evaluation of onsite wastewater management alternatives for unsewered communities.

In rural residential communities, wastewater generated in the household is diverted to an onsite wastewater management system, which consists of a treatment unit and a disposal unit (Figure 1). The treatment unit removes large solids and greases and may provide biological or physical-chemical treatment. The disposal unit is generally a soil absorption system, which provides biological treatment and ultimate disposal of the wastewater through percolation into shallow aquifers or evapotranspiration at the ground surface. Failure of onsite wastewater facilities could cause partially treated wastewater to contaminate groundwater or surface waters and result in potential public health hazards. Onsite wastewater system failures can be prevented through the application of adequate design criteria and proper construction methods.

To determine the feasibility of utilizing onsite systems, both treatment and disposal units should be evaluated with respect to wastewater flows and characteristics, site characteristics, effluent limitations, reliability and economic considerations. Numerous types of treatment and disposal units are available to serve the wastewater management needs of the rural residential homeowner. This chapter provides an overview of available onsite treatment and disposal units, including related design criteria and operation and maintenance requirements.

ONSITE TREATMENT

The most common onsite treatment facility is the septic tank, which was developed in 1881. During the past 50 years, many other types of onsite treatment units have also been developed, including those that provide treatment by biological or physical-chemical processes and treatment units for segregated flows. Onsite units that provide biological treatment include septic tanks, aerobic units and compost systems. Physical-chemical treatment units utilize sedimentation, chlorination and filtration. Segregated flow systems separate the black toilet wastes from the greywater generated in sinks, showers, bathtubs, washing machines and dishwashers. Blackwaste is treated and stored in self-contained toilets, including compost toilets, incineration toilets and privies. Greywater treatment systems are similar to facilities designed for the treatment of unsegregated flows, such as septic tanks.

Septic Tanks

Septic tanks, the most frequently used onsite treatment units in rural areas, are watertight containers in which wastewater is retained to allow solids to settle and partially decompose. Baffles are placed within the tank

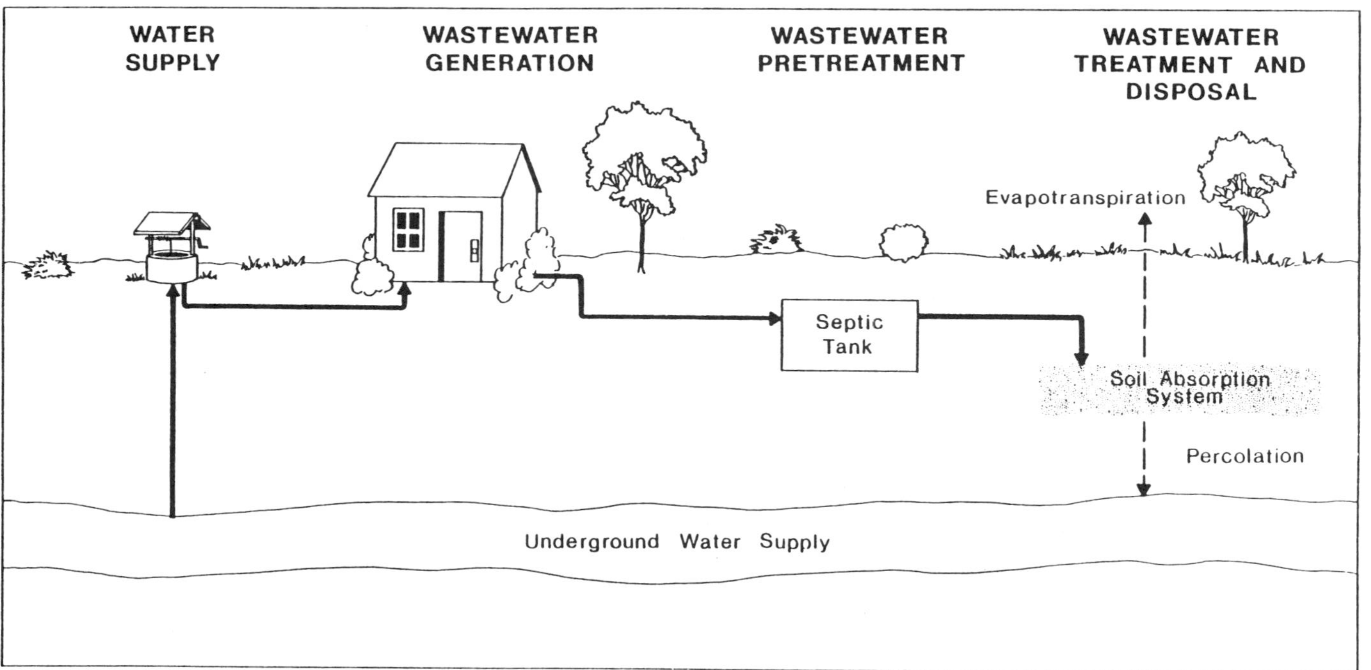

Figure 1. An onsite wastewater management system.

to improve solids settling and to prevent the scum layer of lightweight solids, fats and greases from flowing out of the tank with the effluent. Solids accumulate within the tank and are removed by pumping approximately every three years. The septic tank reduces suspended solids by 40–80% and BOD concentrations by 25–65%.

Aerobic Units

Aerobic systems have been developed to replace or supplement existing septic tanks. Aerobic treatment may be provided by the activated sludge process, submerged biofilters or ozonation. The performance of aerobic units varies with the manufacturer and design, resulting in reported BOD reductions of 85–98%. Reduction of suspended solids concentrations is comparable to that of septic tanks. Ozone systems also provide virus disinfection of effluent and may promote oxidation of solids in soil absorption fields.

Individual aerobic treatment units that utilize the activated sludge process to treat wastewater rely on microorganisms suspended in the wastewater to remove organic material. The treatment units include an aeration chamber, an effluent clarifier for removal of solids, and possibly a primary clarifier to remove solids in the raw wastewater prior to aeration. Septic tanks may be used for primary and final settling chambers; however, many manufactured systems provide complete treatment within one unit. Another type of aerobic unit utilizes microorganisms grown on biofilters submerged in the wastewater to remove organic material. The biofilters may provide more microorganisms per unit volume of wastewater and thereby remove more organic material. Both the activated sludge and the submerged biofilter processes provide oxygen to the microorganisms by mixing air into the wastewater.

To provide more air to the microorganisms, aerobic units have been developed that utilize ozone. The ozone units also include primary and secondary settling chambers to remove solids in the raw wastewater and effluent, respectively.

An aerobic unit will require periodic pumping to remove accumulated solids in the final clarifier. If the solids are not removed on a regular basis, a condition known as "bulking sludge" may occur in the final clarifier in some types of aerobic units, resulting in a high effluent suspended solids concentration. Maintenance requirements for aerobic units depend on the type of system and range from weekly monitoring of pH to occasional replacement of mechanical components. Aerobic treatment units require a continuous electrical energy supply to operate the air compressors.

Chemical Treatment Units

A typical chemical treatment unit disinfects and filters effluent from septic tanks. This system consists of a settling basin, a combination chlorine contact chamber and holding tank, and a cartridge filter to remove fine solids. The effluent may be recycled for use in toilets or discharged to a soil absorption system. Periodic maintenance includes the addition of calcium hypochlorite, replacement of the filter and removal of sludge.

Sand Filters

Sand filters are utilized to reduce suspended solids and dissolved organic materials in the effluent from septic tanks or aerobic units. Two basic types of sand filter systems have been developed: (1) the intermittent sand filter, and (2) the recirculating sand filter. The former consists of a holding tank and an open sand filter. Periodically, wastewater is pumped from the holding tank to the filter at a loading rate of approximately 3–5 gpd/ft^2. The recirculating sand filter is similar, except that 20% of the filter effluent is returned to the holding tank. Maintenance for both types of sand filters consists of raking the sand every four months and replacing the top inch of sand annually to prevent ponding of wastewater attributable to accumulated solids.

Segregated Flow Systems

Segregated flow systems consist of self-contained toilet units for blackwaste treatment and disposal and separate facilities for treatment and disposal of greywater. A variety of commercial blackwaste systems are available, including compost toilets, incineration toilets and privies. Greywater is treated by units similar to those used for unsegregated wastewater flows. Segregated systems may be easily installed in new residences during construction; however, plumbing connections would require retrofitting in existing residences.

Compost Toilets

Compost toilets are self-contained treatment and disposal units for human wastes. Human and sometimes kitchen wastes are transported by gravity or screw conveyors to fiberglass or polystyrene tanks. Small units that serve one toilet are designed to be placed entirely within the bathroom. Larger units are designed to serve several toilets and garbage chutes and are placed under the house in a basement or excavated area. The organic material is composted for a one-year period to produce a humus that may be suitable for fertilizer. The compost toilet unit includes ventilation ducts to vent water vapor and carbon dioxide released by the decomposing wastes. A small fan may be required to supplement natural drafts and remove odors from the tank. In cold climates it may be necessary to install an external heater to provide adequate temperatures in which the microorganisms can survive. Maintenance requirements consist of periodically removing composted wastes to prevent an accumulation of solids. Periodic dilute applications of insecticide may be necessary to control flies; however, application of a concentrated insecticide solution to the composting material may harm the necessary microorganisms in the compost tank.

Incineration Toilets

Commercial incineration toilets are waterless systems that utilize electricity, natural gas or propane gas to attain combustion temperatures within the incineration chamber. By depressing a foot pedal of a typical electric incineration toilet, the human wastes, which are contained in a paper or plastic liner, drop into the incineration chamber. The incineration cycle is completed in 15–20 minutes. The operation cycle of a natural gas or propane gas incineration toilet is similar to that of an electric unit; however, liners are not required and the unit is generally used several times prior to incineration. Exhaust fumes and odors are removed through a vertical ventilation pipe. Maintenance consists of periodically cleaning the waste pan to remove inorganic ash and replacement of liners.

Oil Flush Toilets

Oil flush toilets utilize mineral oil as a carrier fluid instead of water. The wastes and oil are separated by gravity in a storage tank and the oil pumped through a screening and filtration unit. The purified oil is chlorinated before being returned to the toilet tank. A conventional toilet may be used; however, it is recommended that the toilet bowl be Teflon®*-coated because the oil does not produce a scouring effect. A typical residential system would employ about 20–30 gallons of oil. The storage tanks are placed under the house in a basement or excavated area; therefore, this system may not be suitable for existing residences. Maintenance requirements include annual pumping of the solid wastes, addition of chlorine, addition of oil to maintain the proper level, and replacement of oil filters.

*Registered trademark of E. I. du Pont de Nemours and Co., Inc., Wilmington, Delaware.

Privies

Privies are probably the second oldest means of wastewater disposal known to man. A large variety of privies have been developed throughout the centuries; however, in the United States there are currently three major types of privies in use: (1) the dry pit privy, (2) drum privy and (3) vault privy. A typical dry pit privy consists of a stool or squatplate constructed over an excavated pit and covered by a structure to provide privacy. The privy site would be subject to the same siting requirements as a soil absorption seepage pit. Large quantities of water must not be allowed to enter the privy; therefore, the pit is lined with wood and the ground surfaces are graded away from the structure. The dry pit privy is usually abandoned when the wastes accumulate to a level within 12–18 inches of the ground surface. Maintenance of the pit privy includes the periodic addition of dry lime to control odors and insects.

A drum privy consists of a toilet seat placed above a 55-gallon steel drum lined with asphalt or other impervious material and located inside a structure to ensure privacy. To facilitate the compost process inside the drum, approximately 10 inches of sawdust are placed on the bottom of the drum and about two cups of sawdust are added after each use to absorb the liquid from the wastes. When the drum is full, it is sealed with a vented lid and transferred to a disposal or storage site.

The vault privy consists of two permanent compost chambers constructed of concrete and cement blocks with an impervious liner to avoid contamination of the surrounding soil and prevent water from entering the chambers. Each chamber serves one stool or squatplate and can usually be used for six to eight months by four people. When the chamber is full, it is rested for at least one year while the other chamber is placed into operation. After a one-year rest period, the compost is used as soil conditioner or transferred to a disposal site. As with the drum privy, a layer of sawdust is added after each use, and the compost pile is turned with a shovel each month to provide aeration and reduce odors.

Greywater Systems

Treatment of greywater depends on the wastewater source and is similar to the treatment of unsegregated wastewater, which includes blackwastes. The kitchen sink represents about 20% of the greywater flow; however, the kitchen sink is the source of 40–70% of the greywater BOD loading, as well as oil, greases, detergents and cleansers. Washing machines provide 20% of the greywater flow and the major source of phosphorus and nitrogen. The remaining 60% of the greywater is generated in bathtubs, showers and bathroom sinks. A variety of systems have been developed for the treatment of greywater, including septic tanks, sand filters and rack filters, which consist of a rack to support filter media, such as hay or wood shavings, placed inside of a closed 55-gallon drum.

Operation and Maintenance

The operation and maintenance (O&M) requirements for the onsite treatment units discussed here are summarized in Table I. With the exception of periodic inspections of mechanical and electrical equipment under terms of equipment warranties, the homeowner can usually perform routine

Table I. Onsite Treatment Operation and Maintenance

Unit	Operation and Maintenance Requirements	Frequency
Septic Tank	Remove septage	3-5 years
Aerobic Units	1. Inspect warning lights on service panel.	2 days
	2. Monitor sludge characteristics.	2 months
	3. Inspect aeration equipment.	2 months
	4. Remove septage.	
	5. Power requirements (6 kWh/day).	-
Chemical Treatment Units	1. Add calcium hypochlorite.	3 months
	2. Replace cartridge filter.	3 months
	3. Remove septage.	8-10 months
	4. Power requirements (4 kWh/day).	-
Sand Filters	1. Replace top sand layer.	1 year
	2. Alternate filters.	6 months
	3. Power requirements (3 kWh/day).	-
Blackwaste Units		
Compost toilets	1. Remove compost.	1 year
	2. Check liquid levels.	1 week
	3. Power (1-3 kWh/day).	-
Incineration toilets	1. Replace liners if electric.	1 use
	2. Empty ashtray.	3 days
	3. Power requirements (1-3 kWh/day).	-
Privies	Abandon or alternate privy.	6-8 months
Oil toilets	Remove oil.	1 year
Greywater Units	Similar to unsegregated treatment units.	

maintenance. In many rural residential areas, operation and maintenance can also be provided by local septic system contractors. Local regulations generally require that periodic pumping and transport of solids be performed by a licensed contractor.

Summary

The use of onsite treatment units depends on the type of user, wastewater flow, effluent limitations, capital costs, and operation and maintenance costs. The suitability of the treatment units with respect to two different applications, capital costs, and operation and maintenance costs is summarized in Table II.

Table II. Onsite Wastewater Treatment Units

	Suitable Applications			
Unit	Intermittent Use	Stringent Effluent Limitations	Capital Costs[a,b] ($)	O&M Costs[a] ($)
Septic Tank	•		1,500–2,000	25–35
Aerobic Units		•	2,000–4,000	150–200
Chemical Units	•		5,000–6,000	75–100
Sand Filters	•	•	3,000–5,000	100–125
Blackwaste Units				
Compost toilets	•	•	1,000–3,000	0–60
Incineration toilets	•	•	1,500–2,000	50–75
Oil toilets	•	•	3,000–4,000	50–75
Privies	•	•	2,000–3,000	–
Greywater Units	Varies	Varies	1,500–5,000	25–200

[a]Costs based on prices in Northern California, ENR = 3,900.
[b]Capital costs include installation costs.

ONSITE EFFLUENT DISPOSAL

Onsite effluent disposal facilities include leach fields, seepage pits, absorption mounds and evapotranspiration mounds. In a soil absorption system, effluent from the treatment facility flows by gravity or is pumped to the disposal system where the applied wastewater effluent is absorbed by the unsaturated soil particles. After the soil becomes saturated, the liquid moves through the void spaces and may accumulate above an impermeable layer. If this accumulation of liquid is excessive, the effluent may fill the void spaces and cause surface ponding. For a properly operating soil absorption system, the effluent is treated as it flows through the void spaces by a process similar to a trickling filter. Organic material in the effluent is absorbed and oxidized by a slime mat of aerobic microorganisms, which accumulates on the soil particles. As the microorganisms multiply, the thickness of the slime mat increases and eventually clogs the void spaces.

Leach Fields

The most common type of soil absorption system is the leach field, which consists of a series of perforated distribution pipelines placed in trenches or in a shallow bed. A typical absorption trench is about 2–3 feet wide, approximately 2–4 feet deep, and less than 100 feet long. The perforated pipe is placed in the trench on top of gravel or crushed stone, which is also used to backfill around the pipe. The gravel increases drainage and reduces root growth around the distribution pipeline. A minimum topsoil cover of 1 foot is placed over the gravel to prevent contact with effluent, reduce rainwater infiltration and promote evapotranspiration. Untreated building paper is placed between the topsoil cover and the gravel to prevent soil particles from migrating into the void spaces of the gravel.

Seepage Pits

In many cases, the top 3–4 feet of soil are relatively impermeable; therefore, standard leach fields would be impractical. However, if the impermeable soil is underlain with porous soils and the groundwater elevation is low, seepage pits may be utilized. Seepage pits are also used where space for a new or replacement leach field is limited. Seepage pits are cylindrical structures of at least 30 inches in diameter and 9–60 feet deep. As with a trench, both the sidewall and bottom surfaces of a seepage pit are considered to be the effective leaching areas. The ratio of sidewall surface area to bottom surface area is larger for a seepage pit than for a leach field; therefore, the effective size of a seepage pit is larger than a leach field, although the amount of land required for disposal is less.

Absorption Mounds

In the late 1940s, an elevated soil absorption system, the NODAK System, was developed in North Dakota to provide adequate effluent disposal in areas with slowly permeable soils or high groundwater elevations. This and other types of absorption mounds consist of leach fields constructed aboveground using imported permeable soils. Effluent is pumped into the mound and treated as it flows through the layers of imported gravel, sand and soil, The mounds may be planted with ground cover to prevent erosion and become an integral part of the landscape.

Evapotranspiration Mounds

Evapotranspiration mounds provide a "no discharge" alternative for onsite wastewater management. Wastewater and precipitation absorbed through the sandy mound are stored in a shallow-lined bed filled with gravel and sand. The gravel layer provides storage for the effluent during the winter months, and the sand allows the effluent to move by capillary action to the surface of the mound for subsequent evaporation and vegetative transpiration. A mound of sandy soil is constructed above the ground surface over the storage bed and planted with water and salt-tolerant vegetation. To ensure continuous evapotranspiration of the wastewater, the following three requirements must be met: (1) a continuous supply of heat to provide latent heat of evaporation; (2) a vapor pressure gradient between the surrounding air and the mound surface; and (3) a continuous supply of liquid to the evaporative surface. Approximately 590 cal/g of water are needed to evaporate water at 15°C, and the heat may be provided by the heat of the liquid, biological activity or heating coils placed in the mound.

Summary

Onsite disposal units must be designed based on treated effluent quality, soil characteristics, topography, hydrogeology, climate and available soil absorption system capacity. The suitability of the disposal units discussed here with respect to six types of applications is summarized in Table III.

CONCLUSIONS

The use of onsite wastewater systems in rural residential communities is receiving increased emphasis because of the availability of reliable onsite

Table III. Suitability of Onsite Wastewater Disposal Units

Units	Low Percolation Rates	High Groundwater	Steep Slopes	High Rainfall	Small Parcel	No Discharge
Leach Field and Trenches		•	•	•		
Seepage Pits	•			•	•	
Absorption Mounds	•	•		•		
Evapotranspiration Mounds	•	•	•		•	•

treatment units, the development of accurate design criteria, the high cost to construct and maintain central wastewater management facilities, and the support of federal and state agencies for onsite systems. The onsite wastewater treatment and disposal technology described here should be evaluated in detail by land use planners, local agencies, engineers and developers in the planning of all rural residential wastewater projects to provide cost-effective and reliable wastewater management facilities.

7

SOIL FACTORS AS THEY RELATE TO ONSITE SEWAGE DISPOSAL

John H. Long, R.S., District Sanitarian
Land Subdivision and Planning Section
Division of Community Environmental Health
Michigan Department of Public Health
Lansing, Michigan

INTRODUCTION

With increased concern for the environment, particularly for water quality, communities and individuals are being forced to come up with suitable alternative solutions to the wastewater disposal problems; however, the cost of conventional municipal sewer collection and disposal systems is increasing to the point that many communities cannot afford to install them.

In facilities plans, the U.S. Environmental Protection Agency (EPA) is asking for alternatives to be considered, yet we lack the necessary data to fully evaluate those alternatives. Research institutes and private industries are to be commended on their efforts to achieve suitable alternative solutions to onsite wastewater problems. Unfortunately, many of the products do not address total wastewater disposal, i.e., greywater. When they do, the cost and/or maintenance of such a system is beyond the means of the average person for his home. This problem won't be solved until we have an alternative wastewater treatment solution that is both reliable and reasonable to operate. It must be recognized that not all developing areas can be sewered and that we need to take a harder look at a system that has been with us for many years, i.e., the septic tank–subsurface absorption system. This treatment system has been overlooked too long in the effort to find a magical solution because of the reluctance to admit that something so simple could do the job. Septic tank–subsurface absorption systems may not be the answer in all cases; however, they are worthy of serious consideration because they are reliable in operation, require minimum maintenance, and are normally reasonable to install. With the millions of septic tank–subsurface absorption systems in existence and that will be installed because they are inexpensive and reliable, an effort should be made to improve the septic tank system, rather than to develop sophisticated systems that have a limited market. More research is needed on ways to improve on the septic tank–subsurface absorption system. Suggested areas needing research are size and shape of the septic tank, advantages of two-compartment tanks, benefits of dosing tile fields, advantages of alternating tile fields and flow distribution within the tile field.

ROLE OF SOIL IN SUBSURFACE ABSORPTION

Soil plays an important role in subsurface absorption and has characteristics that must be thoroughly evaluated. The absorption system must be designed to be compatible with the soil conditions. Michigan relies on the soil to absorb the sewage effluent because surface discharge of sewage effluent is not allowed for individual home systems. Since the mid-1960s, Michigan has made tremendous strides in the area of soils evaluation for onsite sewage disposal. The "perc test," utilized for many years as a basis for design of a disposal system, has been discouraged because of difficulties in obtaining reproducible results and interpreting the data obtained. Consequently, it has all but been eliminated as the primary method of evaluating the soil. In cases where soil conditions are so marginal and variable that it becomes necessary to obtain additional data, a *stabilized* percolation test may be utilized. This will provide information concerning the permeability of the soil to determine if it will meet the minimum requirements of the sanitary code and to size the tile field; however, this test is time consuming if properly conducted. The sanitarians and engineers in Michigan are primarily using the soil profile evaluation to determine soil suitability and/or its limitations for onsite sewage disposal. The balance of this chapter will deal with techniques of soil evaluation that can be consistently reproduced by the trained observer.

SITE EVALUATION OF SOIL

To properly conduct a site evaluation, soils data must first be obtained. In Michigan and other states, the major source of soils information would be from the soil survey reports and soils map prepared by the U.S. Soil Conservation Service (SCS). These reports are accompanied by interpretation sheets that explain the various soil factors and their limitations for various uses, including onsite sewage disposal. Additional data may be available from the local environmental health division of the health department, or from engineering firms that may have done soils exploration for the site. In addition to these sources, other agencies that may be of benefit depending on the site circumstances would be the Floodplain Management Section of the local Department of Natural Resources (DNR) office or its equivalent; the Cooperative Extension Service; and possibly water well logs.

The site should be visited to view the topography and perform additional soils evaluation to confirm the data available from various agencies. Unless the data have been obtained personally, it is wise to conduct a minimum of two soil borings in the area of the sewage system and that sufficient soil borings be done to get a good cross section of the soil conditions on the lot. These borings should be done to a depth of at least four feet below the proposed bottom of the sewage system. For an adequate soil evaluation, it is necessary to observe the soil profile in its natural state. To observe a pile of soil that has been dug out with a post hole digger or screw auger is unreliable because of the mixing of soils that occurs. In Michigan, the primary tool used to evaluate the soil is a hand auger or a backhoe cut. Use of the latter leads to complex or questionable soil conditions.

When evaluating soil conditions on a site, four major factors can be observed that have a direct influence on operation of the septic tank system.

1. *Soil Texture.* This includes the relative proportions of sand, silt and clay. The higher the percentage of clay and silt, the slower the permeability of the soil.

2. *Natural Drainage.* This refers to the frequency and duration of periods of saturation or partial saturation during soil formation. Observations of the soil profile and colors can indicate whether the soil was saturated, to what depth, and for how long. In glaciated soils, where the soil is not saturated with water, the soil colors will be bright. In soils where the soil is saturated at various times during the year, the soil material becomes mottled (irregular spots of different colors that vary in number and size). The overall color of the soil will be dull with the gray mottles. In these soils, a saturated condition can be expected in the fall and spring, or during periods of excessive rainfall. During dry periods of the year, deep borings may not reveal any saturated soil to a depth of several feet below grade.

In poorly drained soils, where the soil is saturated to the ground surface for extended periods each year, the soil becomes bluish. These conditions present severe limitations for septic tank disposal systems and normally are unsuitable for proper operation of the disposal field.

3. *Soil Structure.* This is the arrangement of primary soil particles (sand, silt, clay, minerals and organic material) into compound particles or aggregates that are separated from adjoining aggregates. Soil structure plays an important role in the permeability of the soil and needs to be considered whenever a site is evaluated for a subsurface disposal system. It becomes especially critical when working with marginal soils or large systems. Examples of common kinds of structure that will be encountered are:

1. granular or crumb-like–excellent for permeability, normally 1/8 to 1/4 inch in size.
2. blocky–chunks of soil 1/4–3/4 inch in size with smooth exterior surfaces that are good for permeability and more typically associated with loam–clay loam texture.
3. platey–thin 1/8- to 1/4-inch-thick horizontal plates that are poor for permeability because of the horizontal layer restricting the vertical movement of the water, can reduce permeability 20-fold and can be associated with almost all soil textures.
4. massive–lack of structure, which means they are poor for permeability because they lack cleavage planes for transmission of the liquid, and that they are normally associated with loam–clay soil texture.

4. *Slope.* Slope must be considered when evaluating a site for some obvious reasons. The first is ease of construction. Less obvious is the interaction of slope and the soil conditions on the site. By correct location and design of the system, slopes can be used because they can help carry effluent away from the area of the septic tank system. In an area with shallow sandy soil over clay, the slope will help in the overall operation of the system, but sufficient borings are necessary to ensure that there is a sufficient area of sandy soil to preclude seepage out on the ground surface. In areas of clay soil, the slope works against the successful operation of the system because seepage will tend to come to the ground surface.

CONCLUSIONS

The successful design, installation and operation of an onsite wastewater disposal system is about as much an art as it is a science. This is attributable to the endless variables involved with onsite waste disposal–soils, site conditions, installation and use. Of the vast number of septic tank systems in operation, no two are identical. A system cannot be judged without some practical field experience and onsite evaluation.

Soils are one variable that can be reduced by careful evaluation of them and design of the septic tank disposal system. Doing this will increase the odds of the resulting system functioning properly.

8

SOIL MOTTLING AND GROUNDWATER MONITORING

David W. Fredrickson
Environmental Specialist-Soil Scientist
Bureau of Environmental Health
Division of Health
Department of Health and Social Services
State of Wisconsin
Madison, Wisconsin 53701

INTRODUCTION

Properly operating soil absorption systems must fulfill two basic objectives. The system must allow infiltration of wastewater into the soil and achieve purification of the effluent. The occurrence of shallow groundwater or zones of soil saturation can have a dramatic effect on both introduction of wastewater into soil systems and on the adequate purification of the effluent.

The Wisconsin Administrative Code recognizes the effects of soil saturation on system operation by requiring a three-foot separation between the system elevation and the occurrence of zones of soil saturation or high groundwater. Most groundwater systems fluctuate during a normal year. In Wisconsin, the spring season is the period of maximum levels of groundwater fluctuation. Zones of soil saturation also generally exhibit their maximum level of saturation during the spring. This can cause problems in the proper siting of soil absorption systems. People purchase property throughout the year. If soil absorption systems are to be properly sited, a method of soil evaluation must exist that can be used year round.

SOIL MOTTLING

Soil mottling is defined as spots or streaks of contrasting soil colors. Mottles are usually brown, black, red, yellow or gray. If a soil horizon has a matrix (background) color of light brown with spots of red and gray, the red and gray spots are the soil mottles. The brown, red and yellow (brightly colored) mottles are commonly called high chroma. The gray mottles (dull colored) are called low chroma.

The soils of Wisconsin are generally pedogenically young soils of glacial origin. In Wisconsin, soils mottling is almost always a result of a fluctuating groundwater or zones of periodic soil saturation. As a result, mottling is used as an indicator of high groundwater, as defined in the Wisconsin Administrative Code.

The use of soil mottling as a morphologic indicator of soil saturation is not unique to Wisconsin. It is used throughout the world to estimate levels of soil saturation. The *Soil Taxonomy* [1] of the United States Department of Agriculture (USDA) specifies that "mottles that have chroma of 2 or less . . . refers to colors in a horizon in which parts have chroma of 2 or less, moist, and value, moist, of 4 or more, whether or not that part is dominant in volume or whether or not it is a continuous phase surrounding spots of higher chroma. If either the minor or major part of a horizon has chroma of 1 to 2 and value, moist, of 4 or more and there are spots of higher chroma, the part that has the lower chroma is included in the meaning of 'mottles that have chroma of 2 or less.' The part is excluded from the meaning if all the horizon has chroma of 2 or less or if no part of the horizon has chroma as low as 2. The phrase also means that the horizon that has such mottles is saturated with water at some period of the year or the soil is artificially drained." The terms chroma and value refer to variables used to describe color.

Many persons outside of the field of soil science and related disciplines feel the interpretation of soil color patterns is a somewhat mystical procedure. Research during the last several decades has documented the reactions that occured within a soil to lead to the formation of soil mottles. With improvements in laboratory procedures, it was found that the compounds of iron and manganese that color a soil are also the compounds found in soil mottles. Vepraskas and Bouma [2] used the scanning electron microscope to determine the iron and manganese concentrations of soil mottles as related to the matrix material of a soil profile. They found that red mottles were rich in iron relative to the soil matrix material. Bloomfield [3] used acid ammonium oxalate to extract iron from mottles and the surrounding soil material. He found that mottles contain as much as four times the concentration of iron as did the whole soil. Similar results were found by Rathburn [4].

Red mottles are iron enriched. Black mottles are enriched in manganese. Gray mottles are areas deficient in iron (where compounds of iron have been removed) or are attributable to the presence of iron in a reduced state. The latter is usually associated with a gleyed soil condition.

MOTTLE FORMATION

Mottle formation includes both chemical and biological reactions. To fully describe the pathway of mottle formation is beyond the scope of this chapter. The Wisconsin *Soil Tester Manual* [5] provides a general description of the processes of mottle formation.

> The chemical reactions that cause soil mottles to form are complex.
> Mottle formation includes both chemical and biological reactions. The chain of events that result in the formation of soil mottles is as follows. With temperature above 40°F (4°C), 2 basic types of bacteria are the agents which decompose or oxidize organic matter in the soil. Aerobic bacteria are the primary agents as long as there is some air in the soil. As infiltrating water and/or a rise in groundwater completely fills all the air spaces and the soil becomes saturated, air and gaseous free oxygen are excluded, dissolved oxygen is depleted and anaerobic bacteria become the primary decomposers. They utilize insoluble manganese and iron compounds for respiration instead of oxygen. In the chemical reactions that occur, soluble compounds of manganese and iron are formed from the otherwise insoluble oxide and hydroxide compounds and begin to flow with the soil solution. Because this action removes iron, a color reduction occurs in those areas tending to turn them gray or white. When these compounds again encounter oxygen in aerated pores, they recombine with oxygen to form yellow and rust colored concentrations. Manganese compounds are reoxidized and form black concentrations.

Several factors must be present to cause soil mottles to form. The first and most important is that the soil must become saturated with water. Soil is a three-phase system consisting of solid, liquid and gaseous phases. With saturated conditions, the air in the three-phase system is removed. Secondly, bacteria in the soil use up the oxygen in the soil-water solution, which results in anaerobic conditions. Now other bacteria use the compounds of iron and manganese in the soil for respiration. When these bacteria use the iron and manganese compounds, they cause these compounds to become chemically reduced. In a reduced form, iron and manganese compounds are soluble and no longer stable and begin to move in the soil-water solution. When a soil drains, the large pores drain first. The iron and manganese in the soil solution are oxidized when they encounter oxygen in these large, air-filled pores. When they are oxidized, they form spots that are enriched in iron (red spots) and manganese (black spots) that can be seen.

Other conditions also must be present. The temperature in the soil must be high enough to allow biological activity and begin the chain of events. Biological activity occurs above a temperature of 40°F (4°C), which is called biologic zero. If a soil is saturated with water but the soil temperature is below 40°F (4°C), soil mottles cannot be formed. Mottles cannot be formed because bacteria will not be active. Rathbun [4] reported that several sites he monitored with wells showed water levels above the level of soil mottling. Temperature measurements in situ indicated that the depth of mottling correlated well with the level of observed water after the temperature was above 40°F.

The soil also can be saturated with water, the soil temperature could be above 40°F, but the soil-water solution could have enough oxygen present to allow bacteria to operate without using compounds of iron and manganese. This can happen when aerated groundwater is moving at a very fast rate. If anaerobic conditions are not present, mottles will not form.

Another factor important to the formation of soil mottles is the pH of the soil. The ease with which soil mottles can form depends on having the correct range of soil pH. Very alkaline soils (high in lime), such as the calcareous glacial tills in southeast Wisconsin, may not exhibit easily recognizable soil mottles, even though they are seasonally saturated. A high pH can prevent redox potentials from becoming low enough to reduce iron and manganese [4]. Even if reduced, the solubility of iron compounds possibly could be much lower in an alkaline soil-water solution.

Fortunately, most wet soils in Wisconsin do exhibit soil mottling. Some soils do not have enough iron and manganese to allow the formation of soil mottles. Some very clean, light-colored sands do not have coatings of iron and manganese, so when these chemicals are not present, mottles do not form in response to high groundwater conditions.

Many different groups have attempted to correlate mottle expression with moisture regime characteristics; however, such research has not been able to relate length and degree of saturation to mottle size, contrast and abundance. Essentially all we know is that gleyed (bluish-green or gray matrix colors) soils indicate that the site is extremely wet almost all year long. High-chroma (red) mottles have been the subject of controversy as to the validity of using such mottles to estimate soil saturation. In many soils, high-chroma mottles may be the only observable evidence of saturation. In light-colored soils or highly calcareous glacial tills, high-chroma mottles are all that an observer may be able to see. In Wisconsin, certified soil testers (CST) have been instructed to utilize both high- and low-chroma (gray) mottles in estimating high groundwater.

RESEARCH INTO SOIL MOTTLING AND OBSERVED GROUNDWATER

Many studies have been conducted within the last 20 years on estimated water levels using soil mottling, versus observed water levels in observation wells. Rathbun [4] found that observed water levels tended to be slightly higher than the depth to mottled soil. Shimek [6] studied several sites with sandy soils in central Wisconsin and found good correlation between high-chroma mottles and groundwater levels, except where the site was artificially drained. Simonson [7] determined that groundwater positions were estimated satisfactorily by using soil mottling in a study in the Pacific Northwest. In Pennsylvania, Latshaw [8] concluded that soil interpretations based on depth to mottling were extremely close to observed water levels.

WHEN IS A MOTTLE NOT A MOTTLE?

Thus far, the discussion of soil mottling has supported the use of soil color patterns in estimating soil saturation. Returning to the definition of mottled—spots or streaks of contrasting soil color—it should be clear that not all spotted or streaked soil is the result of saturated soil conditions. Variegated color patterns do occur that are not indicative of soil saturation.

One of the most common color patterns that could be considered mottled is the occurrence of residual sandstone soil material. Residual materials are easily identifiable and distinguishable from mottles attributable to saturation. The color patterns relate to various layers of sandstone present in the stratigraphy of the bedrock. Observation of the surrounding landscape or of sandstone fragments around the site will usually reveal the color patterns that should be expected in the residuum.

Some soil testers have been confused over the color patterns associated with Spodosols, a soil order in the soil taxonomy that has an albic horizon (whitish horizon that has had iron removed) over a spodic horizon (a reddish horizon that has been enriched in iron). Confusion also has resulted over the observation of tongued soils (soils with tongues of albic material extending into underlying horizons). Again, these conditions are easy to explain in the field. Wisconsin's Department of Health and Social Services does offer continuing education courses for CST's in at attempt to explain these color patterns.

Research in Wisconsin has also addressed the specific soil problems caused by deep silty loess deposits over sandy soils [9]. In such soils, a mottled zone can occur immediately above the textural boundary between the silts and sands. On the basis of this research, Wisconsin has instituted what is called the one-foot rule. Soil testers are allowed to disregard a mottled layer less than 12 inches thick that occurs in the silty soils at the textural boundary. If no mottling can be found in the underlying sands for a depth of 4 feet below the textural boundary, a system may be installed in the sandy soils. Experience to date with this rule has been positive.

The subject of relict mottling in Wisconsin almost always emerges in discussions of soil mottling. Relict mottling is inherited from a paleoenvironment. Mottling that has been effected by artificial drainage is not considered relict. If the drainage system is altered or destroyed, water levels do return to their morphologically predicted levels. Cases of relict mottles have been documented in Iowa.

GROUNDWATER MONITORING IN WISCONSIN

Soil mottling is one of the most important tools available to persons involved in the siting of onsite liquid waste disposal systems. As previously cited, however, the general public sometimes feels the use of soil colors to estimate soil saturation is a mystical procedure.

As a result of problems with calcareous soils in southeast Wisconsin, and a general misbelief in soil mottling, the Department of Health and Social Services was asked to institute code sections on monitoring groundwater levels. Guidelines for monitoring procedures were issued in February 1977 and have since been incorporated into the Wisconsin Administrative Code. The Code is currently being revised, with only minor changes proposed for the sections on groundwater monitoring. Before reading the following sections, it is necessary to explain the institutional procedures used in Wisconsin for programs on private waste disposal.

The rules and regulations for onsite liquid waste disposal are found in Chapter 145 of the Wisconsin Statutes and in Section H 62.20 of the Wisconsin Administrative Code. Permits for the installation, repair, alteration or replacement of a soil absorption system are required and must be obtained prior to issuance of a building permit.

Permits are issued by local government. Recent statutory changes now mandate that private waste disposal programs will be a duty of county government only. Additionally, the statutes list minimum training requirements for county staff and the responsibilities of the county program. The code subsections dealing with onsite liquid waste disposal in Wisconsin are uniform statewide.

The Department has primary responsibility for administration and enforcement of the code. The cooperation between counties and the state is excellent in most cases. This constitutes a background for a discussion of groundwater monitoring procedures.

PROCEDURES FOR GROUNDWATER MONITORING

The best way to present these procedures accurately is to include the code subsections dealing with monitoring. Chapter and section numbers may change in the near future because of a code revision now in progress; currently, however, groundwater monitoring is found in Section H 62.20 (3) (f). Minor changes that are proposed in the procedures will be discussed later.

"(f) Soil mottling and monitoring groundwater levels. 1. A property owner or developer has the option to provide documentation that soil mottling at a particular site is not an indication of seasonally saturated soil conditions or high groundwater levels. If the option to provide documentation is made, water levels observed by monitoring shall apply. Acceptable documentation will result from successful monitoring according to the following procedures:

"a. Monitoring shall be done in a near normal spring season. A near normal spring season is when the precipitation received at a local station equals or exceeds the amount historically received in Wisconsin 2 out of 3 years for both the periods September 1st to March 1st and March 1st to June 1st. These amounts are 8.5 inches and 7.6 inches respectively. In addition, where sites are subject to broad regional water tables, such as large areas of sandy soils, the fluctuation over the several year cycle must be considered.

"b. Areas which are monitored shall be carefully checked for drainage tile and open ditches which may have altered natural high groundwater levels. When such factors are involved, information on the location, design, ownership and maintenance responsibilities must be provided.

"Clear assurance shall be needed to show that the drainage network has an adequate outlet, and can and will be maintained.

"c. Monitoring shall be done by a certified soil tester.

"d. The certified soil tester shall notify in writing the local sanitary permit issuing authority, or in the absence of such, the department, of intent to monitor. It is expected the local authority or department may field check the monitoring at least once during the time of expected saturated soil conditions.

"e. At least 2 locations shall be monitored at a site for a proposed system and replacement. If in the judgment of the local authority or the department, more than 2 monitoring sites are needed, the certified soil tester will be so advised in writing.

"f. Observation wells designed as shown in the following sketch shall be constructed for monitoring. In general, they should extend to a depth of at least 6 feet below ground surface and shall be a minimum of 3 feet below the designed system depth. However, with layered mottled soil over permeable unmottled soil, some wells shall terminate within the mottled layer. Site conditions may, in some cases, require monitoring at greater depths. It will be the responsibility of the certified soil tester to determine the depth of the observation wells for each specific site and if in doubt, they shall request the guidance of the local authority or in its absence, the department" (Figure 1).

"g. Observations shall be made at the following frequency:

"1. The observations shall be made within 2 weeks after the frost is absent and thereafter every 7 days. Observations shall continue until June 1st or until the site is determined to be unacceptable, whichever comes first.

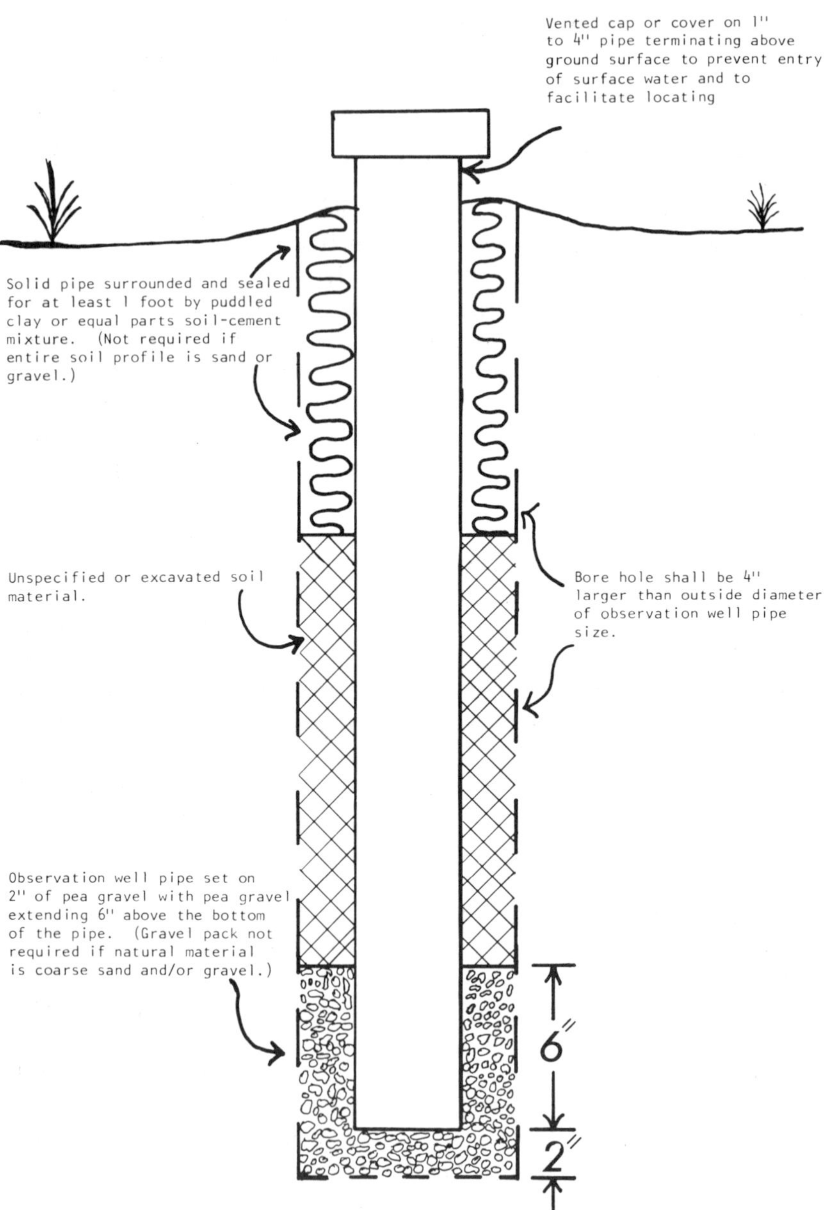

Figure 1. Observation well for monitoring groundwater.

"2. If water is observed after the frost is absent, or at any other time, an observation shall be made one week later. If water is present at both observations, monitoring can cease because the site is considered unacceptable.

"3. If water is not present at the second observation, monitoring shall continue until June 1st. If any 2 successive observations show the presence of water above the critical depth, the site is unacceptable and the department shall be notified in writing.

"4. The occurrence of rainfall(s) of $\frac{1}{2}$ inch intensity or more during the monitoring period may necessitate observations at more frequent intervals.

"5. A site which is saturated above the critical depth for more than 7 consecutive days of a near normal spring season is an unacceptable site.

"h. Submitting data:

"1. When monitoring shows saturated conditions, data giving test locations, soil bore hole or pit descriptions, soil series if available from soil maps, dates observed, depths to observed water and local precipitation data (monthly from September 1st to June 1st and daily during monitoring) shall be submitted in writing, with 2 copies sent to the department and one to the local authority.

"2. When monitoring discloses that the site is acceptable, documentation including location and depth of test holes, soil bore hole or pit descriptions; soil series if available from soil maps; dates observed; results of observations, local precipitation data (monthly from September 1st to June 1st and daily during monitoring) and information on artificial drainage shall be submitted in writing with 2 copies to the department and one to the local authority. A request for a variance to install a soil absorption system must be made to the department."

The design of the monitoring wells corresponds closely to the design used by the Soil Conservation Service. For research wells, the bentonite cap is usually placed immediately above the gravel pack to ensure isolation for the depth of sampling. This is unnecessary for our purposes. Installation is much easier with the cap at the surface, as is inspection of the installation.

Proposed changes for the procedure are the use of three wells per site and a change in the date by which monitoring must begin. This will incorporate a specific date by which the monitoring must begin. In some years, the date of the frost leaving the soil is difficult to determine. Additional writing may be added to make clear that sites with agricultural drain tile artificially lowering water levels will not be acceptable.

REPORTING OF DATA AND EXPERIENCE TO DATE

Problems have been encountered with the reporting of data. A form has been prepared for these reports that has eliminated some of the problems encountered in the first years of monitoring. The major problem is in securing reports for all sites. Reporting is required on all sites, both passing and failing. Not all reports have been filed, however, especially on failing sites. This can give misleading data on whether soil mottling is indeed a valid indicator of soil saturation. As an example, district staff from the Department observed all wells in several counties in southern Wisconsin and reported that 80-90% of the sites had observed water above the critical depth for system installation. Reports filed by the soil testers indicate that approximately 50% of the sites passed.

Field work by departmental staff at several sites with wells that passed monitoring has revealed that the sites were not mottled with a color pattern indicative of soil saturation. Residual soil colors, depositional color patterns and other variegated soil colors were present that were mistakenly called mottles indicative of wetness. From a regulatory standpoint, it is encouraging that licensed persons are being cautious, yet politically these passing sites lower the confidence in the use of soil mottling.

Additionally, the problems with calcareous tills in southeast Wisconsin has prompted some CST's to monitor all sites that are soil mapped as having highly calcareous tills. Many of these sites could have been determined to be suitable without groundwater monitoring.

Another problem has been the reporting of incorrect data. On several occasions within the last two years reports have been received from soil testers that do not correspond with measurements made by county or district staff. As a result, the Department will probably take action to revoke the licenses of several CST's who filed erroneous results.

To date, one site approved by the Department has had that approval rescinded because water was observed in an open boring at the time of the preinstallation inspection. In the future, the Department hopes to be able to inspect systems that have been installed after passing monitoring.

In some cases, mottles may form when the soil is 95% saturated [2,9]. In such cases the site is probably too wet to allow a system long-term successful operation, yet monitoring will not reveal saturation. The department is trying to arrange to have tensionmeters installed at three or four monitoring sites this spring. We are interested mainly in the actual moisture regime of mottled deep silts. Several of these sites have passed monitorings, yet there is concern that system life in these soils will be short lived.

CONCLUSIONS

Monitoring groundwater can be extremely useful in areas with highly variable soil conditions that are marginal for system installation. The Section of Platting, Recreational and Environmental Services has found monitoring data useful for delineating suitable areas in land being platted. The objective of all monitoring studies should never be to discredit the use of soil mottling. Rather, it should be to delineate acceptable versus unacceptable areas.

There is strong evidence for the use of soil mottling as the criterion for determining site suitability with respect to saturated soils. History repeatedly has demonstrated that to ignore nature can result in disaster. Soil profiles do not deceive the knowledgeable observer but are an accurate reflection of the reality of nature.

Monitoring will remain in the Wisconsin Administrative Code, as will the use of soil mottling. As time and experience dictate, some changes may be made in monitoring procedures. Through education, a better understanding of soil mottling may make monitoring a less commonly used procedure.

REFERENCES

1. Soil Survey Staff, Soil Taxonomy, Agriculture Handbook No. 436, U.S. Government Printing Office, Washington, D.C. (1975), pp. 48, 49.
2. Vepraskas, M. V., and J. Bouma. "Model Experiments on Mottle Formation Simulating Field Conditions," *Geoderma* 15:217-230 (1976).
3. Bloomfield, C. "The Distribution of Iron and Aluminum Oxides in Gley Soils," *J. Soil Sci.* 3(2):167-171 (1952).
4. Rathbun, G. J. "Soil Morphological and Moisture Regime Studies of Three Wisconsin Toposequences," M.S. Thesis, The University of Wisconsin–Madison (1979).
5. Bureau of Environmental Health Staff. *Soil Tester Manual*, 2nd ed. (Madison, WI: Department of Health and Social Services, Bureau of Environmental Health, 1979).
6. Shimek, S. "Relationship of Soil Morphology to Observed Groundwater in the 'Sand Plain' of Central Wisconsin," M.S. Thesis, The University of Wisconsin–Stevens Point (1977).
7. Simonson, G. H., and L. Boersma. "Soil Morphology and Water Table Relations: II. Correlation Between Annual Water Table Fluctuations and Profile Features," *Soil Sci. Soc. Am. Proc.* 36:649-653 (1972).
8. Lathshaw, G. J., and R. F. Thompson, "Water Table Study Verifies Soil Interpretations," *J. Soil Water Cons.* 65-67 (March-April 1968).
9. Vepraskas, M. J., F. G. Baker and J. Bouma. "Soil Mottling and Drainage in a Mollic Hapludalf as Related to Suitability for Septic Tank Construction," *Soil Sci. Soc. Am. Proc.* 38:497-501 (1974).

9

TWO ONSITE OPTIONS FOR PROBLEM SOILS

Michael J. Hansel
Staff Engineer
Minnesota Pollution Control Agency
Roseville, Minnesota 55113

INTRODUCTION

If all rural lots were level, with deep water tables, good permeability and no bedrock near the surface, designing and constructing onsite sewage treatment systems would be a straightforward task. Unfortunately, because much of this type of land has already been developed (or is being preserved for agricultural purposes), builders are moving more and more to land that is only marginally suited for onsite sewage treatment. Soon both existing homes with onsite problems and new developments with potential problems will begin to crop up continually.

Many local and state governments view this development with mixed emotions. While not wanting to put a moratorium on building in these areas, they do not want to cope with massive onsite system failures. To be sure, the standard septic tank–drainfield will not work in soils with high groundwater or bedrock, or slow permeabilities, but what is the alternative, short of very expensive centralized sewers or holding tanks? In most cases, local and state codes only provide for the standard system.

Fortunately, there are solutions to this dilemma. For many marginal soil conditions there are onsite sewage systems that will treat and dispose of wastewater at a reasonable cost. Many have been used in Minnesota and are described in the literature[1]. These systems have also been included in the state design standards for onsite systems [2]. This chapter describes two of the most often used alternative systems: pumping stations and mounds.

Specific design and construction standards and specifications, which are based both on the latest research and actual field experience, are discussed.

PUMPING STATIONS

There are many instances in which a house or building is located so that gravity drainage of the plumbing system is to a poor area for sewage treatment (low spots, slowly permeable soils, areas with shallow bedrock, etc.). Whether because of ease of construction, desire for a particular view or orientation, or lack of planning for an onsite sewage system (which is usually the case), the use of a pumping station to move the sewage to a better location often can solve the problem.

An example of this is shown in Figure 1. Houses on lakeshore lots are most often situated as close as possible to the lake for the view and easy access for water recreation. Frequently, however, there is not enough elevation above the lake level (and corresponding groundwater table) to install a sewage treatment system and maintain the necessary three feet of unsaturated soil necessary for treatment. Often, the lot is such that higher ground can be found behind the house, nearer the road. In most cases, a pumping station can lift the sewage or septic tank effluent to the better location and solve the sewage treatment problem.

In other cases, when a group of houses may have a similar problem, or where lots are too small to accommodate an onsite system, the sewage may be pumped to a different site using a pressure sewer system (Figure 2).

In the past, most homeowners have been hesitant to install pumping stations for their sewage systems, fearing malfunctions, even though they

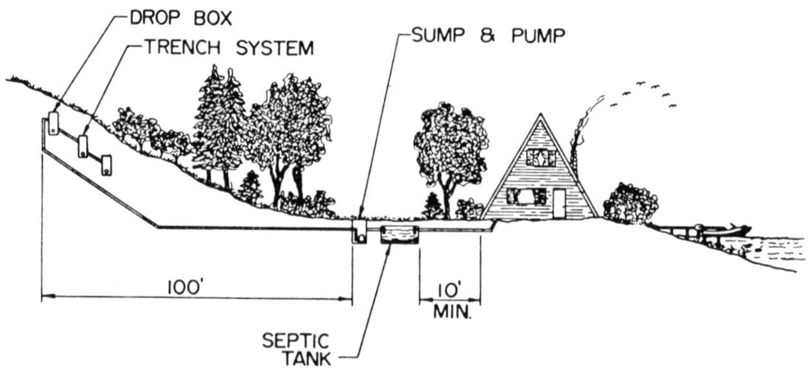

Figure 1. Sewage treatment system [3].

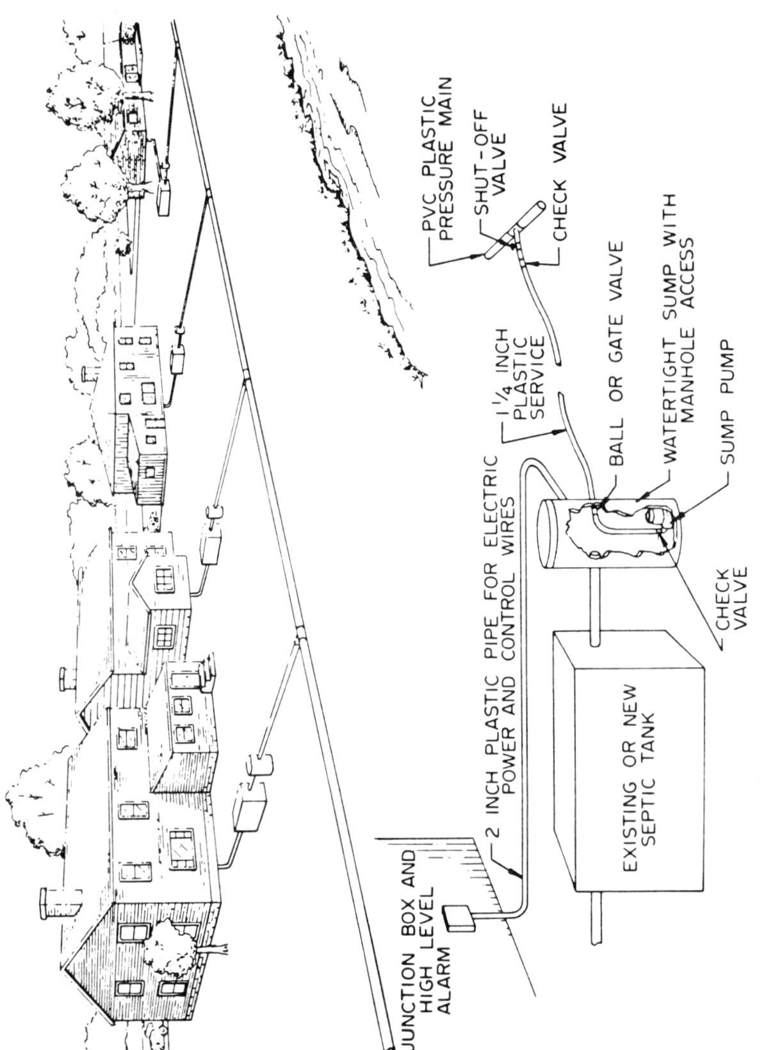

Figure 2. STEP (septic tank-effluent pump) pressure sewer system [3].

do not hesitate to put pumps several hundred feet below the ground in wells, or drive an automobile (which depends on several different pumps) into very remote areas. The reasons for their fears often are reports from friends or neighbors of failures. On examining these reports, most often the cause for failure is improper design, construction or equipment. Most major pump manufacturers now make very dependable low-horsepower pumps and controls, however, and by applying sound concepts of design and construction, home pumping stations can provide years of service with minimum maintenance. Indeed, although no exact counts are available, conservative estimates of the number of homes or small business pumping stations in Minnesota is well over 5000.

APPROACHES TO PUMPING SYSTEMS

Basically there are two approaches to small pumping systems: one can pump either raw sewage (solids along with the liquid) or settled sewage (or septic tank effluent). Both have been used with success in different applications. Each has advantages and disadvantages that must be carefully weighed for each case.

SOLIDS HANDLING PUMPS

Solids handling pumps (or sewage ejector pumps as they are sometimes called) are generally used where there is low elevation to overcome and/or short distances to pump. Figure 3 shows a typical installation of lifting wastewater from the basement to a shallow septic tank and drainfield. Most 0.5- to 1.5-horsepower solids handling pumps can easily transport 2-inch-diameter solids to heads of 12–15 feet and over distances of 10–50 feet.

There are several advantages to this type of pumping approach. The pump is located in the basement where it is accessible for maintenance. The septic tank can be located closer to the ground surface, making pumping of the tank much easier. Finally, the plumbing in the upper floors can still be used, even in the event of pump or power failure.

Disadvantages to this approach include the potential for more maintenance (especially plugging of the pump with solids), less settling in the septic tank because of shearing of the solids and surge flows into the septic tank, noisier operation (because the pump is in the basement), and difficulty of installation in existing structures.

One other type of solids handling pump should be mentioned–the grinder pump, whose use is not recommended because of higher initial and operating

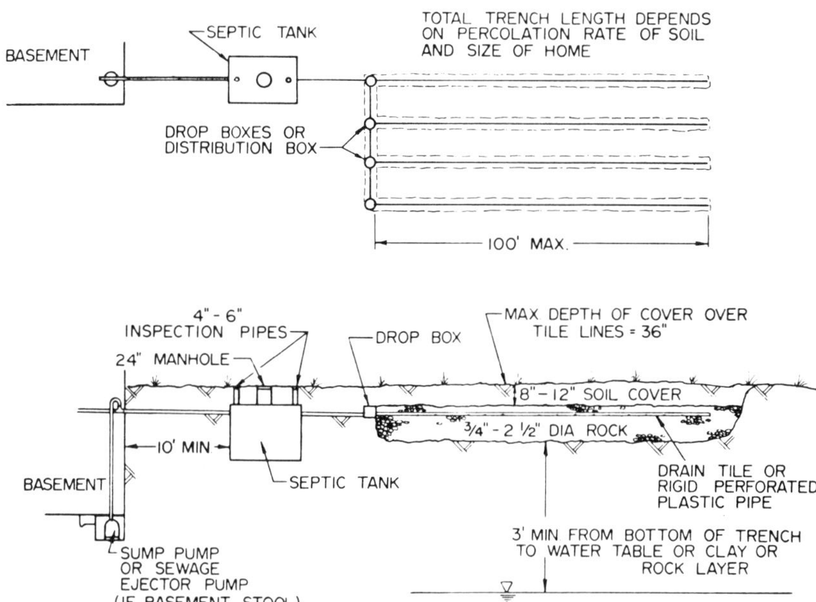

Figure 3. Pumping station for homes (pump in basement) [3].

costs, and much higher maintenance and repair. Although some have been installed in Minnesota, their use has been greatly discouraged by their poor field record.

SEPTIC TANK EFFLUENT

A septic tank–effluent pump (STEP) system is most often used where there is a high elevation or long distance to overcome. Because there are no solids to lift and carry along, effluent pumps can develop much higher heads at lower horsepower. Figure 4 is an example of a STEP system. Another use is shown in Figure 2, where a STEP system is used as part of a pressure sewer system.

The advantage to the STEP system is that settled sewage—essentially liquid—is being pumped so there is less chance of plugging either the pump or the force main. Such an approach allows for better settling in the septic tank, and may help to protect the drainfield in the event that the septic tank is not pumped out frequently enough. Solids carrying over from the septic tank will

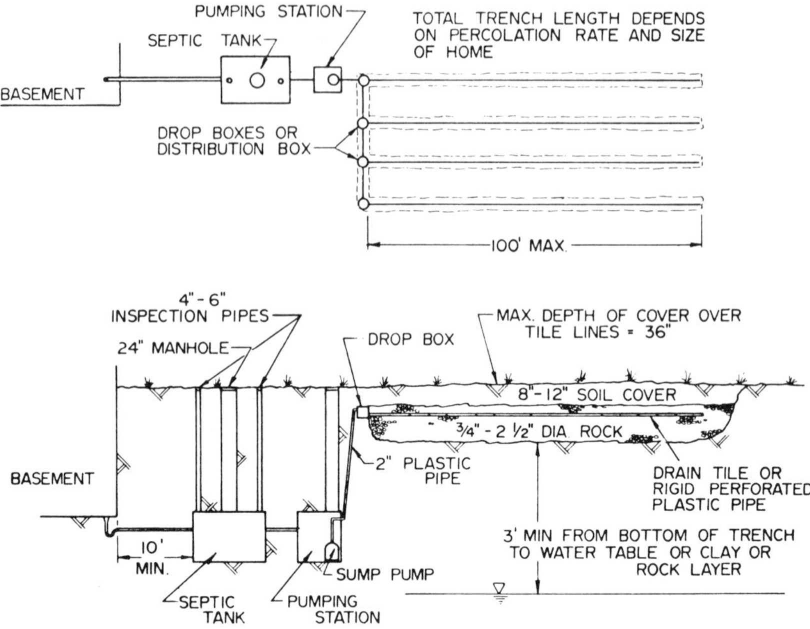

Figure 4. Pumping station for homes (pump in tank) [3].

tend to plug the pump and cause the homeowner to correct the situation before solids are transported to the drainfield.

Disadvantages to the system are that the pump is not as accessible for service, particularly if there is gravity flow from the basement plumbing on a level lot. In this case, the septic tank will also be quite deep, encumbering service of the tank. Using the approach as pictured in Figure 5, the entire house or structure depends on the pumping station. In the event of a pump or power failure, none of the facilities can be used once the reserve capacity is taken up. Finally, in areas of high groundwater, there is the possibility of infiltration and even flotation of the pumping station.

There are a number of variations available that can help to overcome some of these disadvantages. For example, in Figure 6, the use of a self-priming pump located in the basement would solve the problem of accessibility. Figure 7 shows a two-compartment septic tank, which could be used to overcome flotation and, to some extent, the infiltration problem. The first compartment is used as a septic tank (or as a second compartment following another large tank); the second compartment is used as the pumping station. A third possibility (Figure 4) shows a pumping station suspended within a septic tank. The inlets to the pumping stations are located at 60% of the

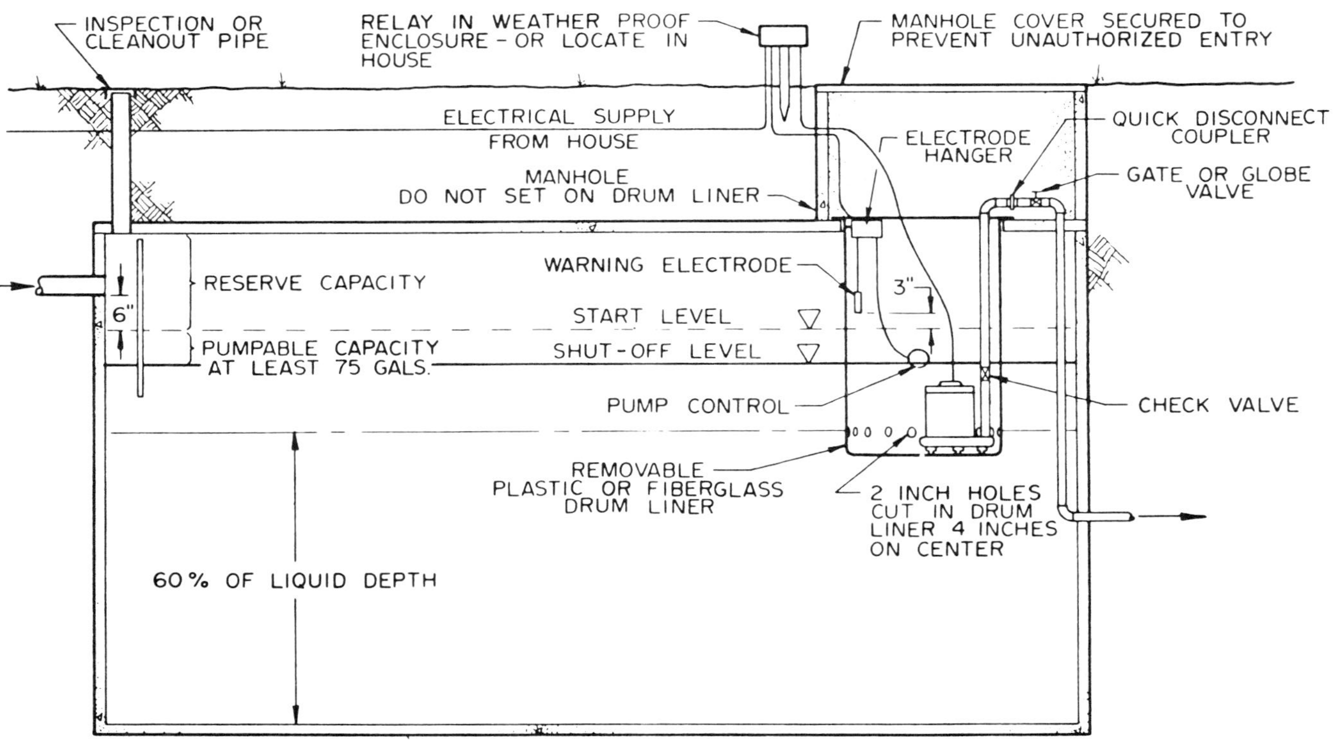

Figure 5. Pumping station within septic tank [3].

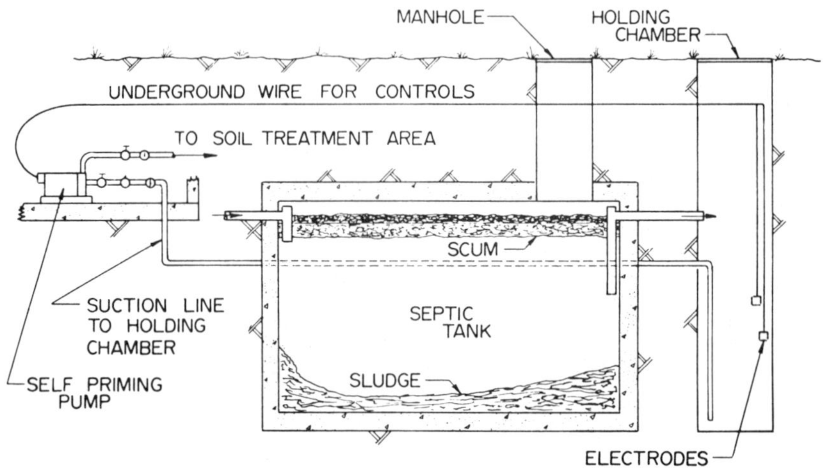

Figure 6. Pumping station with pump in basement [3].

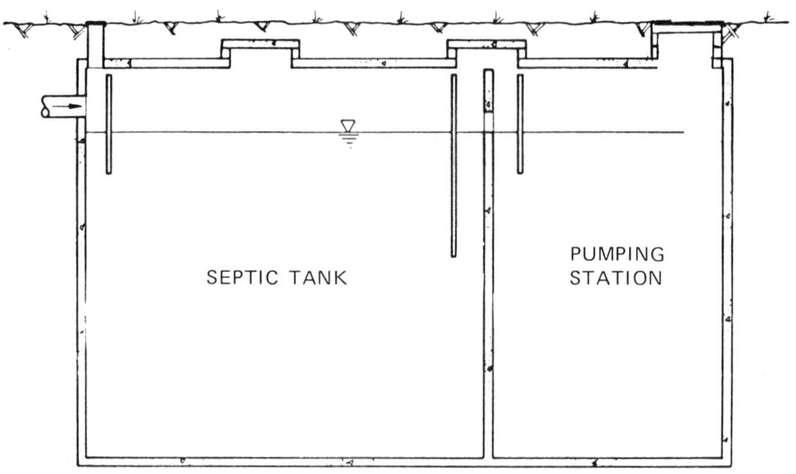

Figure 7. Combination septic tank-pumping station [3].

depth above the bottom, where the liquid is the clearest. Because only 75–100 gallons are routinely pumped out in home situations, the liquid surface will drop only 4 or 5 inches, leaving most of the water in the tank, thus preventing infiltration and flotation. Such a small movement (the tank is designed for a change in elevation of 3 inches) will not appreciably affect the scum layer.

DESIGN AND CONSTRUCTION

The design and construction of the pumping station is crucial to its operation. An advantage to the use of solids handling or sewage ejector pumps is that they are generally sold as a package; sump, pump and controls. However, there are several design parameters that can be controlled.

The size of the sump is important if more than laundry wastes and floor drains are to be pumped or if drainback is involved. Normally, an 18-inch sump will be satisfactory for these two generators, but if a bathroom is added, particularly one that is used often, a larger sump (perhaps 30–36 inches in diameter) will better serve to prevent frequent starts and subsequent wear on the pump.

If it is necessary to drainback the discharge line, the amount of drainback must be carefully calculated. There have been occasions in which a pump in an 18-inch sump was discharging 10 gallons per cycle and 9 gallons were draining back. While the pump was able to remove the water eventually, it quickly burned out. A larger sump would easily correct this situation, or a check valve could be installed to prevent drainback if the pressure line can be protected from freezing.

Solids handling sumps, particularly if they are handling toilet wastes, should be sealed and vented to prevent odors and gases from entering the basement.

The design and construction of STEP systems is somewhat more complicated because they are not readily available as preassembled units. However, all of the components are readily available. Once the principles of design are understood, a STEP system can frequently be assembled for less than prepackaged solids handling units.

Location

The pumping chamber needs to be located where it will be easily accessible for maintenance. A manhole should extend up to the surface and be locked or otherwise secured to prevent unauthorized tampering. The pumping station should not be located in a swale or depression where runoff from surrounding areas could inundate the station and hydraulically overload the soil treatment system.

Materials

The chamber should be watertight, corrosion resistant and flotation resistant. A precast concrete septic tank of 500, 750 or even 1000 gallons is commonly used. Block tanks can also be used, provided they have a poured concrete bottom and are coated both inside and out to prevent infiltration. Concrete culverts set on end with a poured concrete bottom have also been used, as have fiberglass and plastic septic tanks. Metal tanks or metal culverts should not be used, as these generally do not remain corrosion resistant or watertight for long. In areas of high groundwater, precast concrete tanks are the best choice, and in extreme cases, one of the options shown in Figures 5-7 may have to be used. Fiberglass or plastic tanks can be used if they are anchored to concrete slabs or earth anchors.

Capacity

There are really three capacities that must be considered in the design of a pumping station: stilling, pumping and reserve capacities. These are shown in Figure 8.

The stilling capacity, the bottom 12-18 inches of the tank, serves a number of important purposes. First, it prevents turbulence from water entering the tank and entering the suction portion of the pump. Second, it provides additional space for solids to settle in case any are carried over from the septic tank. Third, this area provides cooling for the pump. As can be seen

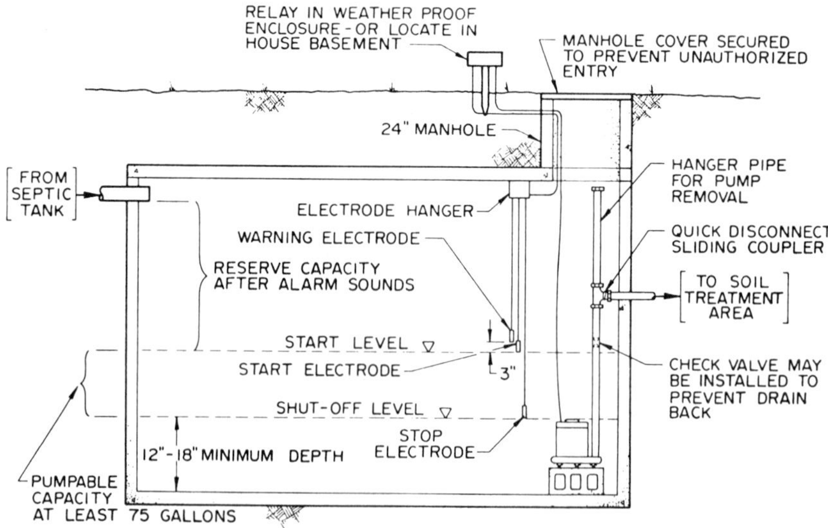

Figure 8. Diagram of the three capacities–stilling, pumping and reserve–that must be considered in the design of a pumping station [3].

in Figure 8, the shutoff depth should be set at the top of the pump casing because submersible pumps are designed to run submerged and depend on water for cooling. For a pump to run exposed in an 18-inch-diameter sump for a few seconds or even as long as a minute will probably not result in a great deal of harm. But if a 600-gph pump needs to pump 100 gallons out of a 700-gallon tank, it may run for several minutes exposed. This will increase the heating of the pump and result in premature burnout.

The pumping capacity is determined after considering two factors: (1) treatment of wastewater in the drainfield, and (2) wear and tear on the pump. Recent research [4,5] indicates that dosing the drainfield several times a day with small doses provides for better treatment by more uniformly loading the soil treatment area and allowing for resting and drying out between doses. Most pump sales and service personnel hold that a pump should not start more often than three or four times a day to hold pump wear to a minimum. A reasonable compromise is to set the controls so that the pumpable capacity is about 25% of the daily sewage flow. However, in no case should fewer than 75 gallons be pumped. Otherwise, there will be insufficient flow to provide for even distribution.

In larger establishments, such as restaurants, resorts and campgrounds, it would be uneconomical to provide such a large capacity. In these situations, the use of dual pumps and 10 or 12 cycles per day (5 or 6 per pump) will keep the pumpable capacity to a reasonable size.

The reserve capacity is needed in the event of a pump or power failure (although in the latter, most rural water supplies depend on the same power source, so the situation is self-limiting). For homes, one day's detention should be allowed (300–500 gallons) so that the pump can be removed and repaired or replaced. For larger establishments, especially where dual pumps are used, a reserve capacity of 25% of the daily sewage flow can be used. Such capacity can be provided by joining two precast tanks, as shown in Figure 9.

Thus, the total capacity for a single-family home would be 100–200 gallons stilling, 100 gallons pumping and 400 gallons reserve, or 700 gallons total. A restaurant generating 3000 gpd using dual pumps would need 200 gallons stilling, 300 gallons pumping (10 cycles, 5 per pump) and 750 gallons reserve, or a total of 1250 gallons.

Pumps

The pump is actually the simplest component of the system. A good quality sump pump should be used, one that is stocked and serviced by a local hardware, lumber or plumbing business. Initially spending about $100

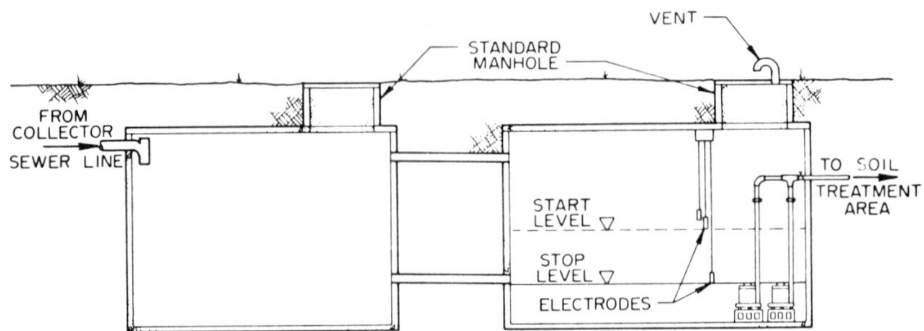

Figure 9. Dual pump and multiple-tank pumping station [4].

on a good sump pump will be far more economical than buying a cheaper model that must be replaced more often.

The pump should be cast iron or bronze, fitted with stainless steel screws or connectors. There are also plastic fitted pumps on the market that could be used. The pump chosen should be able to deliver sufficient quantities of water at the design head. Remember to include friction losses in pipe and fittings as well as head losses. If a pressure distribution system is used (as in a mound), an additional five feet of head should be added to overcome losses at the orifices.

The capacity of a pump for a home installation should be at least 600 gph to handle peak flows and so that the pump does not run too long. The maximum capacity should not exceed 2700 gph at the design head to prevent backup in the distribution or drop box. For other establishments, the pump should discharge at a rate of at least 10% greater than the water supply flowrate, but no faster than the rate at which effluent will flow out of the distribution or drop box. Here again, the use of dual pumps can be economical, as both pumps can be used to handle peak flows.

The pump should be connected to the pressure main using a quick or sliding disconnect, union, dresser coupling or other connector, which allows for easy removal for servicing. A hanger pipe should be brought up into the manhole to facilitate removal, as the chains supplied with most pumps usually corrode quickly and become useless for that purpose. There have been some problems reported using plastic pressure pipe as a hanger pipe, but most installations using Schedule 40 or heavier pipe have experienced little or no difficulty.

A globe or gate valve may be installed after the union or disconnect to throttle down the discharge or to prevent drainback while the pump is being serviced. This is particularly important in pressure sewer applications. A check valve may also be installed to prevent drainback if the pressure line is protected from frost. If drainback must be used, a good rule of thumb is that the drainback quantity not exceed 10% of the pumped quantity. A 1.5-inch-diameter plastic pipe holds about 10.5 gallons per 100 feet, while a 2-inch-diameter pipe holds about 18 gallons per 100 feet. Also, there should be no possibility of water siphoning back from the distribution or drop box and the drainfield. The discharge end of the pressure line should end above the expected water level and be directed against a blank wall to dissipate energy, as shown in Figure 10.

Finally, the pump should not be placed on the floor of the pumping station; rather, it should be elevated on a concrete block 6-8 inches off the floor to allow for storage of settled solids.

Controls

The single biggest problem with home or small pumping stations is with the controls. They have been responsible for more failures than any other single cause and have generally required the most maintenance. However, by following some basic guidelines, most of these difficulties can be eliminated.

The most important caveat is that there be absolutely no electrical-mechanical connection inside the pumping stations. This would include plug-ins, screw-type connections, twisted wires, boxes and relays—anything that requires movement to connect or operate. Such connections and parts should be located either in a weatherproof box aboveground or in the house. If connections must be made, they should be soldered and enclosed in a waterproof (not water-resistant) seal. There are some excellent shrink-on coverings that work well in this application. The problem can be better solved by ordering both pumps and controls with extra long cords, which are almost universally available.

The best controls are those that are available separately from the pump. Usually one can purchase a manually operated pump, i.e., one with no controls, merely a power cord, and separate controls for the same price as a pump with controls in or on the case. Switches on or in the case have several disadvantages. First, they cannot be adjusted (generally) to allow for different pumpout depths and volumes. Second, most are designed so that the pump is exposed through most of the cycle, causing overheating of the pump. Third, the entire pump must be removed to perform maintenance on the controls. Finally, both the diaphragm switch and float-on-case switch are notorious for becoming fouled by the small suspended solids in septic tank effluent.

The best control available, in terms of being trouble-free and providing the best service, is the mercury switch encased in a float. Some are designed

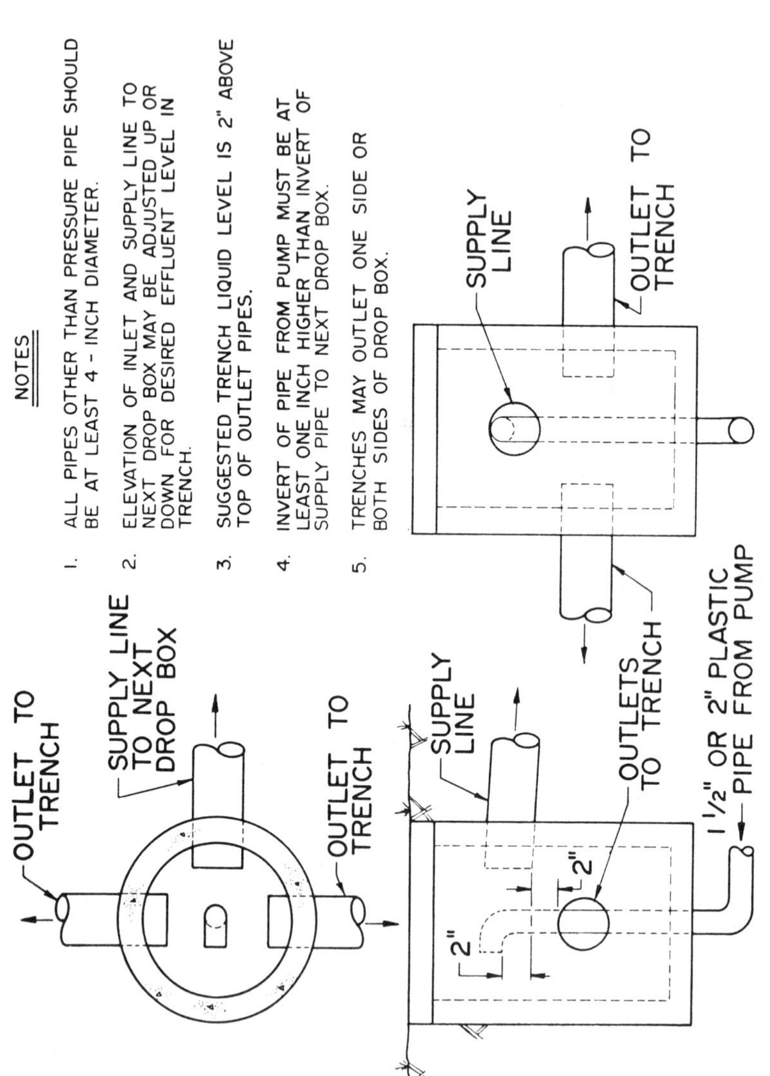

Figure 10. Drop box for pumping effluent [3].

to handle the starting current draw of a 0.5- to 1-horsepower pump directly; the pump is simply plugged into the back of a piggyback plug on the control. Others require a relay. The pumpout depth is set either with an adjustable weight on the cord or by adjusting the connection to the discharge or hanger pipe.

For larger establishments, controls should be used that: (1) alternate pumps on successive cycles; (2) allow both pumps to operate during peak flow periods; (3) warn of the failure of one pump while the other is switched on; and (4) have a high water alarm. While such controls may cost more than the pumps, they are well worth the expense, particularly where the public is involved (e.g., restaurants).

The shutoff control should be set at the top of the pump case to provide sufficient stilling capacity. The "on" control is set above the shutoff to provide a minimum 75-gallon dose and a maximum dose of 25% of the daily flow. The alarm device should be set 3–6 inches above the "on" control to maximize reserve capacity and prevent spurious signals attributable to momentary fluctuations in the water surface during peak flows.

The alarm control should be on a separate electrical circuit because if the alarm were on the same circuit as the pump, and the pump (because of clogging or whatever reason) were to kick out the circuit breaker, the alarm would become inoperable as well. The alarm should provide for an audible signal that can be switched off and a light or other visual signal that remains on to remind the owner to have the pump serviced.

The cost of a pumping system will vary somewhat. For a STEP system, a typical home system cost would be $100–150 for the pump and controls, $500 for the station (installed) and $50–100 for electrical connections, for a total of approximately $750. A typical solids handling pump, sump and controls would cost between $500 and $800, installed. Costs for larger establishments vary much more, depending on the specific installation.

Although pumping stations have been used with all types of soil treatment systems, they are most commonly used with mound systems. In fact, the design and construction of the pumping system generally requires about one-third the cost and about one-half the time for installing a mound system. Once the design and construction of pumping systems is understood, the use of mound systems is a much easier proposition.

MOUND SYSTEMS

Mound systems can be used to solve a wide gamut of onsite problems. By bringing in additional fill soil, mounds can solve problems caused by high groundwater or bedrock. By staying on top of slowly permeable soils and not reducing their infiltration capability by excavating, mound systems can be used to treat and dispose of wastes on slowly permeable soils. Even on rapidly permeable soils, excellent treatment can result by using the existing, less permeable topsoil to provide treatment.

Mounds have been used successfully in all parts of Minnesota in all types of problem soils situations. Although an exact count is not available, it is estimated that there are between 2000 and 3000 in operation. One county alone, Aitkin County, has had more than 500 installed in the past five years.

Theory

In the mound there are two restricting layers or zones: the rock–sand interface and the sand–soil interface (Figure 11). The design and construction of the mound depends on the correct treatment of these two zones. At the upper zone–the rock–sand interface–unsaturated flow is established either by growth of the biomat or use of pressure distribution. This zone must be sized and constructed to allow for even distribution and unsaturated flow.

Once unsaturated flow is established, some treatment will occur in the sand layer. The sand layer also functions to distribute the effluent over the entire basal area of the mound so that it can infiltrate the more permeable topsoil. The topsoil, in turn, further treats the effluent and distributes it over a still wider area before it enters the subsoil.

Design

The design of mounds is based on the flowrates through the two restricting zones. The rock area in contact with the sand is sized on the basis of 1.2 gpd/ft^2 (0.83 ft^2/gpd), which is the long-term acceptance rate of the sand with biomat formation or pressure distribution (essentially the unsaturated flowrate). Although the mound could be any shape, experience has shown that a long, narrow mound functions much better hydraulically than a more square or compact design. For this reason, the width of the bed is limited to 10 feet maximum.

The basal area, or area in which the sand fill contacts the soil, is sized automatically by following two design parameters:

1. There must be at least 1 foot of fill beneath the bed; and
2. The slopes of the dike must be no steeper than 3:1.

With 1 foot of sand, 1 foot of rock in the rock bed, and 1 foot of cover, a 3:1 side slope yields an additional 9-10 feet on all sides of the rockbed. For

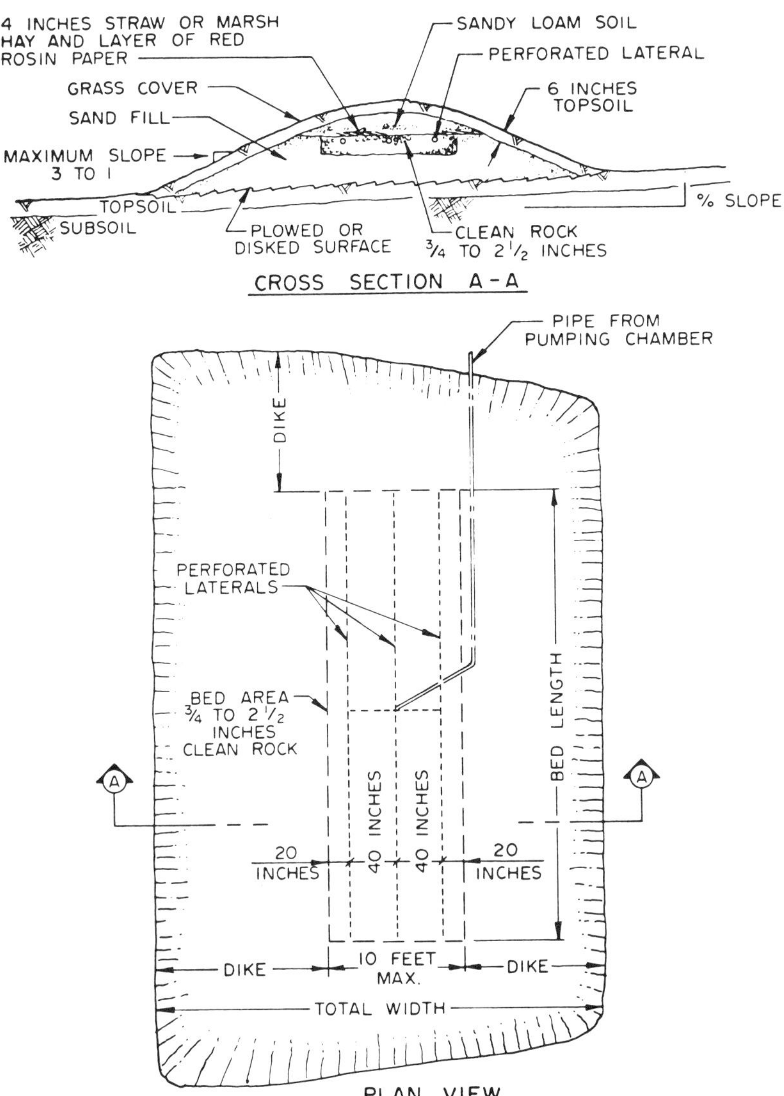

Figure 11. The two restricting layers or zones in the mound—the rock-sand interface and the sand-soil interface [3].

example, a mound designed to accommodate 450 gpd would have a rockbed 37.5 ft × 10 ft. With 3: 1 slopes, the basal area would cover an area 55.5 ft × 28 ft or a total area of 1554 ft^2, resulting in an application rate of 0.29 gpd/ft^2 at the sand–soil interface.

On very slowly permeable soils, a 4:1 side slope is preferred, as this increases the available basal area. For the example above, 4:1 side slopes would result in a basal area of 61.5 ft × 34 ft or a total area of about 2100 ft^2 (application rate of 0.21 gpd/ft^2). By using the entire basal area for treatment and absorption, a much lower application rate results that is acceptable even on very slowly permeable soils.

Location

Mounds cannot be built on every imaginable site. Where there is no soil (i.e., exposed bedrock) or where the topsoil has been removed and a slowly permeable subsoil graded or disturbed, it is impossible to build a mound and have it function hydraulically. Organic soils such as peats and mucks, which subside beneath fill, should not be used for mound construction.

Beneath the sand fill layer, there needs to be a 2-foot layer of soil in place. Some of this can be fill soil, provided it is properly settled, but not all. The maximum permeability of this 2-foot layer can be no faster than 5 minutes per inch (mpi) as measured by the standard percolation test. The reason for this restriction is so that this soil layer can act to treat the effluent which enters it, especially in removing nutrients such as phosphorus.

The minimum permeability of the 2-foot layer depends on the slope: the steeper the slope the more permeable the 2-foot layer must be to prevent all the effluent from running out the bottom slope of the dike before it can be absorbed by the soil. The following rules apply:

Slope (%)	Percolation Rate (mpi)
0-3	Faster than 120
3-6	Faster than 60
6-12	Faster than 30

For natural slopes greater than 12%, mounds should not be constructed because the possibility of side slope seepage is too great. Steep slopes must not be graded to meet these limits, as this will disturb the soil structure and lead to failure. Mounds should be located on crests of hills wherever possible. The second best location is along the contours of convex slopes. Mounds should never be located in drainageways (i.e., concave slopes) or in depressions that collect runoff from surrounding lands. Especially on the steeper slopes, surface runoff water should be diverted around the mound by swales or ditches.

Distribution

Two methods of distribution can be used within the mound: pressure and gravity distribution. Gravity distribution is generally used only when it is possible to bring effluent to the mound by gravity (i.e., when the mound is at a lower elevation than the house). In most instances, however, a pump is necessary to lift the effluent to the mound. As long as a pump is available, the pressure distribution system should be used because it provides for much more even distribution within the mound and for better treatment earlier on [3]. In fact, several cases of localized overloading within the mound have been corrected by using pressure distribution. With pressure distribution, unsaturated flow is set up immediately because effluent is applied at the unsaturated flowrate of the sand fill. With gravity distribution, there is or can be a waiting period of up to several months before the biomat becomes established, leading to less treatment during startup. This can be particularly important for seasonal residences and establishments such as campgrounds.

The design of a pressure sewer system is shown in Table I and Figure 12. Pipe of 1–1.5 inches in diameter is used, with 0.18- to 0.25-inch holes spaced 30–36 inches apart. The maximum length of the pipe is limited to provide less than 10% variation in flow from the first hole (nearest the header pipe) to the last. Joints are glued, ends are capped, and holes must be pointed downward to prevent surfacing of effluent.

Construction

Once the mound has been designed and the location established, the construction should begin on a day when rain is not likely and when most

Table I. Required Pumping Rates and Maximum Perforated Lateral Lengths for Various Perforation Sizes and Pipe Diameters [3]

	Perforation Spacing 30 inches				Perforation Spacing 36 inches			
		Pipe Diameter				Pipe Diameter		
Perforation Diameter	gpm/100 ft²	1 in. (ft)	$1\frac{1}{4}$ in. (ft)	$1\frac{1}{2}$ in. (ft)	gpm/100 ft²	1 in. (ft)	$1\frac{1}{4}$ in. (ft)	$1\frac{1}{2}$ in. (ft)
$\frac{3}{16}$ in.	5.0	34	52	70	4.5	36	60	75
$\frac{7}{32}$ in.	7.0	30	45	57	6.0	33	51	63
$\frac{1}{4}$ in.	9.0	25	38	50	7.5	27	42	54

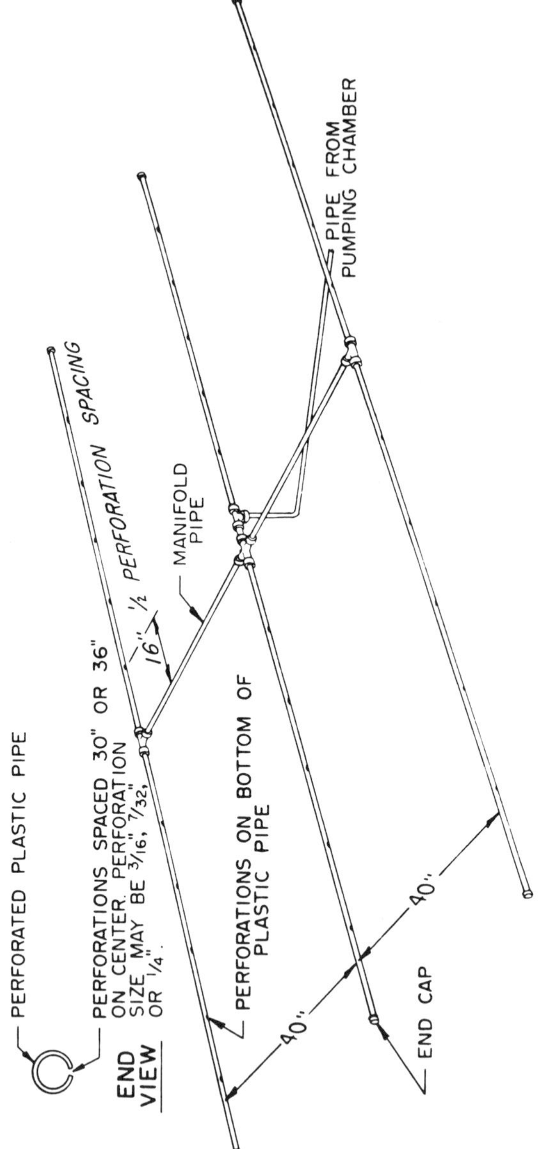

Figure 12. Layout of perforated pipe laterals for pressure distribution in a mound [3].

of the construction can be completed that day. The first step is to install the pressure main from the pumping station and backtamp the trench to prevent effluent from following the trench back from the mound. Next, the entire area of the mound and the rockbed should be staked off and areas designated for stockpiling sand and gravel. Trucks and other heavy equipment should be routed around the mound area.

The single most important construction detail is to rough up the sod or surface vegetation over the entire basal area, either with a plow (a mold-board or chisel plow, or in lighter soils a disc) or with a backhoe to reach out and rough up the surface (the backhoe itself should not be driven on the mound area). Under no circumstances should the sod or any portion of the topsoil be removed.

The purpose of this plowing or roughening is to prevent the vegetation from lying over and rotting, forming a relatively impermeable barrier leading to surface outbreaks. It also serves to increase the actual contact area between the sand fill and the in-place soil, forming a better bond. A number of early mound failures have been traced to either removing sod/topsoil or failure to roughen the topsoil.

After the surface has been broken up, there should be absolutely no vehicle traffic on the mound area. Even foot traffic should be kept to a minimum. Clean sand is then dozed in from the sides using a track-type tractor to minimize compaction. There should be at least 6 inches of the sand fill beneath the tracks at all times.

The sand should be medium to coarse sand, with fewer than 10% of the particles smaller than 0.05 mm, fewer than 50% between 0.05 and 0.25 mm, and at least 25% greater than 0.25 mm. Because the size of the rockbed is based on an assumed percolation rate of the fill of less than 5 mpi, using a finer fill will result in a lower long-term acceptance rate. This ultimately results in insufficient area at the rock–soil interface, leading to overflow of the mound. On the other hand, using a material that is a very coarse sand will not provide sufficient filtration of the septic tank effluent before it reaches the sand–soil interface, which can result in the formation of a clogging layer at that interface and subsequent leakage.

The sand fill should be at least 1 foot thick beneath the rock bed (thicker if more elevation is needed above bedrock or groundwater), extend to the top of the rockbed on the sides, and be feathered out to the edge of the dike. In other words, the entire basal area is covered with sand. Most contractors fill the area beneath the rockbed with 2 feet of sand and excavate 1 foot for the bed. The sand under the rock bed *must* be level; this is crucial for even distribution within the rockbed.

Next, at least a 9-inch layer of rock, 0.5–0.75 inches in diameter, is placed in the area of the rockbed and leveled, again using the track-type tractor to minimize compaction. The pressure distribution network is laid out as described above and covered with at least another 2 inches of rock.

Next, a 4- to 6-inch layer of hay, straw or leaves is placed on top of the rock followed by a layer of untreated building paper. The purpose of these two layers is to prevent any soil from filtering into the rock and plugging it, while allowing liquid to pass through. Neither the hay nor the building paper by itself will completely do the job. The hay or straw, even if carefully applied, contains gaps and crevices, while the building paper is easily punctured by the rock. So by using the hay and straw to cushion the building paper, a satisfactory cover is maintained. In some installations, a filter fabric of spun-bounded plastic or fiberglass has been used successfully. This is usually much more expensive than the straw and building paper method, however.

Next the mound is covered with a layer of sand or other soil. There should be at least 12 inches of cover at the edges of the rock bed, and the mound should be crowned to a depth of 18 inches in the middle to promote runoff of precipitation. The sand or soil should be feathered onto the dikes to result in a 3:1 slope.

Finally, at least 6 inches of topsoil is placed over the entire mound including the dikes, and the mound is seeded or sodded. This last step should be done as soon as possible after completion of the mound to prevent erosion. If the mound is located on a slope, particularly on steep slopes, a diversion ditch or swale should be constructed upslope of the mound to prevent surface runoff, as shown in Figure 13.

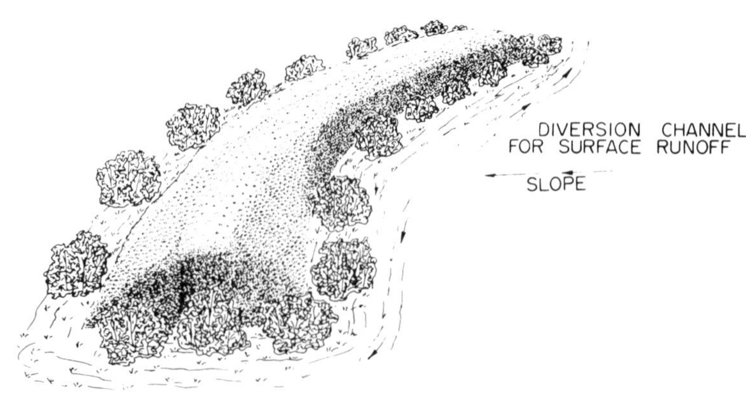

Figure 13. Sewage treatment mound on contour [3].

Summary

Mound systems have been used very successfully in all parts of Minnesota and on all problem soil conditions. While there have been some failures, particularly earlier on, these have been traced to hydraulic overload, improper construction or pumping system failure. The most common causes of improper construction are improper preparation of the sand–soil interface: either smearing, compacting or failing to roughen the surface. Failures have also occurred because of using too fine a sand for fill, building on too steep slopes, or because of soil filtering into the rock from above and plugging it.

The cost of mound systems varies widely, depending primarily on the availability and cost of the sand fill and the experience of the contractor. An entire system, including septic tank, pumping station and mound, would cost anywhere from $2000 to $5000. While considerably more than a conventional septic tank–drainfield system, it is still considerably less, in the long run, than the use of a holding tank, which is often the only other alternative.

CONCLUSIONS

Pumping stations and mounds are but two of the alternatives available to handle onsite sewage treatment problems. Provided they are properly designed, located, constructed and maintained, they can provide excellent treatment for as long a period as a conventional septic tank–drainfield. Complying with these provisions requires not only trained inspectors at the local level who can supervise the construction, but also trained contractors who are familiar with both the requirements and the reasons behind them.

To this end, the University of Minnesota and the Minnesota Pollution Control Agency have cooperated in putting on an annual series of three-day workshops. The Home Sewage Treatment Workshops [3] discuss not only the design and construction of the standard septic tank–drainfield system, but also the construction of alternative systems, including pumping systems and mounds. In 1979 more than 300 participants attended the nine workshops, and a similar number of workshops is planned for 1980. The workshops actually provide for a two-way flow of information because contractors and inspectors can share their practical information and exchange ideas on products and materials, as well as receive information from the instructors.

In these discussions, failures of systems are discussed and possible reasons and solutions. In any new or different type of technology, when a failure occurs there is always the temptation to write that method off. A more appropriate response is to determine why the method did not work as planned and attempt to correct the situation. The first mounds and pumping stations built in Minnesota had a number of problems. Only by analyzing these early mistakes was it possible to revise design standards and construction procedures so that later mounds and pumping systems would be successful. This attitude needs to be kept in mind when trying any new technology.

REFERENCES

1. Hansel, M. J., and R. E. Machmeier. "Onsite Sewage Treatment on Problem Solids," paper presented at the 51st Annual Conference, Water Pollution Control Federation, Anaheim, CA, October, 1978.
2. Minnesota Pollution Control Agency. "GMCAR 4.8040 Individual Sewage Treatment Systems Standards," St. Paul, Minnesota: Documents Section, Department of Administration (1978).
3. Machmeier, R. E., and M. J. Hansel. *Home Sewage Treatment Workshop Workbook*, Office of Special Programs, University of Minnesota, St. Paul, MN (1979).
4. Converse, J. C., et al. "Pressure Distribution to Improve Soil Absorption Systems," in *Proc. Nat. Home Sewage Disposal Symp.* (St. Joseph, MI: American Society of Agricultural Engineers, 1974), pp. 104-115.
5. Otis, R. J., et al. "Effluent Distribution," in *Proc. Second Nat. Home Sewage Treatment Symp.* (St. Joseph, MI: American Society of Agricultural Engineers, 1977), pp. 61-85.

10

A SYSTEM FOR HIGH-SLOPE LOTS

Don Miller
Principal Engineer
Wright and Company
Newport Beach, California 92660

INTRODUCTION

Methodology to handle onsite disposal of domestic wastewater in high slope areas is usually unique. The parcel mentioned in this chapter consisted of a large lot and a single-family residence. Five persons are in residence for a total waste discharge of 400 gpd. The high slope (12°) of the lot prohibited normal leach fields because of surfacing potential.

PROBLEM

Disposing of domestic wastewater on a plot with a slope of 12° from the highway to the rear of the parcel had to be confronted. The local Water Quality Control Board refused a permit based on normal longitudinal leach lines. Therefore, an attempt was made to make use of the gravity flow situation while permitting an effluent that met the water quality standards.

THE SOLUTION

As seen in Figure 1, the elevation differential of 125 feet from the highway to the residential plot is evident. This differential relates to a slope of 12°.

The domestic wastewater is primarily collected in a 1200-gallon fiberglass

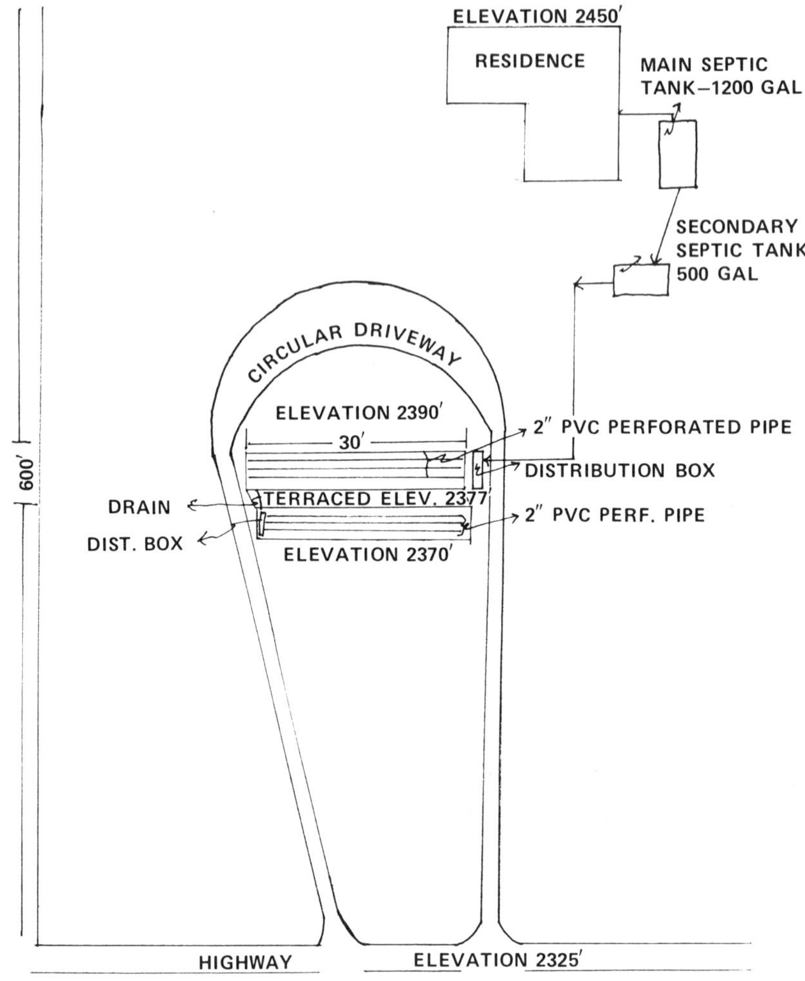

Figure 1. Parcel plan view.

septic tank complete with center baffle, in which it receives a reasonably early treatment for solids. The effluent from the main septic tank is gravity fed into a 500-gallon secondary tank, again with centrally positioned baffle. This secondary or cascade tank further settles the wastewater and then flows to a small distribution box, which feeds the two-inch perforated PVC lines laid in the upper field. Figure 2 shows the construction of the terraced fields.

The 2-inch lines are slightly depressed over the length of the field (2 inches over 30 feet) for gravity flow purposes. It is also necessary to have a similar

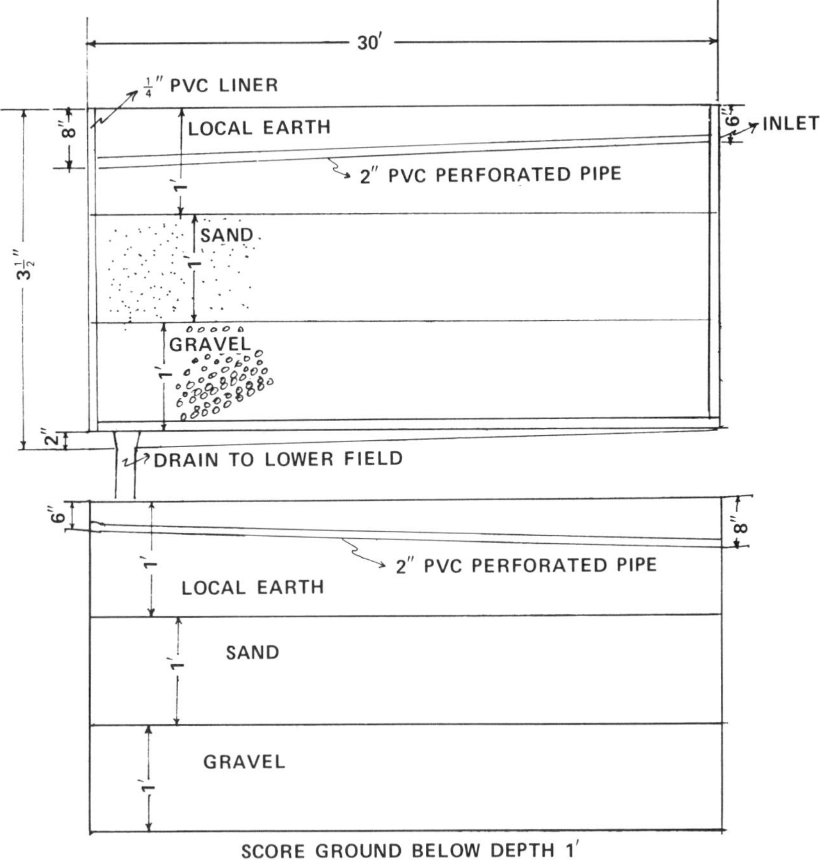

Figure 2. Plan view of terraced fields.

gradient over the whole floor of the upper field. The three dispersing lines are laid on 2-foot centers from the center of the field. This requires that the outer lines be placed 1 foot from the edge of the field for a total width of 6 feet. It is necessary to line the entire upper field with 0.25- to 0.5-inch plastic PVC for collection purposes. A drain is located in the effluent end of the upper field. With the liner in place, the next step is to lay 1 foot of pea-sized gravel on the field area, cover it with 1 foot of good sand, and then cover it with 1 foot of local soil. The dispersing 2-inch perforated PVC pipes are laid at a depth of 6 inches on the inlet end, grading down to 8 inches on the drain end. It is beneficial if shallow root flowers are planted on the surface of the field.

The lower field is fed through a distribution box tied to the upper field drain. A simple scoring of the earth below the lower field will suffice to allow easy entry of the drainage. No liner is required in the lower field and the composition of the lower field, gravel, sand, earth, line placement, etc., is identical with the upper field. The resulting effluent discharged to the attendant soil will meet all quality standards and recycle the wastewater to the groundwater basin without fear of attendant pollution. Naturally, the primary and secondary septic tanks will require pumping every three to four years. The pumped sludge can be transported to a certified dumping site. Also, it is recommended that a small access pipe be attached to the upper distribution box for administration of about 5-10 gallons of hydrogen peroxide (H_2O_2) on an annual basis. This excellent oxidant will keep the terraced fields in good use for many years.

CONCLUSIONS

Onsite wastewater disposal is feasible for single- or multifamily dwellings placed on high slopes. However, each parcel and layout is unique, and care must be taken to make use of available terrain and size and location of the terraced fields. If one looks at each parcel as a total system, influent to final effluent, and installs the components with care, a viable product can be generated. The costs of such a system will range between $2000 and $3000, depending on local construction costs.

11

ENHANCED TREATMENT FOR SURFACE DISCHARGE

Murl G. Teske
Regional Engineer
Office of Environmental Health
Illinois Department of Public Health
Marion, Illinois 62959

INTRODUCTION

Individual onsite wastewater systems with surface discharges are not new and, in most cases, not innovative. Some wastewater treatment systems that have been used for small facilities for many years include waste stabilization ponds, buried sand filters, intermittent sand filters and aeration systems. Many septic tank-seepage field and cesspool systems also have surface discharges that occur constantly or intermittently, depending on the age, size, soil type and flow.

Septic tank-seepage field waste treatment systems have been in use for some time in rural America. A properly designed and installed septic tank-seepage field system in good soil on a large enough lot is probably the most economical, cost-effective system the homeowner can install. A septic tank-seepage field system installed improperly in poor soil on too small a lot is probably the worst headache a homeowner will have.

Many areas of the United States have soil types that are unsuitable for seepage field installation, and where these systems will not work the homeowner is faced with a myriad of problems and decisions as to what he should do for waste treatment. He seldom gets any help from his contractor because the only thing the contractor ever installs is septic tank-seepage field systems. In some rare cases the contractor may be familiar with buried sand filter installation.

WASTE STABILIZATION PONDS

Systems with surface discharges are the next alternative for the homeowner. If his lot is large enough, he can consider a waste stabilization pond, which is probably the lowest cost surface discharge system available to the builder. Waste stabilization ponds require a fairly large amount of land that is free of trees and built in an area where prevailing winds have access.

Algae growth, weed growth (both in the pond and on the berms), odors and safety are all problems associated with waste stabilization ponds. They do not and cannot produce an effluent of good quality without additional treatment. Algae are considered a suspended solid, and prolific algae growth in the ponds spills over with the effluent. If the algae die, they exert an oxygen demand on the stream, they are suspended material, and there is a tendency for some types of algae to form mates, which then die and cause considerable odor problems.

Small children cannot avoid the urge to play in water and, as a result, the waste stabilization pond causes no small problem in terms of safety from both physical and bacterial standpoints. Proper fencing is needed to eliminate this threat.

BURIED SAND FILTERS

Buried sand filters are excellent waste treatment systems with surface discharge of very high-quality effluent. Buried sand filters do have some odor associated with them as a result of the need for venting. Sand size is critical in their construction, and sand in the size range of 1.0–1.5 mm in diameter is best. Sand size as small as 0.6 mm will cause the filter to plug and malfunction.

Buried sand filters should have a minimum bed depth of 24 inches of sand supported by a 3-inch bed of pea gravel. The distribution pipes and underdrains should be bedded in 10-inch layers of gravel in the 1.25–1.5 inch range. The controlling factor for building a buried sand filter is having adequate slope on the land to maintain a gravity system. Dosing should not exceed 1 gal/ft^2/day [1].

AEROBIC WASTE TREATMENT SYSTEMS

Aerobic waste treatment systems provide treatment by contacting the sewage with biologically active biomass being kept aerobic and in suspension by introducing air into the plant. Many different types of systems are on the market, but all use the same basic biological principle.

Aerobic plants work on the premise that all biodegradable material is converted to either biomass or water and CO_2. The biomass continues to build in these systems until it overpopulates the system. Then it begins to carry over with the effluent. Proper wasting of biomass periodically can eliminate this phenomenon. None of the commercially available aerobic units have wasting capability. The inorganic, nonbiodegradable solids in the waste accumulate in the system and/or are discharged continuously in the effluent.

Filtering the effluent from these aerobic systems to keep the biomass and other solids in the system allows a good high-quality discharge. The addition of filtering equipment adds additional maintenance and cost to the system and does not eliminate the need for periodic wasting of a portion of the biomass from the system.

INTERMITTENT SAND FILTERS

Intermittent sand filters provide very high-quality effluent, but have an inherent problem of odors during each dosing cycle. A few simple modifications of this system can eliminate that odor, improve the effluent quality even more, and provide a waste treatment system that can be built almost anywhere and be sized to treat sewage from a single home or for an entire small community of 400 people.

RECIRCULATING SAND FILTERS

Recirculating part of the effluent from an intermittent sand filter back and mixing it with what is dosed onto the sand filter provides the dosed material with enough dissolved oxygen to freshen the sewage and eliminate the odor. Recirculation also improves the effluent quality.

The recirculating sand filter was first designed by R. E. Favreau and M. W. Hines with the Illinois Department of Public Health [2], with the intent of meeting a need in the Southern Illinois area. Their initial design remained simple and effective, and systems with that design are still functioning acceptably.

Modifications to the Favreau-Hines design have taken the recirculating sand filter a few steps farther in control of recirculation and dosing. The recirculating sand filter has three basic components: (1) a septic or Imhoff tank, (2) a recirculating or pump tank, and (3) the sand filter.

Septic Tank

Septic tank design has not changed much since the original *Manual of Septic Tank Practice* was first printed by the U.S. Public Health Service. The septic tank design for the recirculating sand filter system uses this basic design.

Sand Filter

The sand filter design is based on the intermittent sand filter design with some modifications [3]. The filter media is the same as the buried sand filter, using media with 1.0- to 1.5-mm-diameter effective size. Filter bed depth is 24–30 inches, and dosing design is 3 gal/ft^2/day based on raw sewage flow. The underdrains are bedded in graded crushed gravel with a layer of pea gravel supporting the filter media.

Dosing of the filter is done through dosing troughs or pipes spaced no more than 10 feet apart. Holes in the trough or pipe at 12-inch intervals provide fairly even dosing. An even better dosing application would occur using the fixed nozzle principle of the old trickling filters. There are surely other dosing arrangements that would, or could, improve on the pipe or trough concept, and this is one area that could stand additional work. Dosing must be done so as not to cause ponding and scouring of the media. The filter surface should remain level and clear of debris such as leaves, weed growth, mud, etc.

Recirculation Tank

The heart of the system is the recirculation controls and recirculation tank. Recirculation rate must be greater than 3 to 1 to maintain aerobic conditions and keep odor down, but should be less than 5 to 1 to avoid keeping the filter too wet, causing plugging or ponding. Dosing should not occur at intervals more than three hours apart nor less than one hour apart. The entire content of the recirculation tank should be pumped to the sand filter at each dosing period.

To accomplish all of the abovementioned variables requires proper pump sizing, strict control of recirculation, proper recirculation tank sizing, and proper pump cycle controls.

Dosing

The dosing tank should be sized so the entire contents of the tank are dosed to the sand filter during each cycle. Dosing is based on a dosing depth of 2 inches over the entire sand filter surface. For example, a 200-ft^2 filter dosed to a depth of 2 inches would use a volume of 250 gallons. The dosing tank should be designed so that 250 gallons of storage is all that is maintained.

The Pump

The pump should be sized so the recirculation tank is emptied in approximately 10 minutes. In the previous example, a 25-gpm pump would be sufficient. Dosing in this manner would preclude flooding and would ensure even distribution over the filter.

Pump cycle control is critical. The contents of the recirculation tank must be kept aerobic and fresh to avoid odors. Pumping must occur at intervals not exceeding three hours to accomplish this, so the pump must have dual controls. A time clock controller with settings every three hours should turn the pump on. Interconnected with the time clock control should be float controls or some other level of controls that override the time control. The low-level control turns the pump off, while the high-level control turns the pump on and resets the time clock.

The high-level control will handle peak flow period when incoming flow from the septic tank would flood the recirculation tank in less than three hours. The low-level control simply turns the pump off when the tank is empty so the pump does not run dry.

The Flow Splitter

The control of recirculation and discharge is the most critical part of the entire system and design of a good flow splitter is an area where additional work needs to be done. The flow splitter that presently seems to do the best job is the movable vertical gate that is infinitely adjustable and diverts part of the flow to the recirculation tank and part to effluent.

The Complete System

Figure 1 depicts a complete recirculating sand filter system for a home. Figure 2 is the cross section of a sand filter. Figure 3 is the movable-gate flow splitter and Figure 4 is a recirculation tank.

The effluent from a recirculating sand filter that is properly designed and receives routine maintenance is of very high quality. Five-day biochemical oxygen demand (BOD_5) of 10 mg/l, suspended solids (SS) of 12 mg/l and ammonia nitrogen (NH_3-N) of less than 1.0 mg/l are common. Wintertime

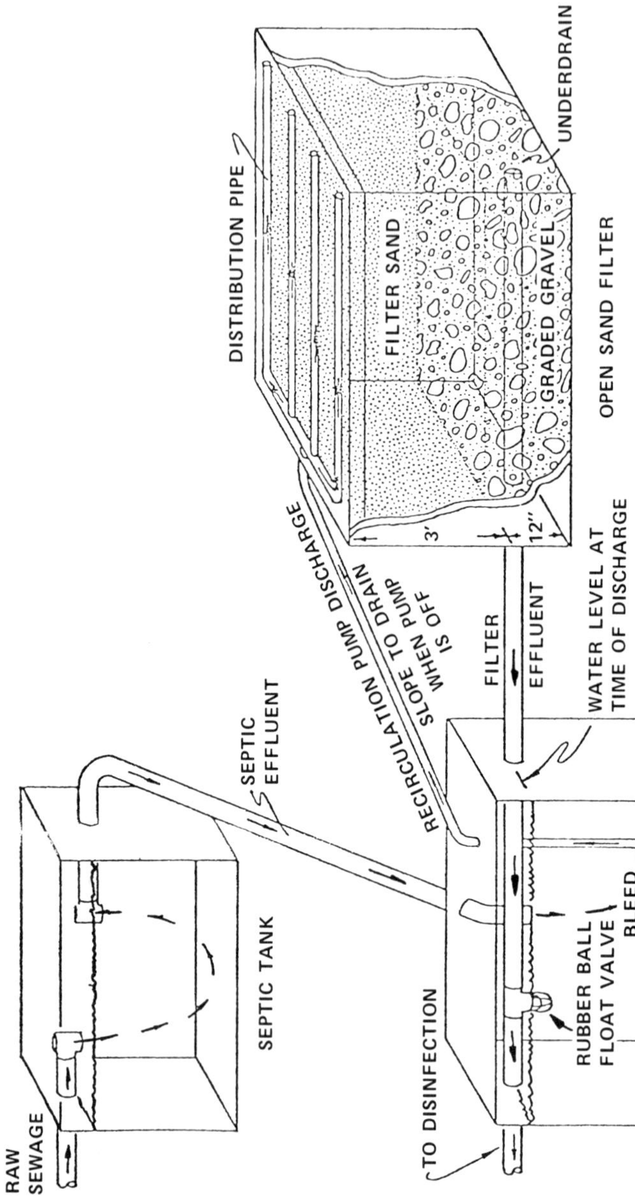

Figure 1. Recirculating sand filter system.

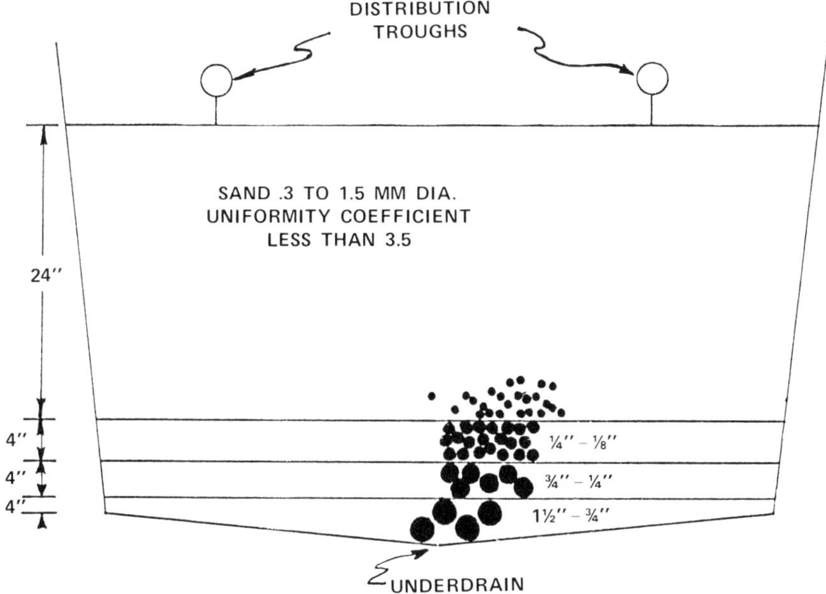

Figure 2. Sand filter cross section.

operation allows NH_3-N levels to go considerably higher because of inactivity of nitrogeneous bacteria, but BOD_5 and SS levels remain very low. Typical sample results from various size recirculating sand filters for 24-month periods are published in the literature [4].

Operation and Maintenance

Operation and maintenance of the recirculating sand filter involves normal pump maintenance and periodic raking and leveling of the sand filter. Sand filters with proper size sand should never require total media removal or replacement. Eventually it may be necessary to remove the top inch or two of the media if it becomes apparent that a buildup of solid material, not degradable, is causing a problem. The septic tank must receive normal maintenance (i.e., periodic pumping) so that solids are not carried over to the recirculation tank.

Keeping in mind that a homeowner will not care to spend very much time with maintenance, the phrase "simple is best" is appropriate. The recirculating sand filter is not the least expensive, lowest maintenance individual waste

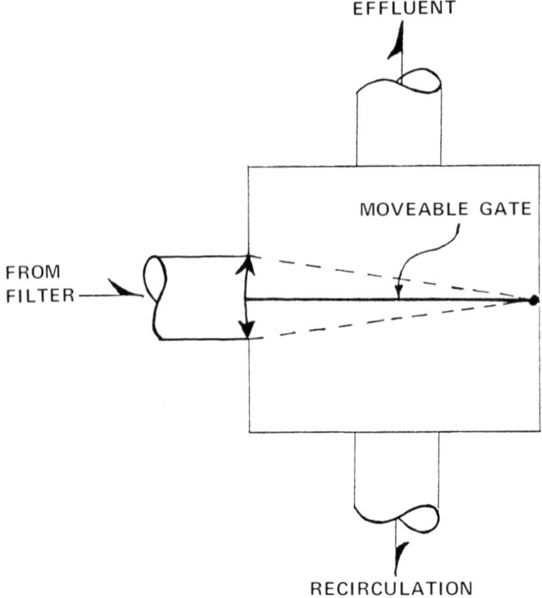

Figure 3. Movable gate flow splitter.

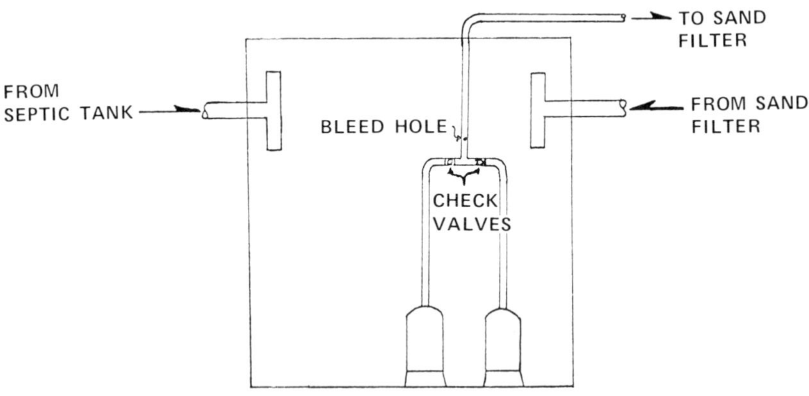

Figure 4. Recirculation tank.

treatment system one can build. It is, however, an alternative that deserves consideration when other simpler systems are not possible. A typical recirculating sand filter system for a home in Southern Illinois now will cost between \$2500 and \$3000, and this involves hauling sand 100 miles or more.

CONCLUSIONS

Individual onsite waste treatment plants can have surface discharges that will be clear, odorless and not cause nuisance conditions to result. Providing for adequate drainage to ensure that the treated wastewater does not pool is important. There is enough nutrient and organic material left in any biological waste treatment plant effluent that would allow algae growth to occur. Lawn or garden watering is a potential use for recirculating sand filter effluent that has much merit because of the nutrients left in the water.

REFERENCES

1. State of Illinois, Department of Public Health. "Private Sewage Disposal Licensing Act & Code," Rules and Regulations adopted in 1974.
2. Hines, M J., and R. E. Favreau. "Recirculating Sand Filter: An Alternative to Traditional Sewage Absorption Systems," paper presented at the American Society of Agricultural Engineers Symposium, Chicago, IL, 1974.
3. Great Lakes-Upper Mississippi River Board of State Sanitary Engineers. "Recommended Standards for Sewage Works" (1978).
4. Teske, M. G. "Recirculation–This Old Established Concept Solves Some Old Established Problems," paper presented at the Water Pollution Control Federation Conference, Anaheim, CA, 1978.

12

EVALUATION OF COMPOST TOILETS–A FIELD AND LABORATORY UPDATE

Dag Guttormsen
Researcher
Institute of Microbiology
Agriculture University
As, Norway

INTRODUCTION

In biological terms, man is often described as a consumer; however, he is also a producer a producer of wastes. Every one of us produces about 1.25 liters of urine and 0.25 liters of feces for a total of 1.5 liters per person per day. If we analyze this material, it amounts to:

- 1.35 liters of water
- 110 grams organic matter
- 12 grams nitrogen
- 2.5 grams phosphorus
- 10^{12} bacteria per gram of feces

These are small amounts, but everything adds up. The solution to this problem has been pipelines and sewage plants. For a scattered population this system is too expensive, and the result has seldom been cost-effective.

ALTERNATIVE SYSTEMS

The population of Norway is 4 million. About 500,000 people use a latrine or have a bucket system; 3.5 million have water closets, but only 35% of these toilets are connected to a sewage system. The rest have septic tanks with an outlet that goes directly to a river, lake or the sea. This, together with other pollutants, has resulted in eutrophication of Norway's lakes, which again results in their decreased value as resource and recreation areas.

What other solutions do we have? We can set up four:

1. Collection systems
   a. bucket
   b. holding tanks with a volume of about 3000 liters
2. Incineration systems
3. Systems with fecal contributions
   a. from a latrine
   b. water closet to a soil absorption system
4. Composting toilets

Collection Systems

These are not usually considered as an onsite system because of the need for a transport system and because the community must have a system for taking care of the wastes. This does not appear to be the optimum solution.

Incineration Systems

Incineration systems are unacceptable because of technical problems and their large consumption of energy.

Drainage Systems

Systems built on drainage, either combined with a latrine or flush toilet, are problematic in Norway. In most places the soil does not have the characteristics necessary for an absorption field. Therefore, the country depends on artificial soil absorption fields.

Composting Toilets

What then is a biological toilet? It consists of a composting unit in which the feces and urine are decomposed under aerobic conditions. The group can be divided into two main types:

1. small toilets, in which the whole unit is on the floor; and

2. large toilets, in which the commode is in the toilet room but the composting unit is below the floor.

Composting is defined as an aerobic process. Feces comprise about 90% water, so are principally liquid. The composting unit must therefore be constructed so that the solids are raised to about 25%. This can be done by: (1) draining the liquid out of the unit; (2) absorbing the liquid, or (3) evaporating the liquid. Drainage requires removal of a liquid containing 2-3% dry solids, mostly salts. And equally important, one can never be sure of the hygienic standard (health safety) of this liquid. If bark or peat is added, excess liquid is absorbed, but the volume requirements of the composting unit will increase. The best method seems to be evaporation.

Evaporation

All composting toilets are vented above the roof. Air is drawn through the composting unit for three reasons:

1. to ventilate the toilet room;
2. to introduce oxygen to the process and remove carbon dioxide (CO_2); and
3. to remove water as vapor.

Some toilets are without a fan and heating element. This can perhaps work in a dry, hot climate; but in Norway, and perhaps also here in Michigan, the fan and heating element are critical.

It is clear, then, that about 70% of the daily production has to be evaporated (e.g., from four people, 4.2 liters has to be removed by the air ventilation system). The amount of water in 1 m^3 of air with a temperature of 20°C and 100% relative humidity is only 17 g. If the air in a toilet room has a temperature of 20°C and humidity of 40%, perhaps one can obtain vented air with a temperature of 25°C and 60% relative humidity. This means that 1 m^3 of air removes 7 g of water. Going back to the need of removing 4.2 liters, 600 m^3 of air must be blown through the composting unit. And a very important factor is that the toilet must not only have the capacity to handle daily use, but also to handle "social events."

How has this problem been addressed? Eleven different models were installed and tested in a laboratory. These were loaded with fresh fecal material daily for six months. The toilets are grouped as follows:

- Small toilets with a grate (Figure 1);
- Small toilets with a mixing device (Figure 2);
- Small toilets with liquid composting (Figure 3);

- Large toilets with a sloping bottom and heating element (Figure 4); and
- Large toilets with separate composting chambers and heating elements (Figure 5).

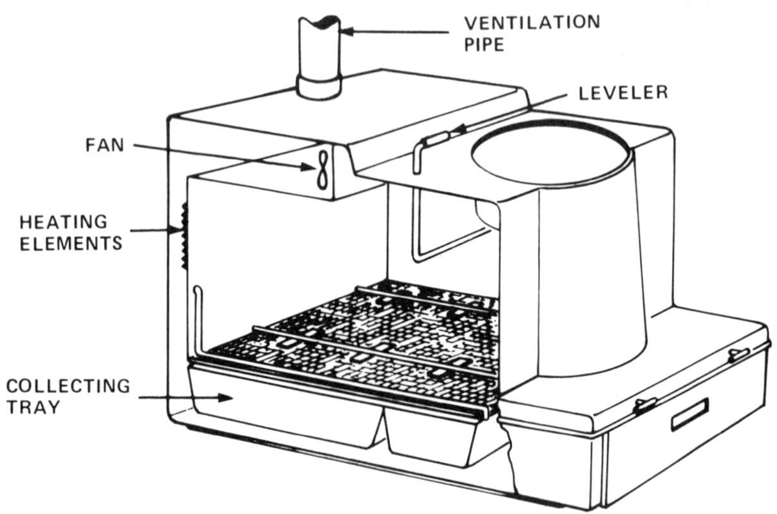

Figure 1. Small toilet with a grate.

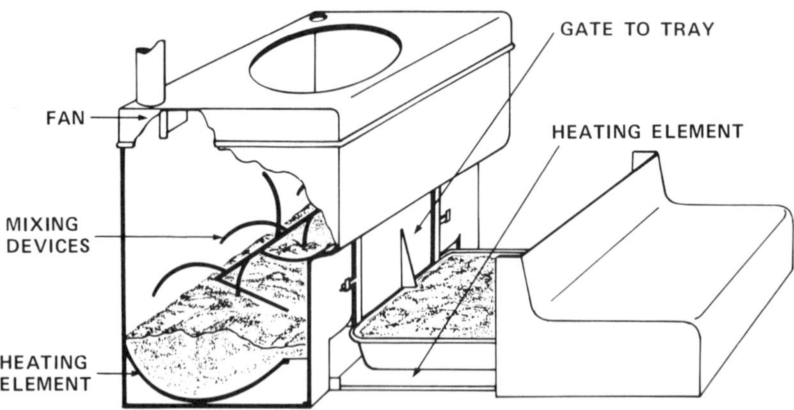

Figure 2. Small toilet with a mixing device.

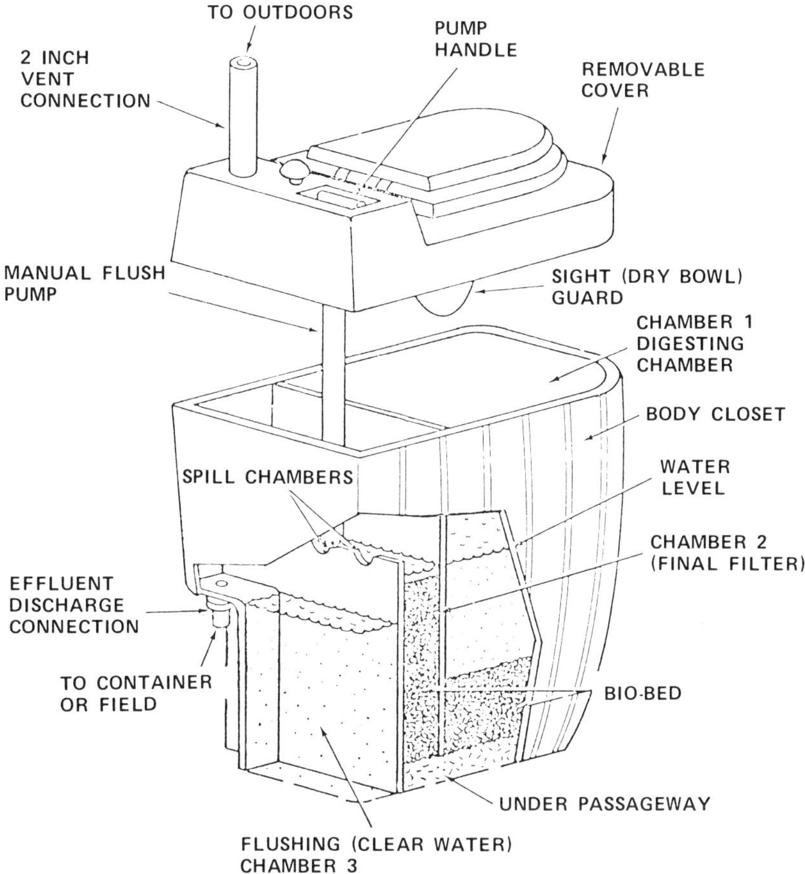

Figure 3. Small toilet based on liquid composting.

The results of the testing are summarized in Table I. It was concluded that most of the models worked if installed correctly and properly maintained. The small toilets had a capacity of two or three persons and the large one (Figures 4 and 5) had a capacity of four or five persons. The toilet in Figure 3 had, at best, a capacity of one person.

After testing the toilets in the laboratory, it was desirable to see whether practical use would yield similar results. It was especially important to see whether the large toilets installed in a cold basement would react other than shown in the laboratory, and to obtain the owners' comments on having a composting toilet in their homes.

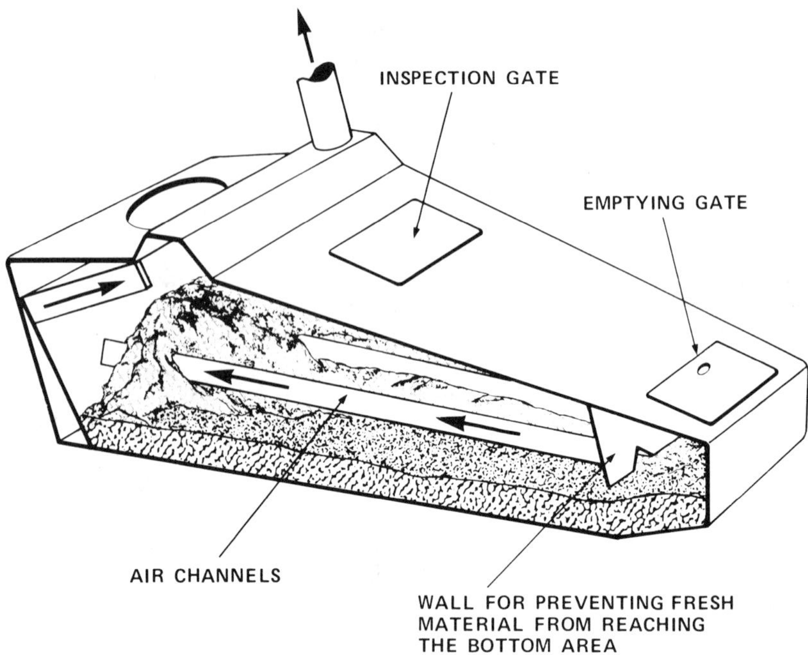

Figure 4. Large toilet with sloping bottom. The large arrows indicate the airstream.

Table I. Some Results Obtained in Laboratory Testing of Different Groups of Composting Toilets

Parameters	Toilet in Figure 1	Toilet in Figure 2	Toilet in Figure 3	Toilet in Figure 4	Toilet in Figure 5
Temperature measured in the middle of the compost, °C	24	45	20	24	22
Amount of air going out of the toilet, m^3/day	750	2000	216	2500	2000
pH of the end product	7.5	8.2	7.7	7.7	7.8
Dry solids in the end product, %	7.0	35	21	25	42
Ash content as % of dry solids, %	45	47	–	40	46
Thermostabile coliforms in the end product, no./g	<20	<20	–	<20	<20

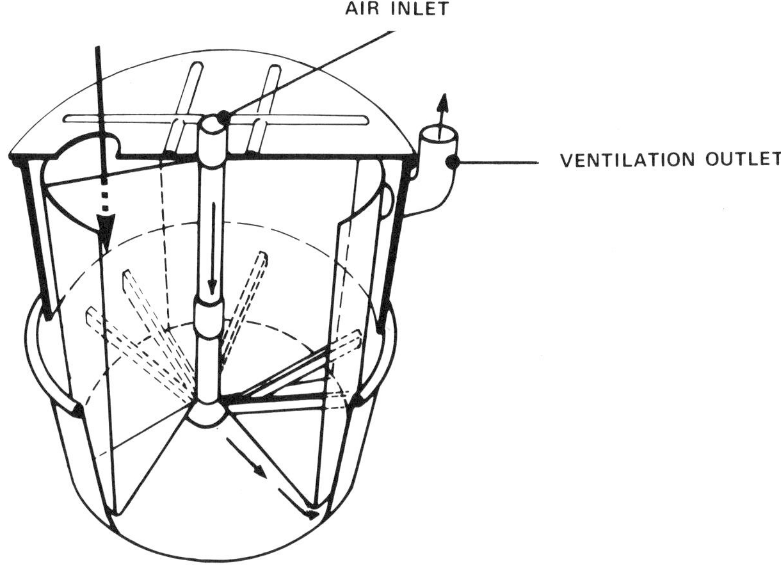

Figure 5. Large toilet with separate chambers. The large arrows indicate the air going through the system.

In 1978 a large project designed to conserve both energy and water and to abate pollution was begun in a community. Ten similar houses were built in a nearby area; all had composting toilets. Five different models were included: Bioloo, Clivus, Toa-throne, Carousel and Comodor. The greywater is discharged via septic tanks to soil absorption fields. To date, the users have shown no dissatisfaction with the toilets; neither have their guests. There have been few problems with the maintenance of the toilets, but problems have occurred with the liquid. In some of the models, the liquid had to be removed. This problem has been solved by increasing the effect of the fan and changing the heating element.

Pollution in the greywater was measured and compared with greywater discharged from houses with flush toilets (Table II). (The levels of N, P and solids were measured before the septic tank.) Converting these data to a percentage, it is apparent that the effect of having a composting toilet is nearly the same as that obtained by having a sewage plant.

There is also a project in the area around the largest lake in Norway—Mjosa. It includes about 90 toilets, mostly in older houses. Last winter was very cold, and there were problems with excess liquid. Most of the users have now changed their heating systems, so this winter's experience will provide more meaningful information.

Table II. Greywater Characteristics [1]

	Greywater Composition	
Parameter	With Flush Toilet (gpd)	With Composting Toilet (gpd)
Dry Solids	107	44
Total Nitrogen	11	1.3
Total Phosphorus	2.5	1.3 (0.42[a])

[a]Using phosphate-free detergents.

CONCLUSIONS

The results of the experiments reported here show the effectiveness of using compost toilets to meet the particular geographic needs of a country such as Norway.

They confirm our previous findings [2] that the compost toilet is the most viable alternative to flush toilets in Norway.

REFERENCES

1. Kristiansen, R., and N. Kloarer. *Vann* 2: 1-6 (1979).
2. Guttormsen, D. "Some Aspects of Composting Toilets with Specific Reference to their Function and Practical Applications in Norway," in *Individual Onsite Wastewater Systems, Proceedings of the Fourth National Conference, 1977*, N. I. McClelland, Ed. (Ann Arbor, MI: Ann Arbor Science Publishers, Inc., 1978), pp. 145-151.

13

LIFE WITHIN THE COMPOSTING TOILET

Daniel L. Dindal
Professor of Soil Ecology
State University of New York
College of Environmental Science and Forestry
Syracuse, New York 13210

INTRODUCTION

Below a composting toilet is an array of life forms–some microbial, others invertebrate animals. They comprise an organized, natural system of tiny living units that physically and chemically digest the ingredients introduced into the facility. This is a microcommunity of decomposer organisms, which, under optimal conditions, function effectively and efficiently. They ultimately produce a reusable humus-like product from human wastes. These organisms should not be destroyed. Establishing optimal conditions in a composting toilet is not difficult, but it requires patience and regular monitoring.

Typical composting of natural debris in open piles has been practiced for centuries in various parts of the world. Such piles are colonized naturally and inhabited by a complex of decomposers, microorganisms and soil invertebrates, which are responsible for the transformation of waste into organic matter. These organisms have been described and basic ecological patterns, such as the food web, of decomposers in compost piles have been shown [1,2]. Many decomposer organisms are the same, and the functional ecological patterns among them within toilet composts are identical to those found in open compost piles. Some people would rather not recognize this fact; however, open piles, as well as composting toilet piles, are artificial accumulations very similar to natural accumulations of vegetative litter and animal debris of forests and fields. Decomposer organisms mediate tremendous decay processes and must be appreciated to understand and manage the alternative technology of toilet composting.

OBJECTIVES

This chapter is intended (1) to provide an awareness of the diversity and functions of the neighboring invertebrate animals common to composting toilets, and (2) to present the final report on the decomposition and fauna associated with natural decay of selected waste items.

METHODS AND MATERIALS

Research Sites

From within four Clivus-Multrum organic waste treatment systems, as described by Lindström [3], decomposer organisms were studied to fulfill the stated goals. Sporadic bulk samples of debris were collected and extracted from three household units in the northeast United States. These units received daily garbage and toilet waste inputs during one to four year periods following use patterns described by Rockefeller [4]. Also, intensive samples were taken for more than a year from a composting toilet facility located along the Long Trail in the Green Mountains of Vermont.

Where practical, composting toilets are ideal for the microcosm study approach to research. The waste materials are generally confined to an impermeable, aerated container, thus being self-contained. Such a relatively closed system permits ready access to the monitoring of waste input, C:N ratio (which is vitally important), decomposer organisms and the eventual output of composted organic matter. The Vermont unit best lent itself to the microcosm approach.

Sampling Methods

Included in the intensive samples taken from the toilet in Vermont were random bulk samples of composting matter and developing humus. Also, selected waste items were introduced experimentally and monitored within nylon mesh bags (1 dm^2) according to the method of Crossley and Hoglund [5]. These so-called "litter bags" were tethered by monofilament lines for relatively easy retrieval. At periodic times spanning a 460-day period, bags were removed, observed and weighed and materials extracted for invertebrates.

RESULTS AND DISCUSSION

Resident Species

Numerous species of decomposers can take up residence and function effectively within the chambers of the composting toilet. Totals of 96 species, representing 70 invertebrate families, were found during this research (Table I). Such diversity of organisms emphasizes the many natural adaptations of decomposer invertebrates for living within a decaying environment. The functional ecological roles of each type of organism within its microcommunity in the composting world are presented as 1°, 2° and 3° decomposers (Table I). First-level (1°) decomposers are any types of organisms that obtain their nutrients directly from the waste residues; in addition to some invertebrates, they include bacteria, fungi and actinomycetes. Second-level (2°) decomposers consume the initial decomposers, while third-level (3°) decomposers are the truly voracious predators within the composting habitat.

Decomposer Dynamics

Microbial Priming

One of the first phenomena apparent on the surface of all experimental waste items was the production of a slime (mucopolysaccharide) coating. Materials with low C:N ratios are coated first, followed later by those having a high C:N ratio. Mucopolysaccharide formation is attributed predominantly to colonies of bacterial decomposers. Colonial deposition of this complex carbohydrate has a priming effect on the appearance of 1°-2° invertebrate decomposers. Fungal colonization of more acidic substrates acts as another type of microbial priming. Primed surfaces are digested by microbes and quickly become grazing areas for invertebrates. Protozoa, rotifers, nematodes and fly larvae feed on bacteria, while mites and springtails ingest fungi and nematodes as the waste is being consumed.

Roles of Secondary Consumers

On a microscale, the transfer of nutrients and energy occurs from the waste substrate to the 1° invertebrates which, in turn, are preyed on by the

Table I. Invertebrates of the Decomposer Food Web Found Within Composting Toilets (Clivus-Multrum Units, Northeast U.S.)

Taxonomic Classification	Decomposer[a] Level
Class ARACHNIDA	
Order CHELONETHIDA–Pseudoscorpions 1 sp	3°
ACARINA–Mites	
Suborder MESOSTIGMATA–Predatory Mites	3°
Family MACROCHELIDAE	
Macrocheles 3 spp	
ASCIDAE	
Proctolaelaps sp	
LAELAPTIDAE 1 sp	
PARASITIDAE	
Parasitus sp	
UROPODIDAE	
Fuscuropoda sp	
PROSTIGMATA–Heterogeneous Mites	
PYEMOTIDAE	2°-3°
Pyemotes bakeri	
PYGMEPHORIDAE	1°-2°
Bakeridania sp	
2 spp	
SCUTACARIDAE 1 sp	1°-2°
TARSONEMIDAE 3 spp	1°-2°
CHEYLETIDAE 1 sp	3°
ERYTHRAEIDAE 1 sp	2°-3°
ASTIGMATA–Mold and Fermentation Mites	1°-2°
TYROGLYPHIDAE	
Caloglyphus 2 spp	
GLYCOPHAGIDAE	
Glycophagus ornatus	
ANOETIDAE 1 sp	
ORIBATEI–Beatle or Moss Mites	1°-2°
TRHYPOCHTHONIIDAE	
Trhypochthonius americanus	
BELBODAMAEIDAE	
Veloppia sp	
ORIBATULIDAE	
Schleroribates sp	
HAPLOZETIDAE	
Xylobates sp	
CERATOZETIDAE	
Ceratozetes sp	
Fuscozetes bidentatus	
ACHIPTERIIDAE	
Parachipteria sp	
GALUMNIDAE 1 sp	
Order ARANEIDA–True Spiders	2°-3°
PHOLCIDAE–Daddy-Long-Legs Spiders	
Pholcus sp	

Table I, continued

Taxonomic Classification	Decomposer[a] Level
THERIDIIDAE–Cobweb Weavers	
Theridion sp	
Achaearanea tepidariorum	
LINYPHIIDAE–Sheet-Web Weavers	
Pityobyphantes phrygianus	
MICRYPHANTIDAE–Dwarf Spiders 1 sp	
AGELENIDAE–Funnel Weavers	
Tegenaria domestica	
ANYPHAENIDAE	
Anyphaena celer	
DICTYNIDAE–Hackled-Band Weavers	
Argenna sp	
Class CRUSTACEA	
Order ISOPODA–Sow Bugs and Pill Bugs	1°
TRICHONISCIIDAE	
Trichoniscus sp	
ONISCIDAE	
Trachelipus rathkei	
Class DIPLOPODA–Millipedes	1°
JULIDAE	
Anuilus sp	
Class INSECTA	
Order COLLEMBOLA–Springtails	2°
SMINTHURIDAE 1 sp	
PODURIDAE 2 spp	
ENTOMOBRYIDAE 3 spp	
PSOCOPTERA–Barklice 2 spp	1°
HEMIPTERA–True Bugs	
NABIDAE–Damsel Bugs 1 sp	2°-3°
ANTHOCORIDAE–Minute Pirate Bugs	2°-3°
Lyctocoris campestris	
COLEOPTERA–Beetles	
HISTERIDAE–Hister Beetles	2°-3°
Margarinotus sp	
Hister sp	
Geomysapiinus sp	
PTILIIDAE–Feather-Winged Beetles	2°
Acratrichis (?) sp	
LEPTODIRIDAE–Small Carrion Beetles	1°-2°
Prionochaeta opaca	
STAPHYLINIDAE–Rove Beetles	2°-3°
Staphylininae	
Philonthus sp	
Quediinae	
Quedius sp	

Table I, continued

Taxonomic Classification	Decomposer[a] Level
Aleocharinae 1 sp	
Omaliinae	
Eloneum sp	
SCYDMAENIDAE–Antlike Stone Beetles 1 sp	1°-2°
DERMESTIDAE–Hide Beetles	1°
Dermestes lardanius	
CRYPTOPHAGIDAE–Silken Fungus Beetles	2°
Ephistemus sp	
Anchicera sp	
NITIDULIDAE–Sap Beetles	1°-2°
Cryptarcha sp	
SILVANIDAE–Flat Grain Beetles 1 sp	1°
LATHRIDIIDAE–Minute Brown Scavenger Beetles	2°
Eniemus sp	
Lathridius minutus	
MYCETOPHAGIDAE–Hairy Fungus Beetles	2°
Typhaea fumata	
TENEBRIONIDAE–Darkling Beetles 1 sp	1°
ANOBIIDAE–Death Watch Beetles 1 sp	1°
Order LEPIDOPTERA–Grain Moth 1 sp	1°
DIPTERA–Two-Winged Flies	
PSYCHODIDAE–Moth Flies	1°-2°
Psychoda sp	
CHIRONOMIDAE–Midges 1 sp	1°-2°
ANISOPODIDAE–Wood Gnats	1°-2°
Anisopus sp	
Sylvicola sp	
SCIARIDAE–Dark Winged Fungus Gnats	1°-2°
Corynoptera sp	
SCATOPSIDAE–Minute Black Scavenger Flies	1°-2°
Scatopsa notata	
Coboldia fuscipes	
CECIDOMYIIDAE–Gall Gnats	1°
Dentifibula (?) sp	
Winnertzia sp	
PHORIDAE–Humpbacked Flies	1°-2°
Woodiphora (?) sp	
OTITIDAE–Picture-Winged Flies 1 sp	1°-2°
SEPSIDAE–Black Scavenger Flies 1 sp	1°-2°
SPHAEROCERIDAE–Small Dung Flies	1°-2°
Leptocera sp	
Sphaerocera sp	
CHLOROPIDAE–Fruit Flies 1 sp	1°
ANTHOMYZIDAE–Anthomyzid Flies 1 sp	1° (?)
MILICHIIDAE–Milichiid Flies	1°
Leptometopa latiper	
DROSOPHILIDAE–Pomace or Fruit Flies	2°
Pseudiastata sp	
Zygohrica sp	

Table I, continued

Taxonomic Classification	Decomposer[a] Level
ANTHOMYIIDAE–Anthomyiid Flies	1°-2°
Euryomma nr *peregrinum*	
MUSCIDAE–Muscid Flies	1°
Fannia canicularis	
CALLIPHORIDAE–Blow Flies 1 sp	1°
Order HYMENOPTERA–Wasps and Bees 1 sp	
CERAPHRONIDAE–Parasitoid Wasps 1 sp	2°-3°
DIAPRIIDAE–Dipteran Parasitoid Wasps	2°-3°

[a]1°–first-level decomposer; 2°–second-level decomposer; and 3°–third-level decomposer.

2°-3° decomposers. Minute fecal pellets from some invertebrates are eaten by other invertebrates. Ultimately, pellets of various sources become aggregated, often held together by mucopolysaccharides and destined to become part of the resultant humus material. Also, invertebrates are responsible for spatial distribution of microbial spores. Some spores that are consumed by decomposer invertebrates are never digested; they are defecated elsewhere and germinate on a new substrate.

Natural Control

As the creatures of the decomposer food web function in their own way, an overriding complex of natural population control is present within the toilet chambers. Stringent competition and antibiosis between microbial components appear to exist. Invertebrates grazing on microbes provide the potential for pathogenic microbes to be destroyed or inhibited. Some decomposer mites and springtails are eaten by predatory mites and pseudoscorpions. Other mites prey quite effectively on various species of fly eggs and larvae. Parasitoid wasps decimate the pupae of other fly species. Spiders and rove beetles prey on still larger creatures.

Colonization and Decomposition Rates

Overall Trends

Colonization and permanent residence within organic debris by all of the decomposers is based on the right combination of a complex of four factors: (1) adequate aeration, (2) ideal C:N ratio, (3) optimal water content, and

(4) degree of surface area exposure of the wastes. Owners of composting toilets should monitor and control these factors constantly for the best mutual existence of user and decomposers. These optimal factors were first suggested in a progress report by Dindal and Levitan [6] based on nylon bag-waste matter assays.

Final results are presented here on colonization trends and decomposition rates of 17 experimental waste items exposed for 460 days (Figure 1). Given enough time, each waste material studied was colonized to some extent by decomposer invertebrates. Even though the longevity of each item appears extended in the figure, within about four months after initial colonization by invertebrates the organic materials lost much of their structural identity. In this outdoor facility, which was not insulated, quick decomposition was confounded by winter's freezing temperatures. However, as the season

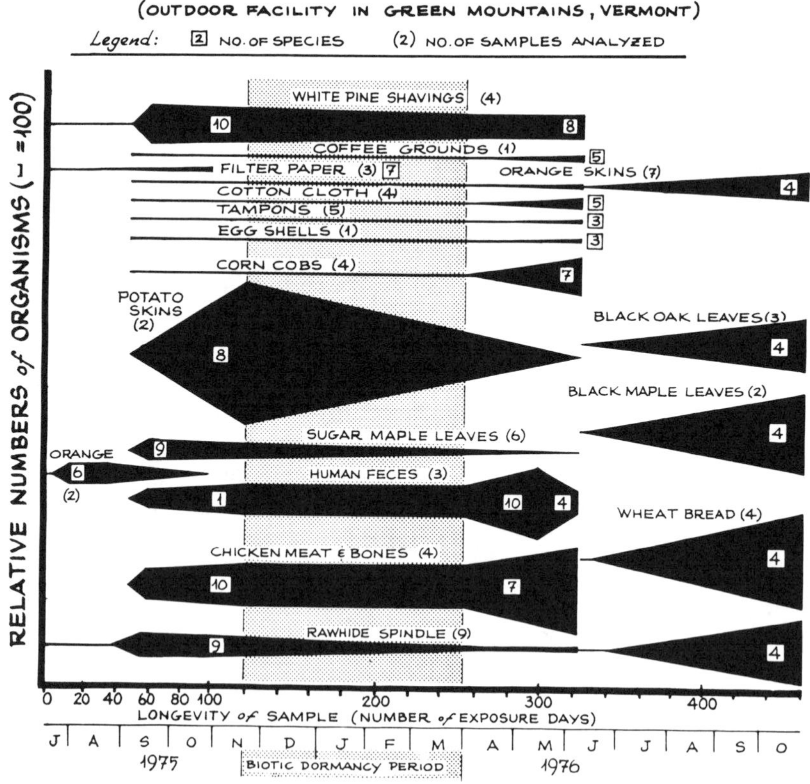

Figure 1. Invertebrate colonization and associated decay rates of residues in composting toilets.

waned, dormancy among the decomposer microcommunity was relieved by higher temperatures and the decomposition processes resumed with vigor.

Impact of C:N Ratio

Most decomposers, wherever they live, survive and reproduce best on substrates that have a C:N ratio ranging from 30:1 to 15:1 [7,8]. In other words, 1° decomposers require an intake of 1 part nitrogen for every 30 to 15 parts carbon they digest and assimilate. Only after this range is attained can the organism function optimally. If the ratio is higher, too little N is present to metabolically process the overabundance of C, so the waste matter is left undecomposed. On the other extreme, so much N is available that after the C source is completely used, the excess N is lost from the decomposing system mostly as ammonia. The initial waste material will be decomposed, but excesses of ammonia trigger unwanted changes in the fine balance of the decomposer microcommunity. Certain invertebrates start to migrate away from the pile, often into the house. This can be disconcerting, so the user must maintain a careful monitoring schedule of the facility.

Carbon and nitrogen content in waste material can be measured quite accurately in the laboratory. Since the average composting toilet operator does not have access to this analytical convenience, several rather simple monitoring evaluations can be made for proper C:N ratio maintenance, assuming ideal levels of aeration and moisture. First, if a waste item remains structurally unchanged for periods of two to four weeks, the C:N ratio of that item is probably too high and an N source should be added. Secondly, if the odor of ammonia appears, too much N is present and a C source such as sawdust, bark chips or shredded paper should be added. The latter case is most frequently encountered because urine and feces, with high N content, are always present in composting toilets, and perhaps not enough garbage* (a fine source of C) is being added.

Although data from experimental waste items (Figure 1) reflect the complex of factors including C:N ratio, the impact of the ratio is very important. For instance, materials with high C:N ratios, such as coffee grounds, filter paper, orange skins, cloth, tampons and egg shells never supported many invertebrate individuals. Paper and cloth are comprised mainly of C compounds, and they support far fewer than 100 individuals per sample. In addition to high C concentrations, other factors causing complexities are as follows:

---

*Composting toilets should be used in accordance with manufacturer's instructions with respect to addition of "garbage."

1. Coffee grounds possess products of the roasting process.
2. Tampons have been sterilized by the manufacturers.
3. Orange peelings contain additional organic acids, all of which may hinder colonization.

Egg shells with some carbonate C are predominantly inorganic, providing very little N and a low source of energy. White pine shavings were not colonized for two months, attributable mainly to the high C:N ratio of about 400:1. After two months the large surface area of the shavings allowed for the absorption of nutritive fluids from the pile; N in these fluids lowered the C:N ratio to a more optimal level, encouraging decomposer colonization. Also, the increased surface area provides numerous spatial niches for a greater variety of organisms.

All the materials with relatively low C:N ratios in the range of 45:1 to 5:1 were colonized almost immediately on introduction. Because potato samples also had some tissue other than skin, colonization by microbial and invertebrate decomposers was extremely rapid. Rawhide spindles with the lowest C:N ratio tested are comprised of the scleroprotein keratin. They exhibited the greatest durability against decay. Also, the spindles provided little nutrition but slowly absorbed fluids, causing them to expand into concentric structures that provided more shelter at an optimal relative humidity for decomposers.

Effects of Increased Surface Area and Moisture Content

Assuming no change in the C:N ratio, any item whose surface area is increased by shredding or finely dividing in some way will be colonized by decomposers more quickly, and will decay more rapidly. The greater the surface area exposed, the greater the number of microsites and the greater the organisms' diversity and activity associated with the substrate.

Moisture levels of 90–95% relative humidity are ideal for most decomposers, and should be maintained for best composting conditions. A dry pile will support few decomposers and the necessary decay will cease; too much water almost always leads to anaerobic conditions. This, in turn, slows the decay processes and causes the generation of putrid gases like hydrogen sulfide. Also, anaerobiosis may stimulate decomposer populations to migrate out of the facility. Reasonable monitoring will alleviate this problem.

Colonization by Artificial Introduction

When first installing a composting toilet, soil and vegetative litter from the local area should be used for the initial substrate on the bottom of the toilet chambers. Peat moss, as recommended for chamber substrate by some manufacturers, is sterile of decomposer propagules, has an acid reaction and may contain concentrations of tannins. Tannic compounds have inhibitory effects on various necessary decomposer forms. On the other hand, native soil has developed naturally within a given locality. Propagules of valuable decomposer organisms will be present because they have also become adapted to the local conditions of microclimate and decomposition.

Of all organisms associated with open compost piles, earthworms and sow bugs are some of the few decomposers that are not easily innoculated naturally into composting toilets. Using native soil will increase the possibility of introducing these efficient decomposers, but if that does not occur both can be innoculated artificially quite easily. Sow bugs feed on paper and dead plant debris and will usually occupy some damp but drier margins of the compost pile. Earthworms will consume almost all types of organic waste items. The earthworm with the greatest potential is the manure worm, *Eisenia foetida*. Also, both earthworms and sow bugs can utilize calcium carbonate from crushed seafood shells or egg shells, and both require a reasonable amount of aeration throughout the pile.

CONCLUSIONS

Valuable decomposer organisms comprise a large component of our world. Under practical conditions, they can be managed for such human benefits as toilet composting. Decomposers respond best to aerobic-moist conditions and substrates having much surface area and optimal C:N ratios. Waste items with low C:N ratios will be completely decomposed in composting toilets (Clivus-Multrum system) in one to four months; materials having a high C:N ratio and possessing little structural heterogeneity may easily remain undecomposed for more than 12 months.

Owners of composting toilets should work in unison with decomposers by adopting a regular monitoring schedule and responding properly to optima that support maximum efficiency of decomposition. A composting toilet is not and should not be a center of filth or a breeding ground for what some consider the invertebrate "misfits" of the world. Much of the human reluctance to accept compost invertebrates is the belief that many, if not all, are disease-laden vectors that spread their ill effects throughout the human race. Certainly some potential vectors exist, but their numbers are relatively small, and if managed properly an entire echelon of competitive and predatory beings will feed constantly on vectors and their products, rendering them ineffective as distributors of disease.

Man's knowledge and educational process have been developed far beyond the day of the outhouse and should lead us into a complete understanding of the ramifications and value of natural waste disposal. Natural waste decomposition systems first evolved on earth between 6×10^8 and 4×10^8 years ago [9] and have since become very effective. It is time to reap some benefits from the past!

ACKNOWLEDGMENTS

Research findings presented here were supported in part by funds provided by the USDA Forest Service, Northeastern Forest Experiment Station–Research Work Unit NE 1601 and also by Clivus-Multrum USA, Cambridge, Massachusetts. (Mention of specific products does not constitute Forest Service endorsement.)

Lois Levitan was the major research assistant on the project. She and R. A. Norton provided invaluable time and assistance in the taxonomic determinations of the decomposers encountered. Invertebrate determinations were verified by J. R. Philips and A. F. Newton, Jr.

REFERENCES

1. Dindal, D. L. *Ecology of Compost*, SUNY College of Environmental Science and Forestry, Syracuse, NY (1971), pp. 6,7.
2. Dindal, D. L. "Soil Organisms and Stabilizing Wastes," *Compost Sci. Land Util. J. Waste Recycling* 19(4):8-11 (1978).
3. Lindström, C. R. "The Clivus-Multrum System: Composting of Toilet Waste, Food Waste and Sludge Within the Household," in *Water Pollution Control in Low Density Areas* (Hanover, NH: University Press of New England, 1975), pp. 429-444.
4. Rockefeller, A. "Toilets That Don't Need Flushing," *Catal. Environ. Qual.* 5(1):15-18 (1975).
5. Crossley, D. A., and M. P. Hoglund, "A Litter-Bag Method for the Study of Microarthropods Inhabiting Leaf Litter," *Ecology* 43(3):571-573 (1962).
6. Dindal, D. L., and L. Levitan. "The Soil Invertebrate Community of Composting Toilet Systems," in *Soil Organisms as Components of Ecosystems*, U. Lohm and T. Persson, Eds., Stockholm, Sweden, *Ecol. Bull.* 25:577-580 (1977).
7. Dindal, D. L. *Ecology of Compost*, SUNY College of Environmental Science and Forestry, Syracuse, NY (1971), p. 5.
8. Alexander, M. *Introduction to Soil Microbiology* (New York: John Wiley & Sons, Inc., 1961), pp. 152-154.
9. Schopf, J. W. "Evolution of the Earliest Cell," *Scientific Am.* 230:111-138 (1978).

14

THE GREENHOUSE AS LEACH FIELD

Abby A. Rockefeller, President
Clivus Multrum Inc.
Cambridge, Massachusetts 02138

INTRODUCTION

The 1977 Amendments to the federal Clean Water Act of 1972 reflect two realizations: (1) that the federal government will be unable to pay for sewering and central treatment of the small, dispersed communities yet in need of "pollution abatement," and (2) that conventional central treatment is not the environmental panacea the 1972 Law imagined it would be. A major corollary to both points is that methods of onsite treatment will be funded up to 85%, rather than the standard 75%, wherever they are "cost-effective" and that they are likely to do less damage to the environment than has central treatment. It is obvious that this promised subsidy will reawaken interest in onsite methods of treatment of wastewater.

In the meantime, however, virtually all the land considered suitable for conventional subsurface disposal that could be wrenched from agricultural use—for it has been largely the prime agricultural land that has been viewed as prime development land—has already been developed. This leaves the so-called "marginal" land—hillsides, areas with ledge or high seasonal groundwater, and swamps. There will necessarily be growing pressure to build on this land with concomitant, and often legitimate, resistance from environmentalists.

Also, during this time standards for onsite treatment have become more, rather than less, stringent, partly as a result of the sewer lobby's interests (bureaucratic and commercial) to force as many people as possible from onsite to central treatment. The result of these pressures and inducements—the scarcity of readily developed land and the higher treatment and groundwater protection standards combined with the bait of the 1977 Amendments—will be to foster the rapid development of alternatives to conventional subsurface disposal. Systems that do not require offsite treatment of a collected effluent or sludge, such as septage, which actually treat the wastes onsite with minimum environmental impact, are bound to look more attractive in the future. Now that 80% of the cost of treatment is in transportation, be it by trucks or pipes, central treatment facilities are becoming unwilling to further burden their already overloaded works with septage and other effluents from outside the sewered district.

LAND USE

Concerning "marginal" land, much that has been considered prime from the point of view of development should have been left alone, and much that is regarded as marginal should have been developed. Agriculture should have first choice of land because it requires certain conditions and because once developed, arable land can never be restored to agriculture. It has been an unfortunate combination of avarice and carelessness that has ignored this. On the other hand, hilly or ledgy terraine can be built on to great advantage with some extra initial expense. In view of the incalculable value of arable land to agriculture, the sacrifice of an initially greater cost should have been made willingly.

OBJECTIVE

This chapter focuses on an approach to the treatment of domestic wastewater developed during the past five years by Clivus Multrum, Inc., a company that believes it can develop much of the now "unbuildable" land and, at the same time, afford better protection to our water resources than is available now from either conventional onsite or central treatment.

DESCRIPTION

Separated Treatment

The first step should be the separation of greywater from blackwastes. This can be accomplished through the use of any type of waterless toilet, the immediate effect of which is to reduce the hydraulic flow by 40%.

This, in itself, has significant implications for the sizing of the wastewater distribution bed. In addition to the water reduction, 90% of the nitrogen, 30% of the phosphorus (much more if phosphate detergents are not used), 70% of the chemical oxygen demand (COD), 50% of the five-day biochemical oxygen demand (BOD_5) and 99.9% of the fecal coliform bacteria never enter the water stream. Where a compost converter of the large type serves both the waterless toilet and as a disposal for the food wastes, complete stabilization of these combined wastes is effected prior to transportation and without energy input. This system also obviates the need for garbage grinders (which are well known to put an intolerable strain on conventional septic tank systems) and keep the solid wastes (trash) from becoming a nuisance because of rotting food. Clivus Multrum, Inc. has continued to promote the large composter for year-round homes over the small box-type units for several reasons:

1. Complete stabilization can be achieved with very little attention to the process.
2. Removal of end product is very infrequent—once every six months to a year for liquid, if there is any, and once every two to five years for compost.
3. Because of the large buffer capacity, nothing happens quickly; it cannot be overloaded suddenly.

Greywater Characteristics

The combined effects of reduction in quantity and improvement in quality of the remaining wastewater—the greywater—make it much easier to treat onsite. Contrary to rumors circulating in the U.S. since the advent of the compost toilet, greywater has been shown to be significantly more, rather than less, treatable in conventional septic tank systems than is combined wastewater [1-3]. In a great many cases it would be feasible to utilize conventional subsurface disposal for greywater alone, where it would be impossible with combined grey and black wastewater. In fact, one of the most likely large-scale uses of the compost toilet is in areas in which septic tank systems have failed because of overloading. In such cases, the use of the waterless toilet will certainly improve the functioning of the septic tank system and will often cause it to recover completely.

The Greywater-Irrigated Greenhouse

Ultimately, this company believes that protection of groundwater will depend on the extent to which nutrients are taken up by plants, something no conventional septic tank system is systematically designed to do. Consequently, for the past three years Clivus Multrum, Inc. has experimented with treating greywater in deep soil beds located in a greenhouse. About ten such systems have now been built of which the company was directly involved with the construction and testing of two.

Design Criteria

Ideally, this greenhouse should be a lean-to structure attached to the house, for it will serve the triple function of solar collection, food production and greywater purification. Soil beds 3 feet deep (a convenient work height and an adequate depth for wastewater treatment) serve as the leach beds for the greywater. In the original test units (built in Spring 1976), these beds were 2 feet wide, so have a single leach line running down the center of each; in the second (built in Summer 1978), the beds are 3 1/2 feet wide (the maximum width for convenient reaching at a 3-foot height), so have two parallel leach lines running the full length of each. These pipes have perforations from 3/16- to 3/8-inch in diameter on the undersides, spaced 1 foot apart. To prevent these small holes from being quickly plugged, the greywater is first passed through a roughing filter consisting of a cone-shaped container filled with 1 inch stones. Hair, lint, food particles and some grease are trapped in this filter, which must be skimmed and back-flushed once every six months to a year, depending on user characteristics. After the filter, the effluent is preferably pumped into the soil beds. Gravity flow is sometimes possible, but will provide a less even distribution in the soil.

The two respects in which we have most radically departed from the norm concerning conventional leach fields pertain to the depth of the leach lines and the characteristics of the soil in the treatment beds.

Depth of Leach Lines

Because there is no danger of freezing in the sheltered greenhouse, there is no reason to lay the leach lines 2 feet or more below the surface, as is customary in ordinary leach fields. Consequently, they were laid no deeper than 4 inches below the soil surface. Besides serving the primary interests of providing as much treatment depth below the pipes as possible and of discharging the nutrients into the root zone where plants can most readily take them up, this shallow depth has other benefits: access to the lines for maintenance or inspection is very convenient, and treatment is likely to be superior because of the greater biological activity and aeration of the soil near the surface.

Soil Type

The second departure from convention pertains to the soil profile and type in the leach beds. Instead of being placed on gravel and surrounded by a biologically inactive subsoil, these lines are laid in an organically rich topsoil. In both greenhouses, 4 inches of coarse (2-3 inches) gravel were placed at the bottom and 2 inches of 1-inch crushed limestone was placed on top of that. A point of uncertainty has been whether to use a layer of sand between stones and topsoil. In the three-year-old greenhouse there was no sand layer, so the topsoil had to be placed directly on top of the stones to avoid what was feared might be the buildup of a slime layer at the interface between sand and topsoil. If this were to happen, there could be a backing up of the greywater and waterlogging of the soil, which would cause root rot in the plants. In the second greenhouse, however, 6 inches of sand were placed between stones and topsoil, and no signs of backing up have been observed during its year of operation. This experience would indicate that a deeper layer of sand would be preferable. It is cheaper than topsoil, would do a better job of filtration, and would prevent silt from the topsoil from leaching out easily.

The company's single most significant observation relative to the use of rich instead of poor soil seems to be that at no time has there been any anaerobic odor, even in the region immediately below the leach lines, although it is here that most of the nutrients are deposited and where the soil may often be soggy. The greywater itself has a characteristic odor that can readily be smelled in the pipes themselves if they are lifted out, but cannot be detected in the soil at all. Therefore, it is evident that the soil has maintained a thoroughly aerobic character. This is believed to be a function of the abundant invertebrate life that thrives in this rich humus soil. Bacteria alone would produce a slime that would eventually cause anaerobic conditions; however, the predacious and decomposing activities of the higher organisms—protozoans, mites, springtails, potworms and earthworms, to mention the major groups—keep the soil porous and free from slime. Earthworms, which thrive in this system, sometimes were found to congregate in large numbers directly in the leach lines, apparently having a taste for their greywater straight.

Plant Growth

Plant growth has been excellent so far, even though there is frequently more wastewater passing through the soil than either the plants need or the soil can hold. The arrangement is something of a hybrid between standard soil agriculture with subsurface irrigation and hydroponics; moreover, it seems to combine the advantages of both methods: the stability of the soil environment (e.g., diseases spread much more rapidly in water than in soil and the necessary range of trace elements is more likely to be present in soil than in water) with the nutritious irrigation and the aeration caused by fairly rapidly percolating effluent. The dosing in these beds occurs whenever a washing facility is used, which may be in quick succession or simultaneously. The surplus effluent will drain through the soil, which acts as a fly wheel, along the sloping bottom of the bed and finally out the drain at the lower end. No fertilizer has ever been added besides what is provided in the greywater. No deficiencies have been detected, although there may be more nitrogen than necessary. Crops are changed twice a year. Cool weather greens and root crops are grown in winter and tomatoes, peppers, cucumbers and other hot weather crops in summer.

Water Purification

The water purification aspect of this setup must, as in conventional leach beds, be largely a function of the ratio of gallons of wastewater discharged per day to the number of cubic feet of soil through which the wastewater passes. The greenhouse soil bed differs from a conventional leach field in that it does not have the limiting factor of the slime layer, which determines how much water can pass through each square foot of soil per day. Wastewater passes through these beds quite rapidly and, apparently, will continue to do so indefinitely. Nevertheless, it is clear that the more greywater that is passed through each cubic foot per day the less effective the treatment will be, and vice versa. There is a total of 54 ft^2 of soil surface in the older of the two greenhouses. Two people use the system regularly. A dishwasher, a shower with a low-flow nozzle, and all sinks are channeled into the greenhouse. This constitutes an average of 25 gpd passing through the soil. The second greenhouse has a total of 150 ft^2 of surface soil. Three people live in the house and produce an average of 150 gpd of greywater from two showers with low-flow nozzles, a washing machine, dishwasher and three sinks.

E. Coli

We have seen the importance of fairly even distribution of effluent through the beds. In testing for the presence of *E. coli* in the postsoil box effluent, numbers up to 100,000/100 ml were obtained when there was a short-circuiting in the leach pipes, so that less than the first third of soil was used. When the pipes were cleaned and leveled, the *E. coli* count was less than 100/100 ml. The presence of fecal coliform bacteria is not to be understood as evidence of the presence of feces because in neither dwelling where these installations were made are there babies whose diapers could have been washed in the washing machine. Rather, these bacteria are known to grow in pipes where wastewater is carried, probably also grow on the stones in the roughing filter, and may even grow in the rich warm soil itself. What their presence indicates in treated greywater remains a matter of controversy.

BOD_5 and Suspended Solids

In five tests of the effluent taken from the bottom drains, BOD_5 ranged from 3–50 mg/1 and the suspended solids from 5–44 mg/1, both averaging about 10 mg/1. This effluent is very light amber in color and odorless, remaining so when stored at room temperature in an airtight jar.

There are several ways in which putting the leach beds in a greenhouse improves its ordinary functions. For example, the deep soil boxes allow even such deep-rooted plants as shrubs and other perennials to be grown. The sheer volume of soil has a very positive stabilizing influence on the temperature, moisture, pH and greenhouse ecosystem.

Temperature

As greywater is usually 10° warmer than combined sewage, it makes a considerable heat contribution to the greenhouse. The soil acts as a heat exchange and recovery medium and, being slower to change temperature than air, maintains a more stable climate for the plants, where there are fluctuations in the air caused by changes outside.

Moisture

Similarly, the plants are protected from the intense drying effects of the sun in a greenhouse by the deep moisture reserve, which induces them to send their roots downward.

pH

The large volume of soil acts also as a buffer to any sudden changes in pH that might occur in the greywater.

Ecosystem

A diverse and balanced population of invertebrates can live in this environment in a manner that it cannot in greenhouses with shallow benches or pots whose microenvironments are subject to great variations in the factors described above. Earthworms, for example, must be able to retreat to deeper, moister levels when threatened by dehydration from above. Moreover, the stability of this environment provides a habitat for the predators of many greenhouse pests as well as for the decomposer organisms so necessary to soil health.

Maintenance

Perhaps the major advantage afforded by the greywater-irrigated greenhouse is the great reduction in maintenance. Ordinarily, greenhouse plants must be watered at least once a day when the sun is out. Because of the automatic subsurface irrigation in this setup, no top-down watering is necessary except to start seedlings. This greenhouse can be left untended for several weeks without danger of dehydration because the deep soil holds a reservoir of moisture that will rise up by capillary action as the surface dries. This maintenance factor could have considerable significance in extending the applicability of greenhouses to a wider group of people than could formerly manage them.

Cost-Effectiveness

The effect of combining the diverse functions of solar collection, food production (or other horticultural use) and greywater purification in one structure should be to make this greenhouse available and attractive to many people, both from an economic and practical point of view. Increasing standards relative to groundwater protection and the scarcity of soils suitable for conventional septic tank systems are making the costs of the latter skyrocket: $5000 is no longer an uncommon figure for a septic tank system. A good-sized greenhouse of the type described could be constructed for this price.

Regulations

The regulatory constraints impeding acceptance of this type of approach to wastewater treatment focus on questions concerning the proper treatment of greywater, more than on the acceptability of the compost toilet. Most states have revised their codes to allow the use of compost toilets, providing a full, or at least half-sized, conventional septic tank system is installed for the greywater. Of the ten or so greywater greenhouses constructed in the Northeast thus far, regulatory concerns have been of two kinds: (1) the safety of irrigating vegetables with a potentially fecal-contaminated wastewater; and (2) uncertainty as to what should be the disposition of the treated effluent draining from the soil boxes. A project of 110 cluster condominiums in northwestern New Jersey has received both state and local approval to utilize the complete system–compost converter for toilet and kitchen wastes and roughing filter and greenhouse for greywater treatment. The postsoil box effluent will be disposed of in drywells. The only requirement not suggested by Clivus Multrum, Inc. is the addition of an ultraviolet (UV) disinfection unit to be installed between the roughing filter and the greenhouse. This project could be a significant demonstration of the feasibility of total onsite treatment for marginal land because one of the design goals is to save the surrounding farmland by building only on the roughest part.

Summary

Conventional onsite disposal systems receiving the combined load of grey- and blackwater are capable only (by almost anyone's standards) of receiving (let alone treating) those wastes in a limited and fast-diminishing portion of the soils in the U.S. Much of the land that remains and which is now classified as marginal could be developed if the anticipated hydraulic and pollutant load were reduced significantly. The treatment criterion of making the effluent percolate at a certain rate and then disappear is no longer acceptable. The new criteria include standards for the protection of groundwaters as well as surface waters. Clean water is in increasingly short supply, both absolutely as we systematically drain the aquifers by the use of central systems that do not return the water to the ground, and relative to the growing number of users.

Separated treatment, implying the elimination of the flush toilet, would save 40% of the domestic water use and more if garbage grinders were also prohibited. The elimination of these two devices would also reduce the pollutant load on the wastewater by well over 50%. The large type of compost system provides a complete, very energy-efficient and economical form of treatment for the organic wastes from toilet and kitchen. The greenhouse-as-leach field could have broad application for greywater treatment for a number of reasons:

1. It can, in combination with the compost converter, provide better treatment than either the conventional onsite or central methods.
2. The demand and advisability of growing at least some vegetables at home is increasing, and the system proposed here is a cost-effective way to do this.
3. Attached greenhouses are becoming increasingly popular because of their heat-producing capability.
4. The functions of plant growth and water purification are symbiotic.
5. Finally, the automatic watering function of the greywater-irrigated soil bed makes the greenhouse-as-food-producer well within the maintenance capabilities of more people than was ever possible before with conventional greenhouses.

CONCLUSIONS

Rational separation of wastes at the source, taking into account the thermodynamic (or real) costs, is the key to the treatment and recovery of all resources that pass through the house and, more particularly, to the treatment and recovery onsite of the organic fraction and wastewater. Onsite treatment is, in turn, the key to low-cost, low-energy, successful recovery of the value of these wastes. Central collection, treatment and disposal of wastewater and its treated by-product, sludge, developed because of the conviction that treatment onsite without groundwater or surface water pollution was not possible. The greenhouse-as-leach field, in combination with the organic converter for toilet and kitchen wastes, is one method that makes it possible. In the not-so-distant future, issues such as that of narrow cost-effectiveness will dissolve in the face of a greater one—the ongoing availability of healthy agricultural land and safe drinking water.

REFERENCES

1. Olsson, E., et al. "Household Washwater," The National Swedish Institute for Building Research, Stockholm, Sweden (1968).
2. Siegrist, R. L. "Management of Residential Greywater," Department of Civil and Environmental Engineering, Small Scale Waste Management Project, University of Wisconsin, Madison, WI (1978).
3. Fogel, M. "Residential Greywater—A Review," Clivus Multrum USA Inc., Cambridge, MA (1979).

15

INTEGRATED WASTEWATER RECYCLING FACILITY

Daniel E. Pavón
President, Eastern Environmental Controls, Inc.
Chestertown, Maryland 21620

INTRODUCTION

The integrated wastewater recycling facility described here differs from all those that have been marketed for commercial and industrial use. The recycling unit that will be presented here is directed toward the individual home or any combination of wastewater flows up to 1500 gpd.

This system is designed to save water, have zero discharge, be non-polluting, cost-effective and hygenically safe. Most systems that have been marketed have depended on membrane filters, activated carbon, oil flush, incineration or any combination of these concepts to achieve some degree of treatment for recycling and discharge of excess waste materials. This concept is designed to utilize the natural biological process (Figure 1).

METHOD

As reported by Bernhart [1], nature has provided specific microbial organisms to be involved in the wastewater treatment process. The key to this system's concept is the aerobic process, to achieve a high degree of treatment in a matter of hours. In this case, the one used is an Eastern Environmental Controls (EEC) advanced wastewater treatment plant ("MINI-PLANT"), which is fully installed in the fiberglass tank (Figure 2).

The microbial activity in the mixed liquor in the aeration chamber creates heat energy, which is in addition to the elevated temperature of the wastewater coming from the home. Additional heat energy is collected by heating

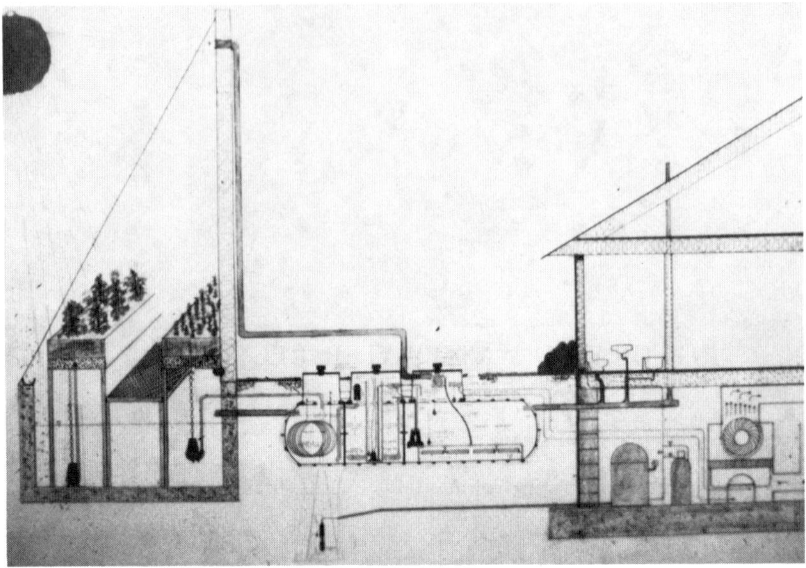

Figure 1. Integrated wastewater recycling facility (residential).

the air that is used for aerobic digestion. This is accomplished by drawing the air through a solar air panel or from a greenhouse. Introducing this warm air into the wastewater stores additional heat energy and, at the same time, creates an ideal environment for high microbial activity.

When the temperature of the mixed liquor reaches 98°F (37°C), a bypass valve opens, allowing the blower to draw air from the atmosphere and prevent the mixed liquor from becoming too hot. The EEC wastewater treatment plant operates as a batch system using very fine bubbling air that is diffused throughout the treatment compartment. The wastewater entering the treatment compartment is accumulated for a period of 20 hours, during which time it is undergoing continuous aeration. The electrical control system is programmed to shut off the aeration at 2 A.M., followed by a three-hour period of quiescent settling. After this period of quiescence, the supernatant is pumped out of the treatment compartment and up through the filter chamber. The very small amount of settled solids that remains is retained in the treatment tank for continued aerobic digestion.

An upflow filter is installed in the second compartment of the tank. The effluent from the MINIPLANT is pumped into a distribution piping system at the bottom of the upflow filter and forced up through the filter media at a flowrate not to exceed 1.5 gal/ft^2. The filtered effluent then flows by gravity out of the filter chamber into the contact tank.

There is a 12-inch polyvinylchloride (PVC) well casing in the filter compartment designed to accept a small backwash pump. After each cycle this pump returns to the treatment compartment any remaining water in the filter media, thereby eliminating the danger of the filter or biomass turning septic.

The disinfection contact chamber is the third compartment. Here the treated wastewater leaving the filter chamber is disinfected, either by iodination, which this author prefers, or chlorination. The contact chamber is also used to house the recycle pump and heat-reclaiming coil. The recycle pump is a standard submersible well pump that pumps the treated effluent into a separate pressure tank in the house. This water is used for flushing toilets, washing cars, watering lawns, etc.* By recycling the water in this manner, water consumption is reduced by 40–50%.

The heat-reclaiming coil removes the heat energy from the wastewater and is then used for space heating the home by means of a heat pump. As Freon® boils at a much lower temperature than water, by this means a considerable amount of energy can be removed from the wastewater. For example, a particular model heat pump operating at an evaporator temperature of 50°F will have a Btu input of 2846 and a total Btu output of 12,296, for a coefficiency of performance of 4.31. If this is converted to kWh, 1 kW equals 3415 Btu; therefore, to convert the 2846 Btu in the abovementioned heat pump, divide by 3415. This equals 0.83 kWh. The output of 12,296 Btu divided by 3415 Btu in 1 kW equals 3.59 kW; therefore, every 0.83 kW will produce 3.59 kW. By means of a circulating pump in the storage tank under the greenhouse, the heat in the contact tank is maintained at or above 50°F. The storage tank under the greenhouse acts as a passive collector storing heat energy, which is then pumped into the contact chamber to be recycled for reuse for home heating purposes.

During the summer months the process is reversed. The heat pump takes the heat out of the house and the heat is released in the water in the contact chamber. From the contact chamber the water travels by gravity to the storage tank under the greenhouse. The water vapors will escape into the atmosphere when the greenhouse windows are open. If the windows are closed, water will condense on the glass and run down into a gutter as distilled water for various uses. This prevents any discharge of pollutants into the environment.

As mentioned previously, the overflow from the contact chamber will flow to a large tank under the greenhouse. The nutrients in the wastewater will be recycled for plant growth using planter boxes.

---

*End use is dependent on regulating acceptability.

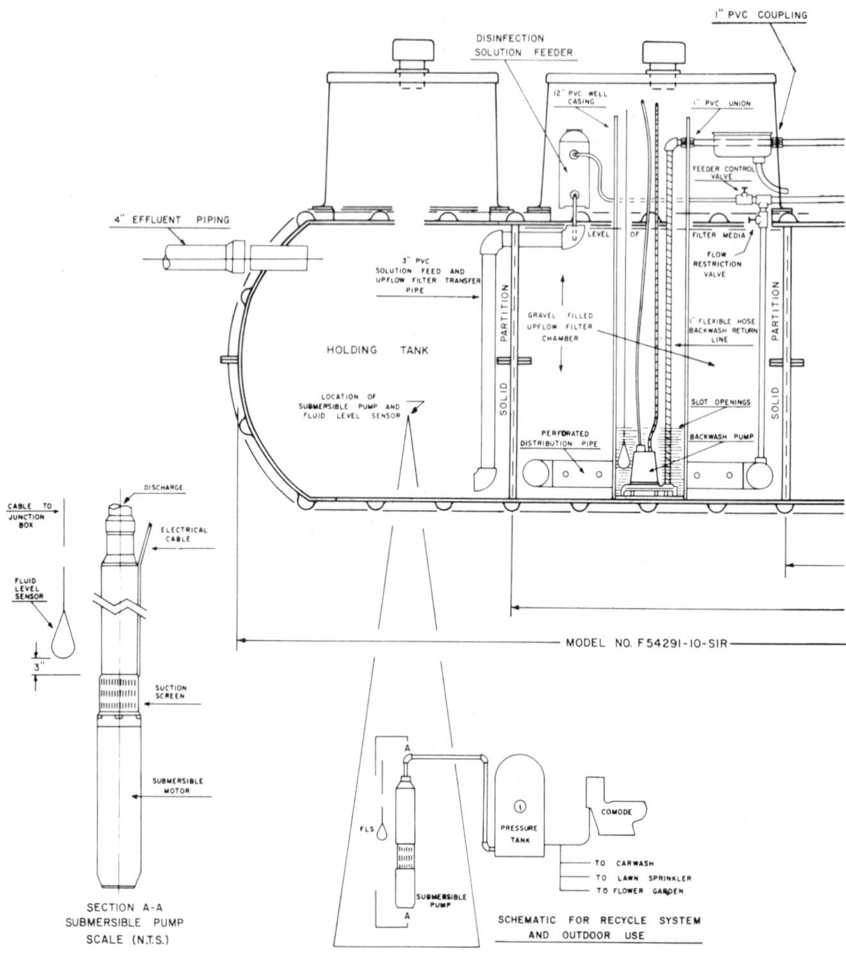

Figure 2. Eastern Environmental Controls

DISCUSSION

Wastewater from the MINIPLANT was tested for phosphorus, chlorides, nitrates and ammonia. As is well known, the amount of nutrients varies from house to house. Referring to Table I, the testing done at the National Sanitation Foundation (NSF) in 1979 presents data that show the average amount of nutrients being discharged from the EEC filter unit to be

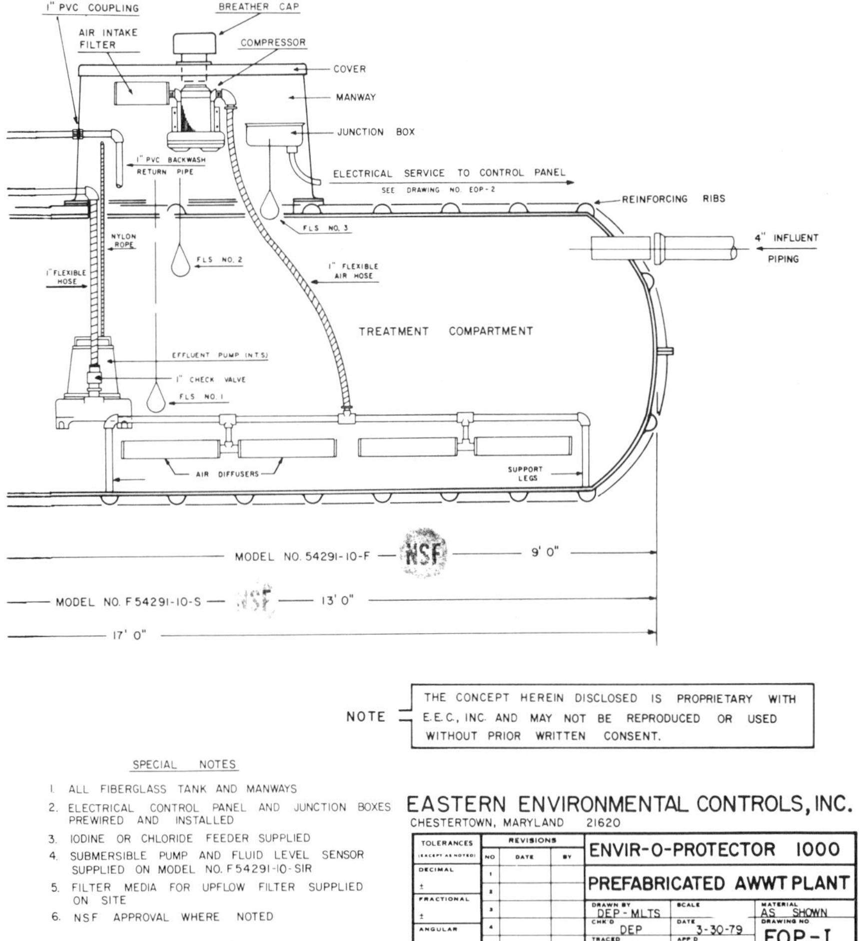

advanced wastewater treatment plant (MINIPLANT).

3.17 mg/l of phosphorus, or 0.026 lb/1000 gal, and 2.85 mg/l of nitrogen, or 0.023 lb/1000 gal of wastewater.

Originally, a hydroponic concept was to be used for the planters in the greenhouse, but this would not have provided sufficient nutrients to support any meaningful amount of vegetable and flower production. Therefore, it was decided to build the planters using a gravel layer under a one-foot-thick layer of sandy loam soil separated by a layer of nylon fabric and using the pea

Table I. Tests as Performed by the National Sanitation Foundation, Ann Arbor, Michigan, Plant 31 - 500 gpd (values in mg/l)

	Phosphorus		Chloride		N as Nitrate		N as Ammonia	
Date	In	Out	In	Out	In	Out	In	Out
9/18/78	5.55	3.50	355	142	0.4	1.9	4.0	0.35
9/19/78	5.15	3.20	355	142	0.4	1.9	3.0	0.13
9/20/78	5.10	2.85	284	142	0.4	1.5	15.5	0.09
9/21/78	5.95	2.85	355	177	0.5	1.7	16.6	0.12
9/22/78	5.35	2.93	355	177	0.5	1.6	10.5	0.12
9/25/78	6.05	3.85	355	177	0.2	4.5	8.4	0.56
9/26/78	6.60	2.75	320	177	0.1	3.5	12.0	0.32
9/27/78	6.55	2.93	355	177	0.2	4.0	7.6	0.60
9/28/78	9.20	3.18	355	213	0.2	4.3	6.8	0.60
9/29/78	10.00	3.68	320	a	0.2	3.6	8.4	a
Average	6.55	3.17	340	169.3	0.31	2.85	9.28	0.32
lb/1000 gal	0.054	0.026	2.837	1.412	0.002	0.023	0.077	0.002
lb/yr	9.855	4.745	517.75	257.69	0.365	4.197	14.052	0.365

[a]Insufficient amount of sample collected to perform all tests required because of sampler malfunction.

gravel layer for subsurface irrigation. There will be some accumulation of settleable solids in the bottom of the greenhouse tank, which can be pumped into a drying pan, air-dried, then placed around fruit trees in the garden.

CONCLUSIONS

The cost-effectiveness of this total systems concept will depend greatly on the amount of heat energy that is removed from the wastewater during the winter months. If a sufficient amount of savings can be realized by recycling the heat energy in the wastewater, by growing vegetables or flowers, or by producing aquatic life in the large tank, this system can be cost-effective. At present it is in the testing stage, but more conclusive information will be available within a year.

REFERENCES

1. Bernhart, A. P. "Treatment and Disposal of Waste Water From Homes by Soil Infiltration and Evapo-transpiration," Ph.D. Thesis, University of Toronto, Ontario, Canada (1973).

16

WASTEWATER RECYCLING IS NOW AVAILABLE

Howard W. Selby, III, Executive Vice President
Robert O. Mankes, Vice President, Marketing
PureCycle Corporation
Boulder, Colorado 80306

INTRODUCTION

The need for water reuse becomes more evident each year. Expanding world population and the inherent increased demand for adequate water supplies have placed water among the earth's scarce commodities. In addition to decreasing water supplies, much of the world is faced with the problem of declining water quality. Therefore, a means of expanding the use of existing water supplies while simultaneously reducing water pollution is becoming not only attractive, but necessary.

PureCycle Corporation has designed and developed a system that recycles all domestic water supplies at the home site (Figure 1). The PureCycle System produces high-quality potable water by removing all the contaminants in the household's sewage and wastewater. The System's original water supply of 1500 gallons is used for all household purposes, collected and purified by the System, then returned to the home for reuse.

The concept of reuse is not new. In fact, intentional reuse of water has been practiced for years. Municipal systems have discharged wastewater into natural waterways which, in turn, become the potable source for a downstream municipality. Another common occurrence of reuse is the septic tank effluent, which is allowed to percolate to subsurface aquifers that are used by neighbors as their source of potable water. The primary problem with these methods of water reuse is the lack of control of the treatment process.

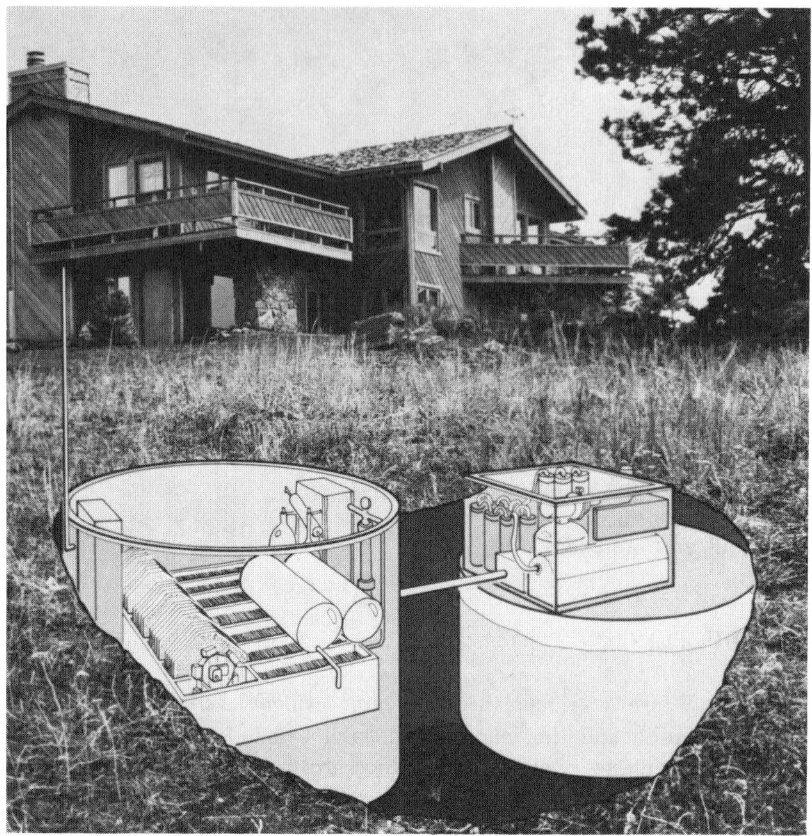

Figure 1. Excessive loading of septic systems causes the development of plumes of poorly treated effluent, which may (1) enter nearby waterways through surface runoff, or (2) move laterally with groundwater flow and discharge near the shoreline of nearby lakes.

DESCRIPTION OF THE PURECYCLE SYSTEM

The PureCycle System provides the maximum control of the treatment process in that each unit is equipped with a microprocessor (Figure 2). This "minicomputer" continuously monitors and controls the System's operation. Water quality data are automatically accumulated and analyzed by the microprocessor. In the event of a malfunction, the microprocessor

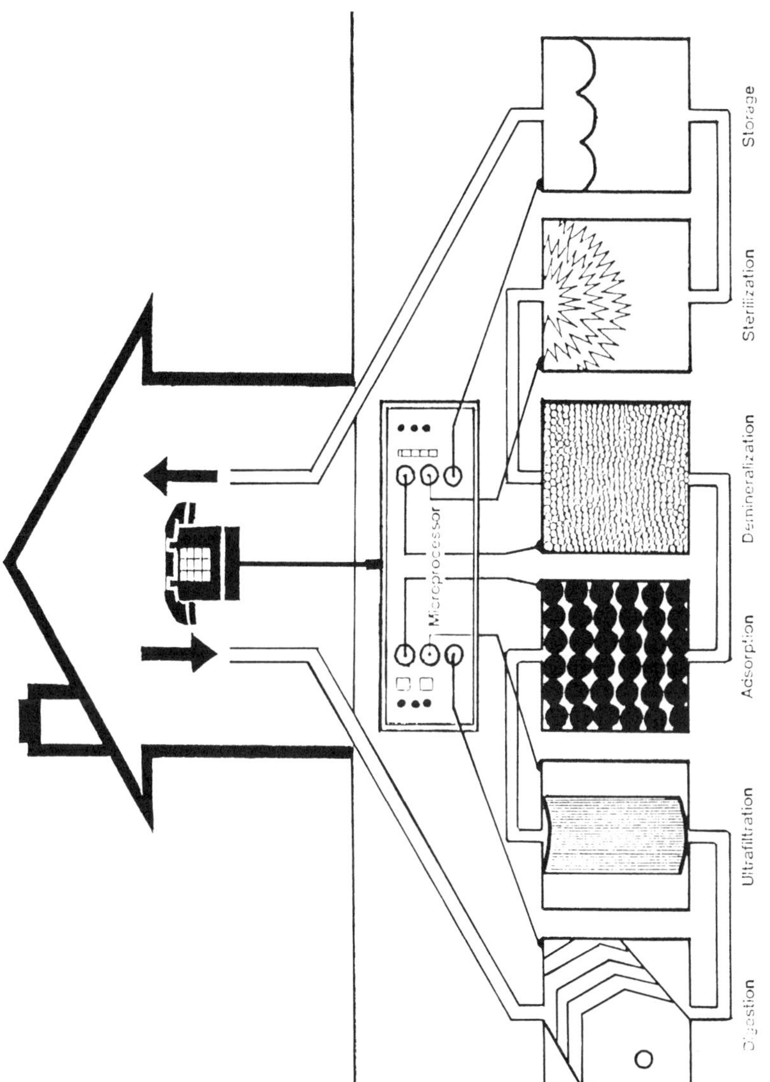

Figure 2. Schematic of microprocessor content of unit processes in PureCycle.

unit is designed to discontinue the water processing procedures and communicate this information to the service center.

The PureCycle System incorporates five well-known and -documented treatment processes to remove the organic, inorganic, suspended and dissolved contaminants in water. These five processes are monitored by a series of sensors and transducers, which report quality or quantity information to the microprocessor. When the sensors detect a quality parameter that exceeds those programmed into the microprocessor, the microprocessor initiates correction and recovery procedures. If the problem is not corrected within a specified time, the microprocessor halts all processing and reports the problem to the service center over the homeowner's telephone line. Discontinuation of water processing prohibits "in-process" water from entering the potable water storage container.

The following diagram illustrates the treatment processes utilized by PureCycle:

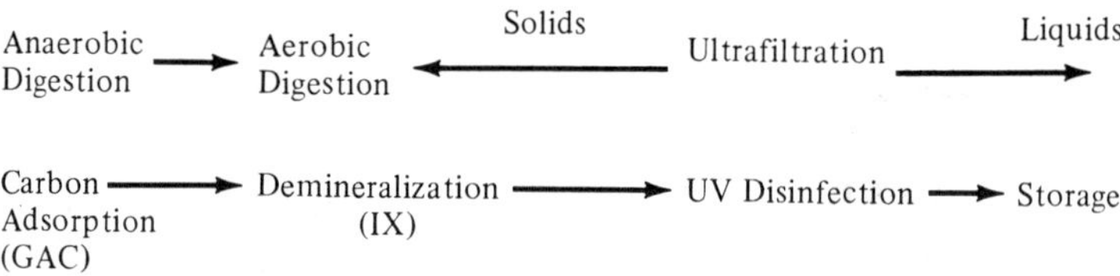

The sensors and transducers reporting data to the microprocessor are as follows:

- Level
- Total dissolved solids (conductivity)
- Turbidity (nephelometer)
- Organic carbon level (ultraviolet adsorption)
- Sterilization (radiation intensity)

In addition to monitoring the quality of water produced, the microprocessor reports information to the service center as follows:

1. *Daily reporting.* The microprocessor is programmed to capture the homeowner's private telephone line and autodial the service center. The unit then relays data for all system parameters. The System can be programmed to call in anywhere from once a minute to once a day.
2. *Service required reporting.* The microprocessor follows the same procedure when a failure occurs and, in addition, sends the problem description data, as well as the amount of clean water available for the homeowner's use.

THEORY AND PRACTICE OF THE OPERATION OF THE PURECYCLE SYSTEM

Contaminants of a domestic residence delivered to a sewage-treating system include fecal matter, urine, laundry waste, dishwasher waste, paper products, food waste, etc. The PureCycle System is designed to treat this wastewater from a domestic residence and, in addition, has the ability to treat the following:

1. Disinfectants
   a. Halogens
   b. Phenolics
2. Water-soluble organics
   a. Acetone, such as nail polish remover
3. Water-insoluble organics
   a. Paint thinner
   b. Floor wax
   c. Pesticides
   d. Antibiotics
4. Heavy metals from metal polishing, photographic solutions, etc.
5. Biological organisms

The System needs to respond by either removing these contaminants or by shutting down and notifying a service center of the shutdown. In either event, no harmful level of contaminant should reach a user of the System.

The mechanism of treatment begins with anaerobic digestion. Spent water is delivered to a 1500-gallon-capacity, 4-inch-reinforced cement tank. The heavy solids settle out and are subjected to anaerobic digestion. The supernatant and some suspended solids are delivered to the aerobic digester, which employs a rotating biological contactor (RBC). The RBC has five separate chambers to ensure that each bath has a reservoir. In addition, each chamber acts as a clarifier to settle solids. These chambers are dumped periodically (under microprocessor control) to subject the settled solids to anaerobic digestion once again. The RBC discs are used as the support to grow and harvest biota for the biological stabilization process.

Each chamber has a dominant type of biota, so that the liquid and suspended solids are subject to particular enzymatic digestion in series. The front end or first disc set biota digests organic material, while the biota on the last set of discs in the series of five is causing nitrification. After the last chamber, the water goes through an upflow gravel bed filter (backflushed periodically under microprocessor control). The influent wastewater has an average BOD_5 of 147 mg/l and the effluent off the gravel bed filter has an average BOD_5 of 22 mg/l. At this point, turbidity is approximately 15 Ntu.

The complete digestion of organic and inorganic compounds is not necessary because following this process is further filtration, organic adsorption and demineralization. In addition, having these subsystems follow digestion means that temporary failure of the digestion process will not impair water quality.

One of the unique subsystems for treating water is the ultrafilter. Ultrafiltration is employed to remove suspended particles. An ultrafilter having a pore size of 50 Å is used. This prohibits the passage of bacteria, viruses and other biological contaminants down to a molecular weight of 50,000, which includes polio, influenza and hepatitis viruses [1]. A backflush system is employed to periodically clean the filter. Should the ultrafilter rupture and allow passage of solids, a nephelometer coupled to the preprogrammed microprocessor will shut the system down at a turbidity of 0.33 Ntu and autodial the service center to report a failure. However, the nephelometer will detect changes as low as 0.02 Ntu.

Nonpolar organic (and some polar) compounds not destroyed in the anaerobic/aerobic digestor not retained by the ultrafilter are adsorbed by the activated carbon in the adsorption system. Although the ability of activated carbon to perform over a broad range of organic carbons is difficult to predict, activated carbon adsorption has been used successfully in this application many times. The U.S. Environmental Protection Agency (EPA) has proposed that some municipal water utilities use activated carbon to reduce the level of trihalomethanes (THM) in water supplies [2]. Indeed, its use to remove taste and odor compounds has been practiced for many years. The monitoring of the adsorption system is done by an online ultraviolet light adsorbance monitor, which can detect organic carbon compounds at less than 100 ppb [3].

Inorganic material and polar organic matter are extracted using ion exchange resins. The hydrogen form and hydroxide form of the ion exchange resins are similar to resins used in commercial applications to provide deionized water [4]. To determine when the resin capacity has been reached and regeneration is necessary, a conductivity cell monitors the effluent of this subsystem. The microprocessor is preprogrammed to regenerate at a reading of 10 ppm NaCl. Regenerate is vacuumed off and held in a separate compartment; water is evaporated off and the salt collected by PureCycle service personnel. Again, the microprocessor controls this function as needed.

UV sterilization is the final treatment of the water in the purification system. Disinfection of waters via UV radiation is dependent on several factors:

1. energy and exposure,
2. transmission of the liquid,
3. liquid flowrate, and
4. attenuation.

UV radiation must hit the microorganism to destroy it, and each organism must absorb a specific amount of energy to be destroyed. Table I gives the

Table I. Effective Amount of UV Energy Necessary to Kill Many of the Common Microorganisms

Parameter	Maximum Allowed	PureCycle Operating Levels
Nitrate (as N)	1	<0.05
Turbidity (Ntu)	0.3	0.15
Chloride	7	1
Fluoride	0.1	<0.01
Iron	0.1	<0.01
Magnesium	0.1	<0.01
Sulfate	0.1	<0.01
Total Dissolved Solids (TDS)	12	2
Zinc	0.01	<0.01
Total Organic Carbon (TOC)	3	<1
Calcium	0.1	<0.1
Sodium	5	1
Ammonia	10.01	<0.01
pH	5–9	6
Phosphorus	0.01	<0.01
Conductivity (μmhos/cm)	25	3
Fecal Coliforms	0	0
Silica	10	0.01
Arsenic	0.05	<0.01
Barium	1.00	<0.01
Cadmium	0.01	<0.01
Chromium	0.05	<0.01
Lead	0.05	<0.01
Mercury	0.002	<0.002
Selenium	0.01	<0.01
Silver	0.05	<0.01
Copper	1.00	<0.01
Manganese	0.05	<0.01
Endrin	0.0002	<0.0002
Lindane	0.004	<0.004
Methoxychlor	0.1	<0.1
Toxaphene	0.005	<0.005
Chlorophenoxys (2,4-D)	0.1	<0.1
2, 4, 5-TP Silvex	0.01	<0.01

effective amount of UV energy necessary to kill many of the common types of microorganisms. The germicidal spectrum of the ultraviolet wavelength is from 2000–3000 Å, with the peak at 2537 Å [5]. The intensity of the ultraviolet radiation is expressed in microwatts per square centimeter ($\mu W/cm^2$) at a given distance. The total UV energy emitted from all sides of the UV lamp is expressed in watts (W). The total exposure of the liquid is a product of energy, time, area and attenuation. The same number of Ultrads can be accomplished with a short exposure at a high intensity of UV or a long exposure at a low intensity of UV.

The amount of energy available to an organism from a given ultraviolet source depends on the UV transmission of the liquid. The transmission of the liquid depends on the quantity and types of dissolved and suspended matter in the liquid. The highly polished water, with an average turbidity of less than 0.15 Ntu, has an absorption coefficient of less than 0.008. The System's UV sterilizer produces enough Ultrarads for sterilization.

After sterilization, the processed water is stored in a 1500-gallon tank and, on demand, pumped to the house for all normal uses, such as drinking, cooking, bathing and laundry.

Table I lists some of the water quality parameters of the water produced by the System.

DATA ON COST AND OPERATION AND MAINTENANCE

A breakdown of the costs of operating and maintaining the PureCycle System, as well as some information on its power requirements, is given below.

Cost Data

The list price for the F03 Plant is $8800, which includes tanks, tops, RBC, ultrafilter, carbon adsorption columns, ion exchange columns, ultraviolet sterilizer, instruments microprocessor, pump and all internal plumbing.

The price *does not* include transportation to the site, taxes, excavation of the hole (30 ft X 20 ft X 8 ft), backfill, 4-inch waste line from house to unit, 1-inch water line from house to unit, or power and telephone lines from house to unit.

The system can be compared to an alternator for sewage treatment *and* water supply. For example, an engineered septic tank and leach field would cost $5000; a 300-foot well would be $5100, giving a total of $10,100.

Service Cost

The service cost per unit is $30 per month, which includes all parts, labor and travel. The service contract will keep the unit looking and working like new. This charge can be compared to the alternatives for municipal waste treatment and water supply.

Power

Power consumption is between 250 and 350 kWh per month. Again the power should be spread over the two utilities–water supply and wastewater treatment, i.e., a central wastewater treatment plant with attendant lift stations, pumps, disinfection equipment, etc., through a water treatment plant having a power demand used to treat and deliver water to the home.

REFERENCES

1. Berg, G., et al. *Virus in Water* (New York: American Public Health Association, 1976).
2. U.S. Environmental Protection Agency. "Economic Impact Analysis of a Trihalomethane Regulation for Drinking Water," EPA Report (1977).
3. PureCycle Corp. Benzoic acid research.
4. Rohm & Haas Co., Diamond Shamrock Co. Commercial Literature.
5. "Water Sterilization by Ultraviolet Radiations," Westinghouse Research Report BL-9R-6-1059-3023-1.

17

INDIVIDUAL AEROBIC PLANT OPERATION AND MAINTENANCE

John Fancy, President
John Fancy Inc.
Waldoboro, Maine 04572

INTRODUCTION

The use of aerobic plants has been extremely limited over the years, and they constitute but a small corner of the total wastewater treatment market. In some areas they have been severely limited, or even prohibited. Under the recent changes in the U.S. Environmental Protection Agency's (EPA) allocation of funds, this could be changed significantly. Although much has been written regarding performance of individual aerobic treatment plants [1,2], there is little in the literature covering their operation and maintenance (O&M). Information on long-term maintenance and operation will be necessary to allow engineers and regulatory authorities to accept a more widespread use of alternative systems.

BACKGROUND

The state of Maine was one of the first to use aerobic systems, partly because of the geographical layout of the state, with its "rock-bound coast." The mixture of rocks and water has been a strong attraction, and a large segment of the states' population lives along the coast. The coastline in a straight line is only a little more than 200 miles long; however, if all of the bays, inlets and peninsulas are measured, it amounts to about 3500 miles of shore. There are few highly developed areas along the northern 75% of the coast. Most of the population is spread quite uniformly along the shoreline. This has meant that few central collection and treatment systems have been built and that many individual homes with poor soil or no soil at all were discharging with straight pipes directly into the ocean in the mid 1960s, when the state began its pollution abatement program.

Because of Maine's unique position, it encouraged the use of aerobic units with disinfection and surface water discharge, along with a number of other alternative ideas. This had advantages and disadvantages. A large part of the problem was solved by individual action, but it also meant that Maine had to put up with some of the early and primitive aerobic systems.

In 1971 the firm of John Fancy Inc. was formed to provide operational advice to municipal and industrial wastewater treatment facilities. It was also contacted, however, by a number of individual aerobic treatment plant owners asking about servicing their units. Many of the first purchasers of this type of equipment were environmentalists, who were concerned about maintaining it once it was installed. It was soon decided that there were enough small plants to justify expansion into this area, and with the growth of the industry, more responsible manufacturers evolved who had a genuine interest in seeing that their equipment was maintained in the proper manner. Also, contributing to the situation was the NSF Standard 40, which, although not perfect in its initial concept, did recognize that servicing was important if the treatment plant were to perform adequately, and required that the first two years of servicing be included with the cost of purchasing.

John Fancy Inc. ultimately made agreements with several of the manufacturers to provide the initial servicing of these facilities directly for the manufacturer, with the owner taking over the cost after the first two-year period. At present, the company services more than 450 units in the home size market, almost all of which are aerobic units providing secondary treatment, with disinfection and discharge to surface waters, mainly the Ocean. Although the company covers the entire states of Maine and New Hampshire, more than 80% of its work is along the coast of Maine. The firm currently employs from four to six employees in small plant servicing, operating primarily in the center of the coastal area. Two further employees work in outlying areas with company vehicles and come to the office only once a week.

INITIAL PLANT ACCEPTANCE

Most of the work comes from service contracts with the manufacturers. The company is usually notified of a new plant installation by one of the suppliers or manufacturers' representatives. An initial inspection is then scheduled by the supervisor of small plant services, consisting of checking the unit over and making sure that it is completely installed, that all parts and equipment are there, and that everything is in working order. Also, a meeting with the new owners is arranged to be sure that they understand the system and how it works, as well as the need to notify the company in the event of an emergency. The servicing is explained to them and certain information is gathered for company records concerning the ownership, their wastewater discharge license, or other permit from the state; and (in the event of seasonally used houses) when a system needs to be started up in the spring and put away again in the fall.

Once this inspection has been completed, a maintenance service contract (MSA) is issued to the homeowner and a bill for services is sent to the manufacturer. Should there be any problem, the company contacts the supplier or manufacturer's representative and asks to have it corrected before the MSA is issued. These problems may be minor, such as an electric line not completely buried or the lock missing, or they may be major, such as the chlorine tank being installed backward, or the entire system installed in a low spot in the ground. One installation at a Coast Guard Lighthouse in Maine was completed at the end of November just before a rainstorm, which turned to freezing rain and left the entire treatment plant under 4 or 5 inches of ice for the entire winter. Another one of their installations was the only concrete tank treatment system known by the company to break up during a heavy storm. When the problems have been corrected, the plant is inspected again. If the system is satisfactory, the MSA is issued. This MSA assures the manufacturer, supplier, installer and homeowner that the unit is considered to have been properly installed, is complete and should work satisfactorily. Hopefully it will not freeze and break up the first winter, wash out during the first heavy rain, have its cover removed by the snowplow or flood during high tide, or any of the other interesting things that can occur.

PAPERWORK

Although the company tries to keep paperwork to an absolute minimum, there must be enough to organize and control the work. The system outlined here seems to satisfy these criteria.

Plant Information Notebook

A page is typed up for each new treatment plant and is put into the looseleaf notebook carried by the service person (see Appendix A). This page shows the owner and location of the treatment facility, with detailed instructions on how to get there. This is essential for seasonal homes, which are often located in outlying areas. The type of treatment facility and the date installed are also listed on the page. Then there is a listing of the equipment in the treatment plant, including the type of disinfection. Also, the page is dated. A new page is typed up for any changes, such as new owners or different equipment. Also included is such information as where to contact the owner if no one is home; the names of the caretakers for seasonal homes; and, if the unit is locked up, if there is a key and where to find it.

This notebook is very important because it prevents a service person from going to work on a unit (particularly an emergency call) without having the correct repair parts. Sometimes modifications have been made to the plant on older units and different equipment used from the original. Even on newer systems, time clocks or other changes are common.

Schedule Cards

A schedule of regular visits is established based on the company's assessment of the frequency needed by the treatment plant, as well as the state license for the particular system and the owner's interest in it. Most people want no part of the operation of their systems or even to know anything about it; however, some are more than willing to keep an eye on the unit and call if there should be any problem.

Normally, visits are scheduled for every other month, or about every eight weeks. This is more frequent than manufacturers recommend; however, almost all of these units have a disinfection unit. This works out to six visits per year for constant use, and normally about five visits per year for seasonally used systems. In practice, it takes about the same amount of time to shut down a system in the fall and restart it in the spring as it does to maintain it year round. This schedule allows the visits to be planned ahead so that each service person can make between eight and twelve visits per day within a specific area. It also enables us to plan out a service person's work a month in advance.

The schedule cards are large cards with notches cut out around the edge indicating the months in which work is to be performed. The cards serve three basic functions:

1. They are used by the supervisor to determine which plants need servicing and to establish the schedule for each of the service people.
2. They are used by the secretary to type up the service report forms.
3. Finally the date of servicing is recorded on the card when the service reports are returned to the office by the field service people.

This provides a quick reference source to determine what date a certain plant was serviced. This is often one of the first questions asked by a homeowner, and even by the regulatory agencies when they call.

Service Agreement

The first two years of servicing are done under a maintenance service agreement or MSA. This provides for John Fancy Inc. to perform all maintenance and servicing on the mechanical equipment, testing of the mixed liquors and the effluent, and general inspection of the system as required to ascertain that the plant is operating satisfactorily and as licensed by the state. A copy of a typical MSA is attached to this report as Appendix B. It also assures that, should any of the mechanical equipment fail during the guaranty period, John Fancy Inc. will replace the equipment at no additional charge to the owner. In this portion of the work, John Fancy Inc. acts as the manufacturer's representative. In fact, the person who sells and installs the plant is usually no longer involved once the plant has been accepted for servicing by the company.

The agreement also spells out that regular inspections will be made of the system and emergency calls will be answered as needed. Currently the price is \$250 for the first two years of maintenance servicing.

After two years, the homeowner has the option of picking up the servicing agreement; however, it is changed slightly in that it becomes a letter of agreement. This provides for the same work to be accomplished but charged out on an hourly basis, rather than on a yearly flat rate. The same as a maintenance service agreement, it holds John Fancy Inc. blameless for damages from power failures, clogging or breaking of either the inlet or discharge piping, misuse of the system by the homeowner, flooding, freezing, crushing of the unit, and fires and accidents unavoidable or beyond company control.

Further, it provides for the replacement of any defective pieces of equipment at the owners' request after he is notified and approves of the need to make such repairs. In neither the letter of agreement nor the maintenance service agreement is the cost of chlorine included, which can be a significant cost to the homeowner.

Service Manuals

Because service is provided to more than a dozen different manufacturers' plants, and because John Fancy Inc. had started in the business before most manufacturers had spent much time on operation and maintenance information, the company has developed its own service manuals over the years. These consist of three-ring looseleaf notebooks with a section devoted to each of the different types of plants operated by the company. Although the material in them varies from unit to unit and depends on the complexity of the system, as well as what information is available from the manufacturer, basically they all contain the following: (1) information on the history of the unit, such as the types and sizes made by that manufacturer, as well as any variations of models; (2) information on changes and retrofitting that may have been done to the units over the years; (3) as much technical information from the manufacturer as possible, such as dimensional drawings, exploded views of components and suggested installation procedures; (4) a section on the actual testing and maintenance to be performed on the units; (5) a section on starting the units up in the spring and shutting them down in the fall, if they are seasonally used; (6) information on disinfection; and (7) information learned from previous experience in servicing, which is recorded for future reference.

These manuals are always carried by the service people. The purpose of this is to provide a high degree of uniformity, not only among units of the same manufacturer, but also between the different types of units in the results that are reported. How this is accomplished is outlined in the following section.

Service Reports

These are printed on three-part NCR paper and are divided into four basic parts. The top of the page has a place for the name and address of the owner, the location of the plant (town or area in which the plant is located), the type of plant and its capacity. This information is typed in before the service person sees the form. In the field, the service person will fill in the other three parts and put the date and his initials on the top of the form. The second section is reserved for field tests of both the effluent and the mixed liquors. There is also a space for the results of any laboratory tests that are done later. The next section of the form provides an area to note the observations regarding the operation, appearance and equipment, as well as any comments on the work performed. The last section of the report is for listing the equipment and chemicals used in the servicing, as well as the time required for the work.

This three-part form is returned to the office when completed. One copy is filed after a record of the service date is put on the schedule cards. Two copies are mailed to the owner, with one being for his own records and one copy available for forwarding to the regulatory authority. This service report shows the owner when and what was done and any costs involved.

FIELD WORK

Very little has been published regarding the work actually done by service people in the field [3], so this chapter will outline in some detail a typical inspection visit, keeping in mind that no amount of written detail can compensate for common sense on the part of the service person working on his own in the field.

Typical Service Visit

The service work is organized to the point where it makes no difference which of the service people performs the actual field work. Although an attempt is made to keep the same people in the same area, this may not be possible, particularly during emergency calls. Regardless of who is performing the actual work, all of the servicing is done exactly as outlined in the service manual. The service person will arrive at the site with two important items: (1) the service manual, which tells how to do the work; and (2) the service report form to record information for a permanent record. A copy of a service report is attached to this report. The service person also will have with him the necessary tools to perform the work and any parts or equipment needed in the work.

Using the service report form first, the service person records the date, his initials and time of arrival, along with data on whether this is a scheduled visit, a startup, shutdown, or an emergency visit. The next step is to follow the step-by-step instructions in the servicing procedure outlined in the service manual. For instance, for one well-known brand of aerobic plant the inspection procedure is given below.

Inspection Procedure

Fill out report form 201 for each visit to a unit. Some installations have more than one treatment plant feeding into the same chlorinator. In this case, a separate form 201 must be filled out for each unit (except when only one unit is being worked on) and careful note made of which unit is which. Please make a complete record and keep careful notes of the inspection. This procedure is for surface discharge units; for subsurface, follow same procedure except disregard chlorination references.

1. Remove cover and note general appearance of unit. Inside of aeration unit, walls, pipes, etc. should be dirty (covered with black spongy material) but this should not be more than 1/4 inch maximum. Note odor as soon as cover is removed.
2. Remove cover from chlorinator. Note general appearance of unit (should be almost clean) and of effluent in unit.
3. Collect a sample of the effluent from the discharge side of the chlorine tank (end opposite chlorinator) and put 1000 ml in the Imhoff cone. Check

the chlorine residual (as described elsewhere in this manual) on this same sample. Record chlorine residual on report. Put 0 if there is no chlorine residual, but there is chlorine available. If there is no chlorine, mark report "out of chlorine." If test is not done, mark report "not done."

4. Collect 1000 ml of mixed liquor and put in graduated cylinder. Check temperature of this sample and time settling for one-half hour. Also note floc formation and settling rate. Floc should group together in a very few minutes to settle quite rapidly. Rate floc OK or poor. If settleability is less than 600 in 10 minutes, the settling is slow; if between 400 and 600, OK; if less than 400, fast. If unit has just been started up or has a problem, it may have no floc. Be sure to note color, which should be a rich brown.

5. Check the chlorine tablets in the holders and add enough so both tubes are at least 75% full. Record number of tablets used if from the owner's supply. Put this information under "Special Notes."

At least once a year the complete chlorinator should be removed and cleaned by washing it (if no outside water is available, wash it in the ocean). Remove the two tubes and the plastic top of the chlorinator. The body can then be lifted at the discharge end and slid off an inlet pipe. All parts should be washed.

6. If the water in the chlorinator is black or has scum or sludge on it, the unit should be pumped out. The tank holds 67 gallons so it can be bailed out with a pail if no electricity is available. The best way is to use a small electric submersible pump. This small quantity can be disposed of by putting it on any spot that will not create a mess. Be sure to rinse and clean tank completely.

7. Check the motor-blower set to be sure it is running and lay your hand on it to check the temperature. It should be quite warm but you should be able to hold your hand on it. Listen to be sure it is running smoothly. Check alarm by pinching tube to it while watching the indicator. The color should change from green to red and then go back to green when you let go. Note any problems on report.

8. Check foam in main unit and scum in clarifier ring. If scum is less than 1/4 inch it is OK. If more, remove with net and note this on report. Hose down main unit if necessary and possible. Note if aeration unit is not aerating as much as normal in this model.

9. Remove the air pipe to the diffuser by disconnecting the union near the center of the tank. Check the pipe for wearing or cracks and clean and check the diffuser. Repair pipe if necessary. Put oil or grease on threads on union so it can be removed regularly.

The inspection procedures for mechanically aerated units and, of course, other brands of diffused aeration units, are similar in the sampling and testing; however, they vary depending on the type of equipment that is installed.

Emergency Servicing

Emergency calls have been one of the more complicated problems dealt with during the years of servicing small plants. One reason for this is that the owners themselves want very little to do with the treatment plant and are even reluctant to look at an alarm so that they could at least notify the company should there be problems. Generally, the first indication is an unpleasant odor, and a service person is quickly requested to come over and fix it. Unfortunately, in a fair number of these cases the problem was that the unit had been shut off inside the house by the owner, who then forgot that it had been turned off. The company has been fairly successful in educating people to leave the unit's controls alone and let the service person do the adjusting.

Another problem encountered was that regardless when the treatment plants broke down, many people never seemed to remember to report them until Saturday night, yet were most anxious that a service person should come down immediately and fix them. To eliminate as many of the weekend problems as possible, one of the service people works on Saturdays, especially during the summer months. Also, an answering machine has been installed so that telephone calls can be monitored several times during the weekend.

Although most servicing is provided on eight-week frequencies, there is, of course, someone in the area more often than that. Some places with a high concentration of treatment plants are visited at least once per week, and sometimes two or three times. This means that any emergency calls normally can be taken care of within two days. Of course if the plant is a batch-type operation, the service must be rendered as soon as the call is received.

In the early days of servicing, calls were received from about half the service plants between the regularly scheduled visits. Over the years, by improving servicing methods and upgrading some of the older treatment plants with newer equipment, emergency calls have been reduced to the point where more than 90% of the plants will operate the entire year without any emergency visits.

Personnel

Through the years different types of people have been hired to service wastewater treatment plants. A number of individuals had state certificates for operating municipal or industrial treatment plants. For the most part, however, these people tended to be very dissatisfied with working on the smaller-sized units and few stayed more than a couple of months. The company has trained some of its own personnel, starting out with someone who had a background in mechanical work or sufficient chemical or biological training.

Both male and female people have been employed in servicing, and there has been no difficulty with the female service people as far as their ability to perform the work. There is an occasional heavy lifting task involved, such as trying to remove a submersible pump from the pit under the porch. However, for the most part this has not proved to be a difficulty. There are some people, however, who have complained about a woman servicing their system and who feel that they are not getting adequate work if she is doing it. By the same token, however, this has worked in reverse where people preferred to have a woman around their property.

One particular person completed a two-year wastewater treatment operator's course then found that he preferred to service the smaller units, working on his own with very little supervision. He keeps excellent records and will invariably repair the problem before he returns, rather than just come back and report that something is not working correctly. Some of the important traits of people hired for servicing include: (1) the ability to work alone without supervision; (2) the ability to get along with the homeowner and communicate with them where necessary; and (3) a basic understanding of wastewater treatment.

COST OF SERVICING

To provide a better picture of the servicing costs, the records of 22 plants serviced during the last 2- to 4-year period have been reviewed. These plants represent three distinct groups. First, four of the units are older, diffused air-type systems, 5- to 8-years old, which are representative of the earlier aerobic units. Generally they were constructed of metal. Six are of the newer type diffused aeration units, with ages ranging from 3 to 6 years; basically these are the present generation of diffused aeration equipment and are of fiberglass construction. The remaining 12 plants are representative of the newer mechanical aeration type equipment and have been in service from 3 to 4 years. These are typical of the fiberglass and concrete units now being constructed.

Ten of these units are used year round, while 12 are used seasonally. All except one is overboard discharge into surface waters. These plants represent approximately 5% of those serviced by the company and are roughly in the same proportion of types of units and types of uses as in the total number of plants serviced.

These plants were visited a total of 240 times, which is broken down into 215 regular visits and 25 emergency calls, or repairs that could not be scheduled into regular visits.

Viewing all 22 of the plants and breaking the cost down among three different factors–labor, parts and chlorine–shows that labor costs varied from a low of $49.50 to a high of $214.50 per year. The mean labor cost for all 22 plants was $83.54. Some of these plants did not require any parts or equipment; however, the maximum was $121.93 and the average for all plants was $41.51. Chlorine was not required by some of the plants, but one plant used a maximum of $99.77 worth. The average again was $38.16. This gave an average operating cost for the 22 plants of $163.21 (Table I).

Table I. Average Operating Cost of Different Types of Aerobic Units

Labor	Parts	Chlorine	Total
	Four older units (diffused aeration)		
$106.43	$67.85	$38.16	$212.44
	Six newer units (diffused aeration)		
$100.98	$19.86	$38.16	$159.00
	Ten newer units (mechanical aeration)		
$111.65	$10.75	$38.16	$160.56

As can be seen by breaking down the costs for servicing by each of the different types of units, the older units tended to have the highest cost for repair parts, $67.85, while the newer units dropped down correspondingly to a lower level. One surprise is that labor costs tended to be in the same range for all plants, regardless of age. From this table it appears that the only variable in operating the systems is the cost of the repair parts themselves.

It should be remembered that these costs represent the actual field cost of servicing and maintenance and do not include any costs for long-term debt reduction or debt servicing. Also not included, as they were not available from company records, are the electrical costs.

CONCLUSIONS

The satisfactory long-term operation of small aerobic treatment plants, assuring not only an acceptable effluent but also minimizing emergency calls and problems for the homeowner, can be accomplished by a planned and controlled program of servicing, as outlined here. It should make no difference whether this program is carried out by a public staff or private firm, and this should be a matter of economics. When planning an alternative system, adequate provision must be made in projecting the operating costs, as it is easy to use unrealistically low figures.

APPENDIX A

WASTEWATER TREATMENT PLANT SERVICE REPORT

Invoice # ________

JOHN FANCY INC.

P. O. Box F
14 Jefferson Street
Waldoboro, Maine 04572
(207) 832-7584

Contract # ________

Time Arr. ________ Total ________

Location ________ Date ________
Type of Plant ________ Capacity ________ By ________

( ) Scheduled visit
( ) Start up
( ) Shut down
( ) Emergency ________

SAMPLE
B.O.D. ________
Fecal Coliform ________
Suspended Solids ________

Effluent - Cl_2 Residual ________ D.O. ________
Settleable Solids ________
( ) Clear ( ) Slightly Cloudy ( ) Cloudy

Mixed Liquors - ½ hr. Settle ____ Temp ____
D.O. ____ Floc ____ Settling ________
Color ________ Odor ________

OPERATION

General Appearance - ( ) Very Good ( ) Good ( ) Poor ( ) Unsatisfactory
Scum and Grease Build up - ( ) None ( ) Some ( ) Heavy ( ) Cleaned
Electric Motors and Blowers - ( ) OK ( ) Not Working ( ) See Note Below
Controls - ( ) OK ( ) See Note Below ( ) Checked Complete Cycle
Chlorination - ( ) Ok ( ) Adjusted ( ) See Note Below
Pumps - ( ) Ok ( ) Not Working ( ) See Note Below
Special Notes ________

Quan.	Item	Price

____ Total Billable hrs. X Labor Rate per hr. $ ________ = ________
Sales Tax ________
Total Amount ________

White copy for owner's records.
Yellow copy may be sent to the appropriate regulatory authority.

Form 201-A

Please pay by this invoice

APPENDIX B

MAINTENANCE SERVICE AGREEMENT

Between JOHN FANCY INC.(Servicer) and ____________________________(Owner)

covering a _______ G.P.D. wastewater treatment located at

_____________________. This treatment plant is a _________________model

as manufactured by ______________________________. This agreement covers a

_________year period beginning ____________________. The cost is _______per year paid in advance. This agreement is null and void if not accepted within 30 days of above date. This copy is for your records.

____________________________	__________	____________________	__________
Owner	Date	John Fancy	Date
New _________ Renewal ______		MSA________	

The servicer agrees to perform all maintenance, servicing, testing, and inspection as required to ascertain that the plant is operating satisfactorily and as approved by the appropriate regulatory authority. This work includes:

A. Maintenance, cleaning and adjusting to all parts, including controls of the unit, as needed.
B. Testing of the operation of the plant and the final effluent to assure proper operation and compliance with license or approval.
C. Testing of the chlorine residual, replenishment of the chlorine supply and regulation of the chlorination (if plant has chlorinator). *NOTE: the cost of chlorine is NOT included in this agreement.*
D. A written report to the owner of each visit, plus a copy which may be forwarded to the appropriate regulatory authority.
E. Inspection of the facility as needed to insure satisfactory operation.
F. Emergency calls are limited to two (2) calls per year. Calls exceeding this number will be billed at our standard rates for labor and mileage.

If it should be necessary to replace any parts of the equipment, the servicer shall immediately notify the owner of such need and at the owner's request, shall make such replacements without further charge, except for the parts and materials required if not covered by a guarantee.

When the servicer indicates the need for sludge removal, as determined by testing, the owner shall make provision to have the plant pumped out. *The cost of such pumping is NOT covered by this agreement.*

Renewal of waste discharge license with the regulatory authority concerned, or any reports required, are the owner's responsibility. A copy of the servicer's report should be forwarded to the appropriate regulatory agency, and for most plants this will cover the reporting requirement in the license, if any.

Service calls resulting from the following reasons are not covered by this agreement and will be billed at the standard hourly rate and mileage charges:

A. Power or fuse failure.
B. Clogging, breaking, crushing, or freezing of either inlet or outlet piping.
C. Discharge of any material, liquid or solid, into the unit which it was not designed to receive.
D. Flooding, freezing, tank settling, or crushing of unit from overload on ground above.

The servicer is relieved of any further responsibility if at any time during the term of this agreement the owner permits any other person or employees of any other company to render any service or make any adjustments or changes to the equipment, except when instructed by us. We will not be responsible for any direct or indirect damages arising from failure of system and/or equipment, but undertake, under the terms outlined in this agreement, to do such overhauling and adjusting as may from time to time be necessary.

The servicer will not be responsible for damages resulting from fires, accidents, and delays unavoidable or beyond our control.

The owner agrees to permit the servicer to use and release the information obtained on the operation of the plant at his discretion.

The cost of this agreement includes the shutting down in the fall and the starting up in the spring of seasonal plants. These plants will be visited regularly only when in operation. It is the owner's responsiblity to notify the servicer at least four (4) weeks in advance of the desired date of the spring reactivation of the system.

JOHN FANCY INC.
BOX 152
WALDOBORO, MAINE 04572

FOR SERVICE CALL 832-7543

REFERENCES

1. Hutzler, N. J., et al. "Performance of Aerobic Treatment Units," in *Home Sewage Treatment*, Proceedings of the Second National Home Sewage Treatment Symposium, ASAE Pub. 5-77, St. Joseph, MI (1978), p. 54.
2. Glasser, M. B. "Garrett County Home Aeration Wastewater Treatment Project," report prepared for the Environmental Health Administration, Bureau of Sanitary Engineering, Maryland State Dept. of Health and Mental Hygiene, Baltimore, MD (1976).
3. Cover, A., and F. Lucician. "An Operator's View of Performance: Sanitation District #3, Boyd County Kentucky." In *Individual Onsite Wastewater Systems*, Proceedings of the Fourth National Conference, N. I. McClelland, Ed. (Ann Arbor, MI: Ann Arbor Science Publishers, Inc., 1978), p. 135.

18

EVAPOTRANSPIRATION–THE CHESAPEAKE BAY STUDY

Kenneth M. Lomax, Assistant Professor
Lois S. Lane, Biologist
Horn Point Environmental Laboratories
Center for Environmental and Estuarine Studies
University of Maryland
Cambridge, Maryland 21613

INTRODUCTION

This chapter addresses the problem of operation and maintenance (O&M) of evapotranspiration systems. Evapotranspiration (ET) as a method to dispose of wastewater may be one part of an onsite wastewater system. As a part of the home wastewater system, the evapotranspiration unit by itself must be considered prior to discussing the O&M of an entire onsite system utilizing evapotranspiration. Evapotranspiration as a disposal method was studied at Horn Point Environmental Laboratories (HPEL) for approximately five years (Table I). According to these studies along the Chesapeake Bay, grass as vegetation will move water at approximately 3.5 mm/day (0.08 gpd/ft^2 of bed) on an annual design average [1]. To achieve this disposal rate with grass, design, construction, vegetation and water quality must be considered. The term "ET bed" will be used here to mean one unit of the disposal system. The ET beds installed at HPEL in 1975 were designed on the basis of Alfred Bernhart's publication [2].

DESIGN CONSIDERATIONS

The width and depth design recommendations of Bernhart seem to be supported by observations at HPEL. According to that publication,

Table I. ET System Summary, Horn Point Environmental Laboratories

Identification Number	Bed Size, Width Length (m)	Waste Treatment	Liner	Construction Completed
375	6 × 27	Aerobic	Natural polyethylene	November 1975
378	6 × 27	Aerobic	None	August 1975
379	6 × 27	Aerobic	None	September 1975
380	6 × 27	Anaerobic	Black polyethylene	October 1974

the recommended depth at the sidewall is about 45 cm, based on observations that a shallower bed would have insufficient storage, and that a deeper bed would be a waste of material. In one lined bed with little or no wastewater added, precipitation appeared as free water at the bottom of the bed for a short period (1-3 days) and then would disappear. A deeper bed would not move the water as quickly. There were no observations that would suggest that a shallower bed would have benefits. A bed width of 6-8 meters is substantiated by the following observations.

1. Construction is easier if the bed is not too wide. Construction of the bed, which usually involves hand labor to distribute sand and gravel within the bed, is made easier if machinery can place the materials to most parts of a bed. Also, a narrower bed can be kept flatter and more level than a wider bed.

2. Placement of multiple beds on a given home site may be easier than one large equivalent-area bed. Thus, if the width and depth of the bed are established, the only other variable in bed size is the length, which can be varied to achieve the required surface area. It should be noted that multiple beds are not only easier to construct and maintain level, but also flow of wastewater can be divided among beds to achieve maximum disposal.

Another characteristic of ET bed design is the liner. According to our studies, a plastic liner is an important aspect of the total ET bed. Without a liner separating the bed from the surrounding soil, water can move from the bed into the soil during low groundwater periods, starving the vegetation of its needed water. If the vegetation were not watered well in the summertime and should die back, then it would not be healthy enough to retain the transpiration rate that is so critical in the late winter and spring. The liner needs to be installed to keep the vegetation healthy. It seems that 10-mil-thick polyethylene is a satisfactory liner when sand is placed on either side of the polyethylene to protect it.

The next design characteristic to be discussed is distribution of the wastewater within the bed. There is a layer of gravel about 15 cm deep in the bottom of the bed, which contains the 4-inch perforated sewer pipe. Both the pipes and gravel allow the wastewater to spread evenly to all parts of the bed. In each of our first beds, a distribution box is connected to the four pipes that run the length of the bed, but in the second beds no distribution boxes were installed. With a distribution box, the velocity of energy of the pumped wastewater is dissipated by the box, causing the water level in the box to rise. The water level rises until sufficient head is created to move the water through the entire pipe system. In three of the four "first" beds, the water level in the distribution box has risen above the box lid, occasionally appearing on the bed surface. There has been no surface water on the second beds as a result of water pumped from the first to the second beds. These experiences suggest that a distribution box can create the unwanted operational problem of wastewater on the ground surface. Some of the pump-dosing problems that have been observed and were thought solvable by increasing the frequency of dosing and reducing the length of dosing, tend to be an effect of the distribution box. Without a distribution box the importance of more frequent pumping is reduced, but several pumpings per day are still preferred to occasional large doses. Based on this characteristic, we recommend no distribution box be used within the evapotranspiration bed.

Another recommendation not particular to our study is that the grain size of the sand in the ET bed be relatively large to allow for water and organism movement within the sand [3]. The last part of the bed in construction sequence is the topsoil needed to start the grass seed and establish the vegetation on the top of the bed. We would like to know whether a silt-loam soil might improve the runoff potential relative to a sandy loam topsoil, but have not had the opportunity for comparative testing. The design characteristics mentioned above are only as good as the bed construction that follows the design.

ET BED CONSTRUCTION

Bed construction with supervision is certainly a part of management, just as operation and maintenance. Construction has a very strong impact on the necessary maintenance of the system. The primary construction characteristic we emphasize is that the bed needs a firm foundation. Although this may seem obvious, one bed at HPEL was installed in soft soil, with the result that the ET bed sank after construction, and seems to continue to sink with all of the heavy gravel, sand and water on top of the soft foundation. Along with a firm foundation, the bed must be constructed with a flat bottom: flat within a 2-cm tolerance on survey of the bed bottom. The sand and gravel placed in the bed during construction are moved by hand. Not only is this procedure costly, but also it must be supervised to ensure that it is done according to design. Future construction techniques with widespread use of ET systems may allow for special machinery to install the sand and gravel in the beds.

Another construction characteristic is that the bed must be finished and vegetation established prior to loading the bed with wastewater. If the ET system is being installed to repair a failing septic tank system, this means that the ET system has to be installed and have grass growing on the bed before the old system is eliminated. For new construction, the house should avoid loading the bed until the vegetation is established, meaning that the bed must be constructed before the house is constructed. This sequence is the reverse of common practice of installing the septic tank system after the house is complete. The necessity to establish the bed prior to loading reflects the importance of the vegetation.

Vegetation on the bed must be healthy for the system to work properly. Grass that dies back in the summer will not be vigorous for winter transpiration. The importance of vegetation was obvious on system #375, which was completed in November 1975. For the next several months the bed surfaces at 375 were just soft mud with dormant grass seeds, until warmer weather allowed the seeds to germinate and establish a uniform stand of Kentucky 31 fescue. During the next cold season, the bed surfaces remained firm with a relatively green color to the grass. Bushes are often planted as a vegetation for ET beds because the increased leaf surface area should increase the transpirative capacity of the bed. Bushes also have another benefit in that they reduce personnel impact on the bed. It is more difficult to play football among bushes—an activity that is detrimental to the grass-covered ET bed.

WATER QUALITY MEASUREMENTS

Water quality data comprise the last information to be presented about the beds per se. Water quality which we measured going into and within the bed indicated measurable differences between aerobic and anaerobic treatment (Table II). Parenthetically, no difference in rate of water movement was detected. Dissolved oxygen measurements in situ in the bed substantiate the sensory perception that there is no odor escaping from the beds (Table III). One water quality concern has been that salt might build up from the chloride content of domestic wastewater. Over the years that ET has been studied, there seems to be no measurable

Table II. Water Quality Comparison Between Aerobic (375) and Anaerobic (380) ET Systems with Lined Beds (mean values with numbers of samples shown in parentheses)

	375		380	
	Influent Pump Pit	Test Hole No. 2	Influent Pump Pit	Test Hole No. 2
BOD_5 (mg/l)	106 (48)	[a]	157 (46)	[a]
NFR (mg/l)	59 (47)	[a]	71 (31)	[a]
NO_3-N (mg/l N)	8.7 (50)	3.6 (49)	12.2 (51)	1.9 (29)
PO_4 (mg/l PO_4)	25.7 (36)	9.8 (37)	23.6 (26)	10.1 (27)
pH	7.8 (52)	7.0 (50)	7.4 (50)	7.3[b] (29)

[a]No samples for BOD, see Table III for dissolved oxygen.
[b]Includes some samples from test hole No. 1.

Table III. Dissolved Oxygen Concentration in ET Beds from January 1977 through September 1979 (mean values, mg/l O_2)

	First Bed		Second Bed	
Test Hole	1	2	3	4
System Number				
375 Mean value	0.9[a]	0.5[a]	1.4[b]	1.3[b]
Standard deviation	0.7	0.4	1.3	1.4
Observations	48	45	27	30
379 Mean value	0.9	0.9	2.9	3.6
Standard deviation	1.0	1.0	1.7	2.5
Observations	82	89	32	38
380 Mean value	1.0	1.8	2.6[b]	4.0[b]
Standard deviation	1.1	1.6	2.8	3.2
Observations	107	106	11	10

[a]Average for 1977. Free water below hole in 1978-79.
[b]Free water below hole in 1977. Data obtained from measurements beginning January 1978.

chloride increase (Table IV). In terms of pathogenic indicators, the bacterial flora in the bed and going into the bed are similar to those of other wastewater systems. As desired, the vegetation seems to use wastewater nutrients. We measured a lower concentration of nitrogen and phosphorus in the free water of the bed than in the influent water going to the bed

Table IV. Chloride Concentrations in ET Systems with Lined Beds (mean values per season, mg/l Cl^-)

	375		380	
	Influent Pump Pit	Test Hole No. 2	Influent Pump Pit	Test Hole No. 2
Winter 1977	28	37	24	4[a]
Spring 1977	31	–	38	26
Summer 1977	33	49	54	47
Fall 1978	34	56	30	50
Winter 1978	23	9	38	21
Spring 1978	11	8	37	22
Summer 1978	20	25	65	32
Winter 1979	17	8	17	22
Spring 1979	–	2	49	26
Fall 1979	4	1	20	6

[a]Includes some values from test hole No. 1.

(Table II). These water quality results have helped to describe the functional characteristics of the ET bed as a wastewater disposal unit.

OPERATION AND MAINTENANCE

The next discussion relates HPEL's experience with an entire system for an individual home that utilizes evapotranspiration for disposal. Several problems were encountered, all of which could be solved by management. Some of them are operation and maintenance. It is most important to note that a useful, technologically sound system should not be eliminated just to avoid management problems. A lined bed is recommended so that the vegetation be healthy throughout the year and watered at a regular rate. However, a liner does create some problems. First, there is no flexibility in long-term overload or underload of the wastewater coming into the bed. For an ET system designed to handle 1000 liter/day, a long-term application of 1500 liter/day is likely to cause an overflow failure of the system. Weekend visitors causing a short-term peak water use do not pose a problem according to HPEL's studies; however, a change in the family's size, or the sale of the home to a family with different water use characteristics could result in problems from too much or too little water being applied to a lined ET bed. The problem of an overload causing a visible overflow may be easier to understand than the problem of an underload. For one of the first beds in the study, the free water depth at the influent end of the bed was limited to about 2 cm by the elevation of the overflow pipe. The effect of the lowered water level, like an underload, was that grass roots seeking water entered the distribution pipes and eventually plugged the pipes.

It is recommended that all individual home systems be required to have a water meter indicating the family's water use. If the electric and gas companies require meters, shouldn't the sewage management authority require a water meter? Such a meter would help determine whether the system is receiving the expected volume of wastewater and would eliminate the tendency to blame the sewage system when the family uses too much water. Installing a water meter in rural systems with management is a reasonable low-cost addition to the system and would provide valuable water use information. After all, if a researcher is expected to measure wastewater flow to make a realistic evaluation of the systems (Table V), how can a management authority avoid having such critical data?

What about care of the ET systems? Two major parts of an ET system are the mechanical/physical aspects and the biological aspects. For these systems, mechanical problems have demanded more immediate maintenance response. For low, flat topography, it is necessary to use pumps in the systems to move the wastewater. Each delivery pump from the treatment unit to the first ET bed of the system has needed periodic cleaning for all systems. Several failed and were replaced. The failures caused noticeable wastewater flow reduction in the home and had to be corrected within a few hours. This type of maintenance requirement, which affects the family's water use, would probably have been handled by the homeowner;

Table V. Water Use Data for ET Systems from January 1977 through September 1979 (liter/day/system)

System Number	Mean	Maximum Week and Date	Minimum Week and Date
375	1450	2930 7/5/78	954 2/11/78
378	270	1660 1/13/77	0 3/18/77
379	508	1660 7/31/79	0 2/18/77
380	550[a]	1630[a] 11/11/77	290 8/25/78

[a]Including supplement in 1977.

however, the failure of an aeration system might not receive homeowner attention. For one of the aerobic treatment units, which utilizes a pump for aeration, the pump requires semiannual cleaning to prevent clogging of the intake area. An aeration pump failure on this system during 1978 may have gone unnoticed for about a week, causing a measurable change in the influent water quality to the ET bed. Another example of mechanical problems related to pumping is the level control–electrical switching equipment.

One physical aspect that has needed attention is the stormwater drainage. Swales are required to keep outside surface water from entering the bed and to help the bed surface shed as much rainwater as possible. These swales have filled up in a few places causing runoff to puddle and potentially enter the bed. Another physical maintenance requirement would be repair of the bed crown, should settling occur in the bed. This crown is needed to help shed precipitation and to provide a zone of aerated soil during periods of highest water level in the bed. For one bed of a HPEL system, a crown repair was delayed to observe the effect of settling. Eventually, the bed surface showed ponded water when the bed was full.

An ET bed can be thought of as a fragile ecosystem that will dispose of wastewater only if attended properly. Some activities are detrimental to the biological functioning of the disposal system. For example, use of the bed for gardening would eliminate the more hardy grasses and evergreens so important for late winter, early spring transpiration. Planting trees in a lined ET bed should be discouraged because stabilizing roots cannot penetrate the liner to hold the growing tree against wind forces. Attending this ecosystem also involves regular mowing of the grass to maintain both growing vegetation and a sufficient leaf area for transpiration. Obviously, extremely short or tall grass is not desired for maximum transpiration. A grass height of 8–10 cm on these beds appeared healthy and aesthetically pleasing. These biological aspects require that the homeowner be educated as to proper care of his ET beds. Education is a management requirement particularly necessary when a new family moves to an existing ET system.

The operation and maintenance problems that HPEL encountered with ET systems are not insurmountable and could be covered by an effective management scheme. It is probable that this need for management of ET systems and the lack of a management scheme are together the primary reason that ET systems are considered as a last alternative in home sewage disposal. Another reason they might not receive an equal alternative status is the present high cost of the system, but future relative costs might be lowered by widespread construction of the ET beds for wastewater disposal. Evapotranspiration of wastewater can be a viable alternative disposal method in the Chesapeake Bay area and should be considered in helping to reduce water pollution from home sewage.

CONCLUSIONS

The movement of water into the air by a grass-covered evapotranspiration bed can be an effective means of wastewater disposal in the relatively humid climate of the Chesapeake Bay. Recommended sizing of an ET bed for this geographic area is 3.5 mm/day of water (0.08 gpd/ft^2) for a grass-covered bed. A lined bed for complete evapotranspiration provides for more healthy grass throughout the year, but demands maximum and minimum flowrates of water. Proper bed construction requires a firm foundation and a level flat bottom. The mechanical aspects of the system require regular maintenance and should be the responsibility of a management authority. The transpirative ecosystem so essential to year-round wastewater disposal requires homeowner understanding of the system. Acceptance of ET systems for home sewage disposal to help reduce water pollution depends on satisfactory management of the entire onsite wastewater system.

REFERENCES

1. Lomax, K. M. "Evapotranspiration Method Works for Wastewater Disposal Along Chesapeake Bay," *J. Environ. Health,* 41(6):324-328 (1979).
2. Bernhart, A. P. *Treatment and Disposal of Wastewater from Homes by Soil Infiltration and Evapotranspiration* (Toronto, Ontario: University of Toronto Press, 1973).
3. Bennett, E. R., and K. D. Kinstedt. "Sewage Disposal by Evaporation-Transpiration," EPA 600/2-78-63, U.S. Environmental Protection Agency, Cincinnati, OH (1978).

19

THE MICHIGAN FREEWAY REST AREA SYSTEM–EXPERIENCES AND EXPERIMENTS WITH ONSITE SANITARY SYSTEMS

A. E. Erickson
Professor of Soil Science
Department of Crop and Soil Sciences
Michigan State University
East Lansing, Michigan 48824

J. W. Bastian
Assistant Supervisor of Roadside Development
Michigan Department of Transportation
Lansing, Michigan 48909

INTRODUCTION

Michigan has considered itself a tourist state since the introduction of the automobile back in the early 1900s. The Michigan Department of Transportation (DOT) has long recognized that it must provide not only roadways for the movement of vehicles, but also service to the traveling public. It was no surprise to the Michigan DOT when the National Outdoor Recreation Resources Review Commission revealed that driving for pleasure leads the list for all outdoor recreation, surpassing fishing, hunting, swimming and hiking, nor that more than one-third of all highway travel was either recreation or pleasure oriented. Michigan's expanding tourist economy is based on the travelers who make up these statistics. It is firmly believed that providing good roadways, attractive roadsides and tourist service facilities plays a significant part in the tourist economy of Michigan. Last year more than $8 billion of commerce was generated by the tourist industry in Michigan, second only to the manufacturing economy.

HISTORY

Roadside development in Michigan began during the late 1920s, when picnic tables were placed along a few scenic highways. The Department of Transportation constructed the first tourist roadside park on a state two-lane highway during this same period. A typical roadside park provided for safe parking, picnic facilities, drinking water, an information board and rustic toilet facilities using a 1000-gallon holding tank.

By 1958, 115 tourist roadside parks, 20 scenic turnouts and more than 2000 individual picnic table sites had been established along state trunkline highways.

During 1979 the Michigan DOT opened its 75th Freeway Rest Area to the traveling public. Additionally, 102 roadside parks and 40 scenic turnouts along the two-lane system attract nearly 40 million visitors each year.

FREEWAY REST AREA DEVELOPMENT

The Federal Interstate Highway System was begun in 1956. Michigan's activity in roadside development from 1956 through 1965 emphasized the construction and operation of Freeway Safety Rest Areas. These rest areas evolved from the Tourist Roadside Park System previously developed along the two-lane highways throughout the more scenic areas of the state and provided the same basic services to the freeway traveler. In 1960 Michigan's first three rest areas were opened along I-94 in the Kalamazoo area.

The early freeway rest areas were accepted almost immediately by the traveling public, and the heavy use of the rustic vault toilets made it readily apparent that an upgraded type of sanitary system would be imminently necessary. About 8% of the freeway mainline traffic entered each rest area. On the more heavily traveled routes, a turn-in of this percentage would account for a rest area use of upwards of 750,000 visitors each year, each area being serviced by vault-type toilets.

In 1966 the Michigan DOT discontinued the use of rustic vault toilets at freeway rest areas and adopted a policy of providing flush-type toilets at all new rest areas. A further program was begun that year to retrofit all existing rustic toilets with full flush systems.

REST AREA SANITARY SYSTEMS

Early in the planning stages of the modern rest area program, a policy was adopted to utilize nearby sanitary sewers, if they were available within a reasonable distance. In lieu of entering a sewer system, a septic tank–tile field system would be used on lighter soils and a lagoon system on heavy soils.

Septic Tank–Tile Fields

Early septic tank–tile field design included a three-compartment septic tank capable of at least 24 hours retention with two separate tile fields. A typical deep trench tile field design was used for the most part, with the fields being dosed on an alternative basis to 90% of the capacity of the field tile.

This design worked reasonably well provided the hydraulic absorption capabilities of the receiving soils were not violated. The alternating field design lacked the ability to completely rest a field for aerobic reclamation during the very heavy summer season use and this, it was felt, did contribute to some hydraulic problems and subsequent field failure at a few locations.

Present septic tank–tile field design provides for a three-compartment septic tank, which leads to a distribution box that in turn can feed any of four separate tile fields. Each field can support the entire sanitary requirements of the rest area. This design allows good flexibility in managing the system because it permits the complete resting of three fields while one is being used. Furthermore, the operator can open two fields should he expect very high use in such special situations as a holiday weekend.

The multiple-field design has been used for the last 10 years in Michigan freeway rest areas without one failure.

Lagoon Systems

Early lagoon design provided for a two-cell system capable of operating either in parallel or series. Hydraulic requirements were designed on a projected 20-year anticipated load, with discharge on a seasonal basis to a receiving surface water. Organic loading was well under the recommended maximum of 20 lb/ac/yr of BOD_5 for Michigan.

More recent lagoon design provides for a three-cell system with full flexibility of moving the wastewater to any cell. Either a parallel or series operation is possible, with the effluent usually being polished by an onsite land treatment system with eventual discharge to the water table.

Special Systems

When uncommon geologic or other conditions are encountered that have a bearing on the ability to use a typical onsite system, special systems are designed.

Septic Tank–Leaching Pits

At two locations in the state, inconsistent soils made up of granular pockets in basically heavy soils in association with rugged terrain were encountered. Because of good separation from the water table, a system consisting of a septic tank with several leaching pits located over the granular areas was used at both locations. Except for the failing of three leaching pits, which were located incorrectly in the adjacent clay soils, rather than in the granular pockets, the systems have worked satisfactorily.

Recirculating Oil System (Aqua Sans)

An Aqua Sans Recirculating Oil System is being used at one rest area location where there is a combination of low availability of water and heavy soils. Local opposition to sanitary lagoons excluded their possible use, and the nearest sewer was seven miles away.

As a result of a request by the Michigan DOT, the Aqua Sans system was monitored by the National Sanitation Foundation (NSF) for a period of eight months during 1978. The evaluation covered turbidity, color, odor and total coliforms. In general, the system has worked quite well and showed a coliform count of only 1/100 ml in 68 samples analyzed. More recently, some mechanical and plumbing problems have surfaced with this sanitary unit, but efforts are being made to make modifications to the system that would correct these problems.

RESEARCH

In 1974, as a result of the state DOT's concern for the forthcoming more restrictive effluent discharge standards mandated by the Clean Water Act of 1972, a research agreement was entered into with Michigan State University.

The purpose of this project was to evaluate the effectiveness of existing onsite systems in the freeway rest area system and to design and evaluate land treatment systems that could overcome deficiencies of existing systems. The land treatment systems were used to polish and dispose of lagoon effluents or septic tank effluents where soil conditions did not permit tile fields. A wide variety of conditions of soil, landscape, depth to water table and land availability were encountered. Five of these sites will be discussed.

At all sites the performance of the systems was followed by sampling the wastewater before, during and after treatment; sampling the soil at various depths; and sampling the water tables on, adjacent to and at a distance from, the treatment facility. Water samples were analyzed for total coliforms, fecal coliforms, total streptococci, fecal streptococci, biochemical oxygen demand (BOD_5), total organic carbon (TOC), total phosphorus (TP), inorganic phosphate phosphorus (i-PO_4), total Kjeldahl nitrogen (TKN), ammonia nitrogen (NH_4-N), nitrite nitrogen (NO_2-N), nitrate nitrogen (NO_3-N) and suspended solids (SS), according to methods given in the U.S. Environmental Protection Agency (EPA) *Methods Manuals* [1,2].

Septic Tank–Tile Fields

This rest area has a septic tank system that discharges into four rotational tile drainfields. The soils are loam texture with a water table at 25–30 feet below the surface. Wells for water sampling were placed adjacent to, and on all sides of, the drainfield and at distances from the field.

It was found that i-PO_4, TKN, NH_4-N and fecal coliforms do not appear in the water table. NO_3-N is found in the water table adjacent to the drainfield in an average concentration of 25 ppm. The concentration of NO_3-N varies in the well samples, with the lowest well averaging 3.1 ppm and the highest averaging 66 ppm.

This system, which could be considered conventional, is failing with regard to NO_3-N removal, although this NO_3-N is rapidly diluted as it moves through the aquifer.

Septic Tank–Sand Filter–Overland Flow Evapotranspiration

The Ithaca rest area had a septic tank system in which the effluent was pumped into an elevated sand filter, which had tile drains at the base because the poorly drained clay loam soil at the site would not support a conventional drainfield. A schematic cross section of this sand filter is given in Figure 1. Intensive use of this facility during the summer season caused an overloading of the system, with a breakthrough of N, P and coliforms.

An Overland Flow Evapotranspiration System (OF-ET) was designed as an alternate system for summer use and was placed in the median because the rest area property could not be expanded. The OF-ET was placed in the median between the northbound and southbound lanes. It was 20 feet wide and 1600 feet long, with a uniform slope of 0.3%. Reed canary grass, *Phalaris arundinacea*, was planted on the OF-ET. The septic tank effluent, which had a very short retention time during the summer, was collected in a 1000-gallon tank, which was continuously ozonated to oxidize the volatile organics and control odors. Thousand-gallon batches of ozonated effluent were pumped to the control structure at the top of the OF-ET. The adjustable

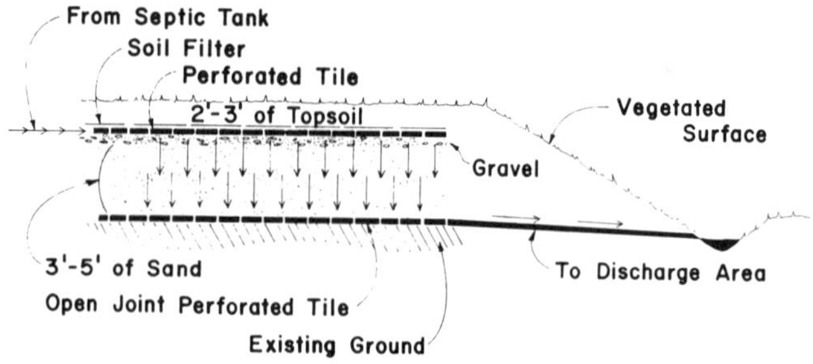

Figure 1. Sand filter section above a clay soil.

notched weir on the control structure distributed the wastewater across the OF-ET. The grass grew well and produced a tortuous path for the shallow flow of effluent. The ozonation and oxidized flow on the EF-ET controlled any potential odor problem.

The system was operated for two months at an average loading of 5000–6000 gpd, which was equivalent to 0.25 inches over the whole OF-ET area. There were peak days in the operation when 12,000–15,000 gpd were applied with no problems.

Measurements of the changes in quality of the wastewater as it moved down the OF-ET showed that all of the parameters except NO_3-N were greatly reduced when the effluent had flowed 400 feet. The NO_3-N concentration peaked at 30 ppm at this distance but declined beyond this point as the grass and denitrification at the soil surface removed NO_3-N from the system. Table I shows the efficiency of both the sand filter and OF-ET in reducing pollutants from septic tank effluent. The sand filter reduced TN only by 28% and TP by 70%, while the OF-ET did better than this at 200

Table I. Percentage Reduction in Pollutants from Septic Tank Effluent Treated by a Sand Filter or an Overland Flow Evapotranspiration System Measured at 200 feet and 800 feet Downslope

Pollutant	Sand Filter (%)	OF-ET (%) 200 ft	OF-ET (%) 800 ft
BOD_5	87	62	91
TP	70	75	89
TN	28	55	98
SS	83		62
Fecal Coliforms	99		99

feet. At 800 feet on the OF-ET, BOD_5 was reduced by 91%, TP by 89% and TN to 98%.

Most of the time the wastewater infiltrated the soil or was evapotranspired so that it never reached the outfall at 1600 feet. During three heavy rains there was some outfall from the system, but only on one was there enough to measure at the weir. This outfall amounted to 1700 gallons, or one-third of one day's application, and had at least a 95% reduction in all parameters.

These two polishing treatment systems complement each other. During the winter season, when the sewage loading is low, the septic tank effluent is one of better quality, and the sand filter satisfactorily polishes the effluent. During the summer season, when the bulk of the sewage is produced, the OF-ET does an excellent polishing of the poorly treated effluent, with little discharge except during heavy rainfall.

Lagoon-Seepage Beds

This system consists of a three-celled lagoon system, which discharges into seepage beds on a level, slowly permeable clay loam soil with a high water table. The water table will fluctuate from the surface in the spring to 5 or 6 feet in a dry summer. This area had adequate space so that the seepage beds could be constructed at the rest area. The seepage beds were designed so that the release of effluent from one of the lagoons would add between 1 and 1.5 feet of wastewater to the bed. This provided good aeration during the seepage process, which proceeded at a rate of 0.5–0.6 in./day.

Sampling wells to reach the shallow water table were placed around the seepage beds and at a distance from them for control samples. Water from these wells was sampled throughout the year and more frequently during discharge. There were seasonal changes in NO_3-N in all of the wells, but never were the wells adjacent to the seepage lagoons different than the control wells.

These lightly loaded seepage beds are filtering the organic matter and microbes, absorbing the phosphate and converting the TN to NO_3-N. The NO_3-N is denitrified in the anaerobic zone just below the flooded soil surface. Because the beds are used only once or twice a year, there is ample time for rejuvenation before recharge. So long as these beds are used during the warm part of the year and when the natural water table is several feet below the surface, this system will perform well.

Lagoon–Overland Flow–Evapotranspiration

This system is on one of the busiest information centers in the state. It is situated in the median with ample land, but with an uneven landscape, variable soils and some soils with high water tables. The system consists of two lagoons with continuous discharge through a sand filter into a ditch that reaches a lake within a half mile. When the continuous discharge was disallowed, an OF-ET was constructed on a 4-acre field that had a soil with 1–3 feet of sand over clay and a slope of 4%. A sketch of the OF-ET is given in Figure 2. The OF-ET had a 23,000-gallon chlorination tank at the top. The chlorinated lagoon effluent was distributed across the top of the OF-ET using perforated flexible plastic drain tile. Six level ditches were plowed across the slope to reduce channeling and to keep the water evenly distributed as it moved down the slope. Reed canary grass was planted over the original wild grasses.

Operation of the system involved operating the lagoons in series, pumping 23,000 gallons of effluent from the second lagoon up to the chlorination tank for overnight chlorination and allowing the chlorinated wastewater to discharge over the OF-ET system for a 6-hour period. The system was usually operated 5 days per week, but could be operated more intensively. Depending on the amount of rainfall, 10–20% of the wastewater added ran off the OF-ET and accumulated in the south catchment for recirculation.

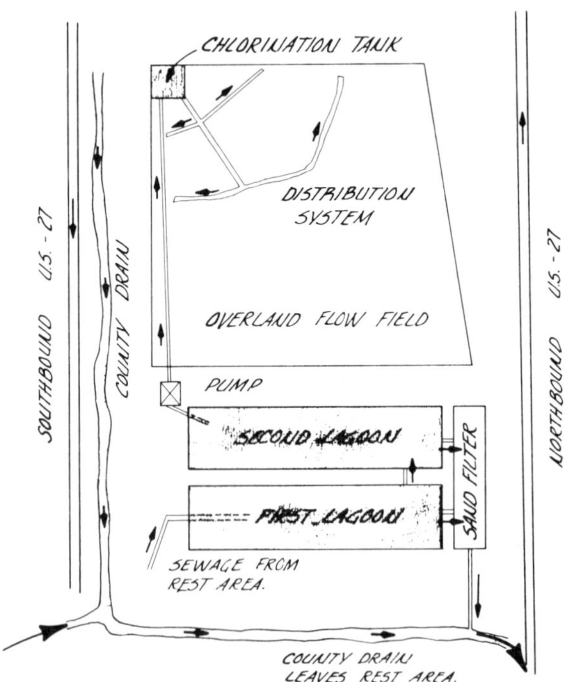

Figure 2. Plan view of overland flow evapotranspiration system.

Water from the ditches, catchments, shallow wells into the perched water table on the OF-ET, and perimeter wells that reached the water table were sampled and analyzed twice a week. The data are summarized in Table II. The concentrations of all the pollutants leaving the OF-ET were very low and the percentage reductions in BOD_5, i-PO_4 and TN were 96%, 97% and 94%, respectively. Only TOC stayed at half its original concentration, but probably was this high only because of the contribution of organic carbon from the dense grass cover. Nitrate-N remained at a constant of about 0.5 ppm, which was probably the limit to which the grass could extract NO_3-N under these conditions. The microbiological studies showed that the lagoon and chlorination had effectively killed those microbes associated with human feces. Any populations in the OF-ET effluent were attributed to wildlife.

For this system to ensure complete evapotranspiration of the effluent, it should be 50% larger; however, the quality of the outfall exceeds any reasonable standards.

Lagoon-Modified Barriered Landscape Water Renovation System

This information center has a two-lagoon system on a sandy loam soil with a water table 3–6 feet below the surface, depending on the season. To eliminate the discharge of the lagoons into a ditch, which leads to a river, a modified Barriered Landscape Water Renovation System (BLWRS) [3,4] was constructed in the highway median using the natural water table as the barrier for the system.

The BLWRS is an efficient land treatment system that uses all the properties of an aerated soil to decompose the organics, nitrify the N to NO_3 and absorb the P. In addition, there is a barrier 4–6 feet below the surface to intercept the water, create an anaerobic environment and direct

Table II. Concentration and Percentage Reduction of Pollutants by an Overland Flow Evapotranspiration System

Pollutant	Concentration (ppm)	Reduction (%)
BOD_5	2.5	96
TOC	32.7	48
i-PO_4	0.09	97
TKN	1.9	97
NH_3-N	0.12	99
NO_3-N	0.45	0
TN	2.35	94
Water		87

the anaerobic water through a trench into which organic matter is placed. In this environment, the denitrifying bacteria will denitrify the NO_3 to nitrogen gas (N_2) and, in this way, remove N from the wastewater. The modified BLWRS as constructed is shown in Figure 3. The natural water table acts as the barrier to direct the anaerobic water through the peat-filled trench as it moves away.

In the operation of the system, lagoon effluent is taken from the second lagoon. The effluent is ozonated continuously in a 12,000-gallon holding tank to reduce the odors. The ozonated effluent is spread on the two-thirds of an acre BLWRS, with low-angle sprinklers operated at low pressure so as not to produce any aerosols. The spraying required 6–8 hours.

Wells on and off the BLWRS were used to obtain water from the top of the aquifer for analysis. Soil samples from the BLWRS were also analyzed to monitor the movement of pollutants through the system. After 10 weeks of spraying during the summer of 1979, there was no change in the C, N, P and microbiological parameters measured in well waters from wells adjacent to, or at a distance from, the BLWRS. All indications are that the system is operating as designed.

CONCLUSIONS

The wide range in conditions at the various freeway rest areas in Michigan has required a variety of onsite treatment systems. Various land treatment

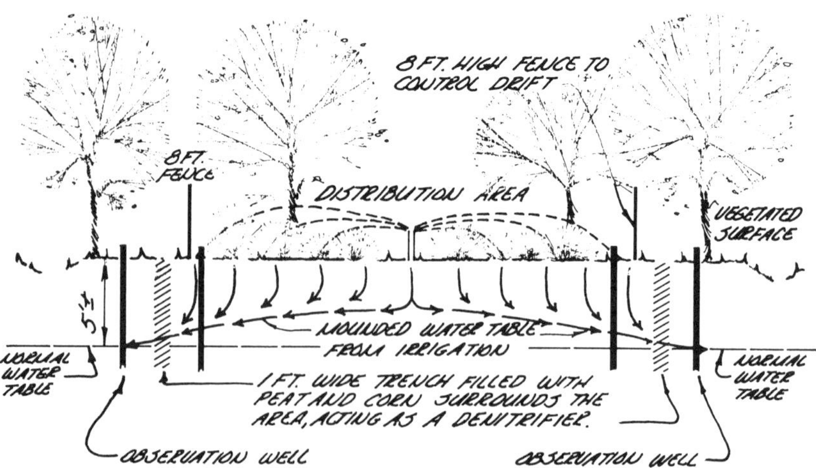

Figure 3. Sketch of a modified barriered landscape water renovation system using a shallow water table as the barrier.

systems have proved useful in treating, polishing and disposing of wastewaters in some cases. The selection of the proper system or combination of systems to match the physical constraints of a particular site can ensure the quality of effluents and dispose of them so that they will not harm the environment.

REFERENCES

1. Office of Technology Transfer, Environmental Protection Agency. "Methods for Chemical Analysis of Water and Waste," EPA-625/6-74-003 U.S. Government Printing Office, Washington, D.C. (1974).
2. Office of Research and Development, Environmental Protection Agency. "Microbial Methods for Monitoring the Environment," EPA-600/8-78-017 U.S. Government Printing Office, Washington, D.C. (1978).
3. Erickson, A. E., J. M. Tiedje, B. G. Ellis and C. M. Hansen. "A Barriered Landscape Water Renovation System for Removing Phosphate and Nitrogen from Liquid Feedlot Waste," *Proc. Int. Livestock Waste Conf.*, Columbus, OH (St. Joseph, MI: American Society of Agricultural Engineers, 1971), pp. 232-234.
4. Erickson, A. E., B. G. Ellis, J. M. Tiedje, A. R. Wolcott, C. M. Hansen, F. R. Peabody, E. C. Miller and J. W. Thomas. "Soil Modification for Denitrification and Phosphate Reduction of Feedlot Waste," EPA-660/2-74-057 (1974).

20

ALTERNATIVE WASTEWATER COLLECTION SYSTEMS FOR SMALL COMMUNITIES

R. C. Jones, P. E. and G. F. DenBesten, P.E.
Williams &Works
Grand Rapids, Michigan

INTRODUCTION

Recently, an increasing number of small communities have undertaken wastewater projects to abate pollution of area groundwater or surface water and/or to comply with state and federal standards. A traditional method of providing public wastewater facilities consists of 8-inch-diameter or larger gravity collector sewers, forcemains, pumping stations and interceptors leading to a central treatment plant. Cost of wastewater treatment is almost always higher for smaller communities because treatment cost is shared by fewer users and collection systems are in areas of lower population density. With the collection (transport) system accounting for 80% of the wastewater system's capital costs, much study has been given to alternative methods. Two alternatives currently receiving considerable attention are pressure and vacuum systems.

The U.S. Environmental Protection Agency (EPA) recognizes financial burdens associated with wastewater systems in small communities. Step 1 Facilities Plans will be carefully reviewed where projected total user costs for wastewater services exceed the following percentage of annual household median incomes:

- 1.5%, when median is less than $6000;
- 2.0%, when median is between $6000 and $10,000
- 2.5%, when median is over $10,000

Federal government incentives that encourage investigation of innovative/alternative methods are (1) an additional 10% federal grant allowance for such systems; (2) a 15% preference for cost-effectiveness; and (3) 100% replacement of defective systems if design goals are not met within two years of completion.

SYSTEM TYPES

Alternative systems receiving the greatest attention are vacuum and pressure sewer systems. Both use small-diameter lines (usually PVC) placed at minimum depth below the frost line. The greatest potential for cost savings occurs where there is a normally high groundwater table and/or scattered home sites, as are frequently found in rural communities, along rural lakeshore areas and in areas of low-lying homes. In severe terrain conditions these may be the only alternatives.

Vacuum System

Of the alternative systems previously mentioned, the vacuum system has been the least popular. Elements of the traditional vacuum system are shown in Figure 1. Vacuum systems depend on a central vacuum source constantly maintaining 15–25 inches of mercury on small-diameter collection mains. A gravity vacuum interface valve separates atmospheric pressure from the vacuum in the mains. The valve can be either in the home sanitary sewer service line or in a vacuum toilet. When the interface valve opens, a volume of sewage enters the main, followed by a volume of atmospheric air. After a preset interval, the valve closes. The packet of liquid, called a slug, is propelled into the main by the differential pressure of vacuum in the main and the higher atmospheric pressure air behind the slug. After a distance, the slug breaks down by shear and gravitational forces, allowing the higher pressure air behind the slug to slip past the liquid. With no differential pressure across it, the liquid then flows to the lowest local elevation and vacuum is restored to the interface valve for subsequent operation. When the next upstream interface valve operates, identical actions occur, with that slug breaking down and air rushing across the second slug. That air then impacts the first slug and forces it farther down the system. After a number of operations the first slug arrives at the central vacuum source. When sufficient liquid volume accumulates in the collection tank at the central vacuum source, a transfer device, such as a sewage pump, delivers the accumulated sewage to a treatment plant.

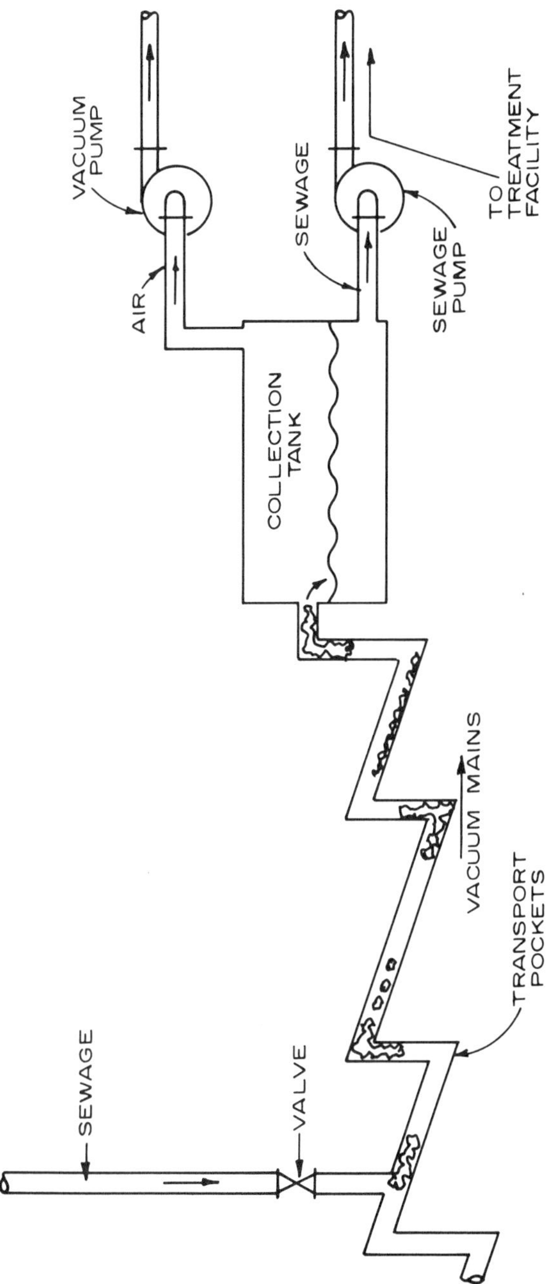

Figure 1. Elements of a vacuum sewage system (courtesy of U.S. EPA).

The problems associated with central vacuum systems are as follows:

1. Malfunction of a household vacuum valve or central vacuum unit can occur, which results in loss of service to a potentially large number of dwellings. If the failure is in the household valve, the malfunctioning valve must quickly be located and isolated. This may necessitate nearly around-the-clock availability of qualified technicians.
2. A potential health hazard exists if the residential vent stack is less than 3 inches in diameter. When the household valve operates it may evacuate traps, allowing gas from local holding tanks to enter homes.

The advantages of vacuum-type systems are as follows:

1. Vacuum toilets use less water, which may affect treatment costs.
2. Standby power may be provided at a central vacuum unit to maintain service during power outages; normally this is impractical where each residence has individual pressure pumping units.

The first vacuum system constructed in the United States was at Lake of the Woods, Virginia. Design and performance of this system have been studied and published by the U.S. Environmental Protection Agency.

The Indiana Department of Natural Resources has reported on a vacuum system constructed at Plainville, Indiana, where the system served a community of 170 homes. The community has experienced high operation and maintenance (O&M) costs and an average of 30 service calls per month. Subsequent remedial work on design- and construction-related problems have reduced these air break service calls to 5 per month.

Pressure Systems

A pressure sewer system consists of two major elements: (1) the onsite pressurization unit, and (2) the transport conduit or pressure main. In all designs, household wastes are collected in the building drain and are either conveyed directly to the pressurization unit or conveyed through a pretreatment unit (septic tank) before entering the pressurization unit. The pressure main can take many forms but generally consists of a single, small-diameter conduit that has numerous feeder lines from each pressurization inlet. This arrangement is desirable because it minimizes sewer retention time. A typical example of a pressure sewer flow diagram is illustrated in Figure 2.

There are two major alternative pressure systems:

1. The first is a pressurization unit consisting of a single grinder pump (GP) (Figure 3) of approximately 10 gpm capacity, in which wastes are received directly from the household and are pumped to the pressure main. These pumps are equipped with cutters on the suction end and are usually of 1.5- to 2-HP

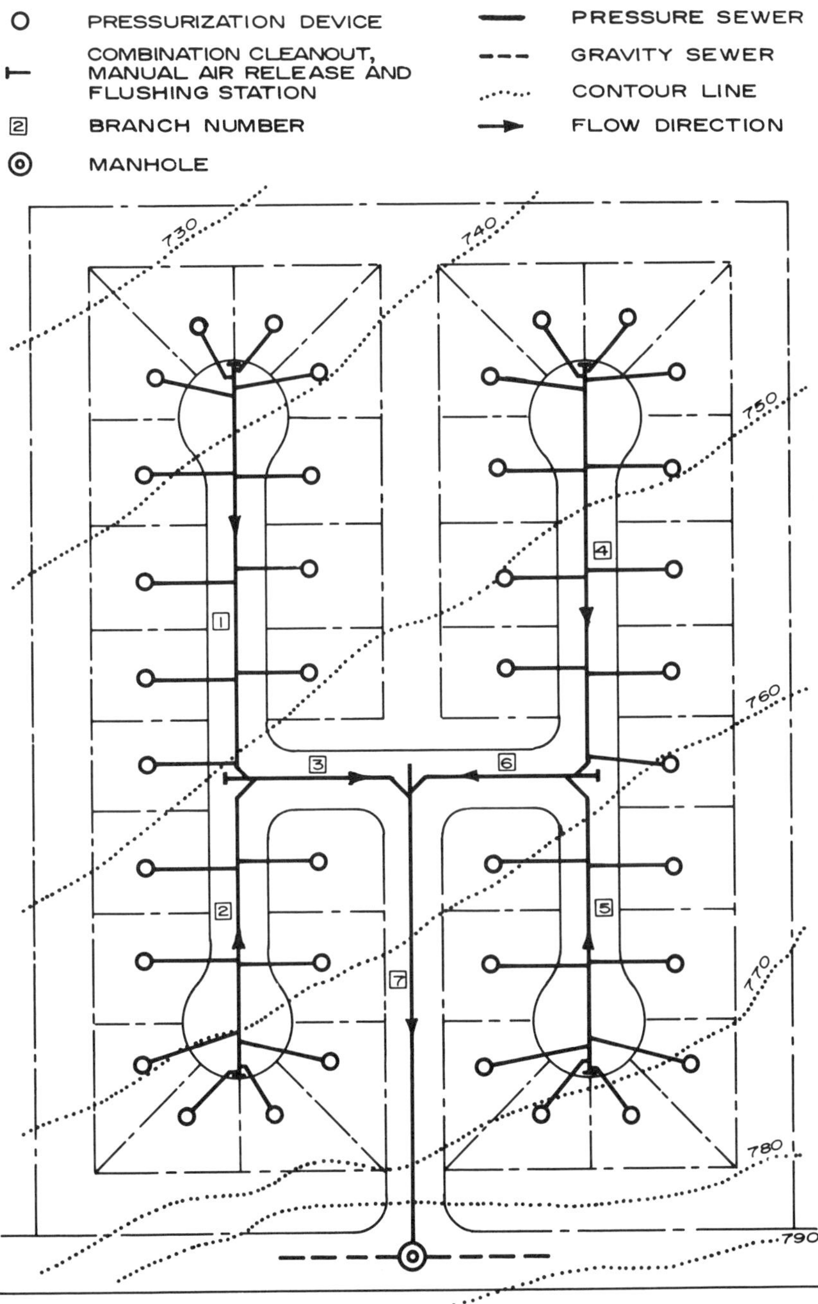

Figure 2. Typical pressure sewer layout (courtesy of U.S. EPA).

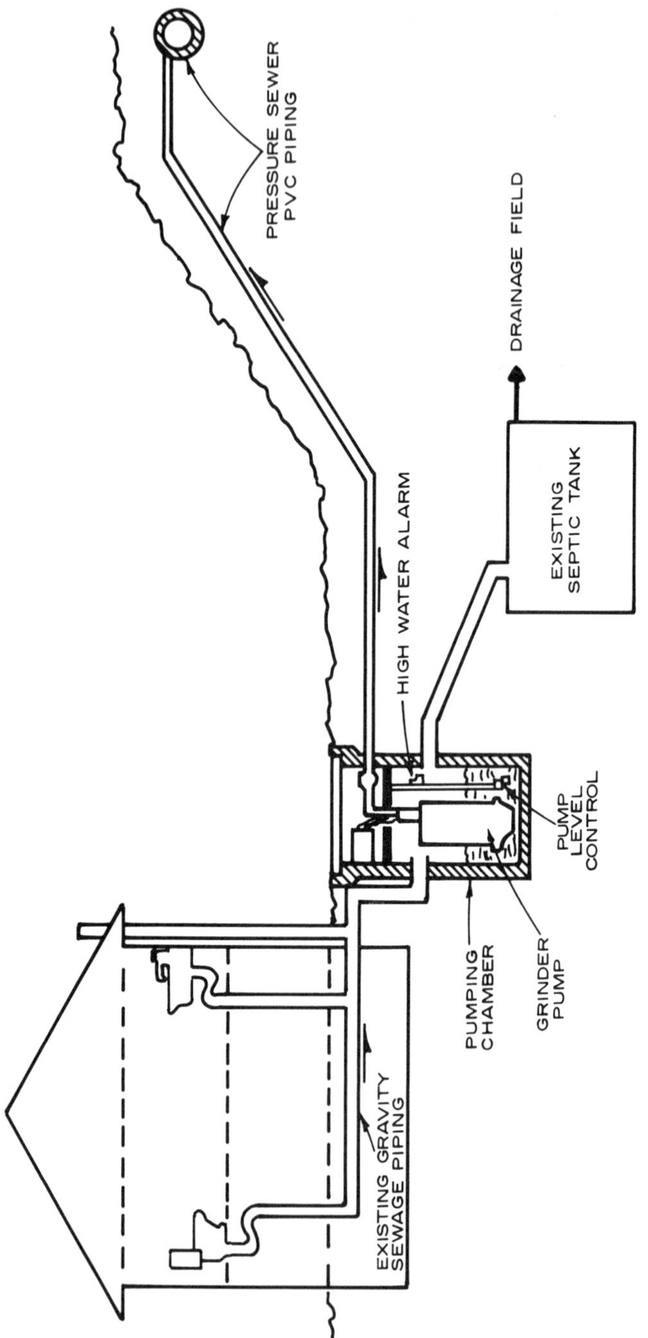

Figure 3. Typical grinder pump installation (courtesy of U.S. EPA).

range. They shred the solids to a size that can pass through the small-diameter pressure line. These types are used to pump to gravity collection systems where terrain requires an individual pressure unit to serve isolated, low-lying homes. The unit is installed in a belowground prefabricated chamber with possible overflow to an existing septic tank for additional storage during power outages. In areas of high seasonal groundwater tables, care must be taken to ensure that overflows are located high enough to prevent groundwater inflow.

2. The second is a pressurization unit consisting of a single septic tank effluent pump (STEP) (Figure 4) of approximately 10 gpm capacity where wastes from an existing or replaced septic tank are pumped to the pressure main. These pumps are normally inexpensive sump pumps, not equipped with solids cutters. They are capable of passing 0.5- to 1-inch solids and usually range from 0.33–0.5 hp.

Both systems normally consist of an easily removed pumping unit. Piping includes isolation and check valves in a fiberglass (FRP) pumping chamber. A second check valve is recommended at the main pressure line or at the property line to provide redundancy and allow servicing of individual pressure lines.

Control is provided normally from mercury float switches to energize and deenergize the pump and to energize an alarm for high water conditions. The control panel is usually mounted on the house exterior and contains pump control and alarms; a combination audio/visual alarm is recommended. Power is provided from the homeowner's existing 220-volt electrical service; an exterior circuit breaker permits maintenance in the homeowner's absence. Power costs are included in the homeowner's monthly power company utility bill and conservative power usage costs for both STEP and GP units are usually from 20–50 cents per month. It is recommended that spare pumping units and controls be available so that equipment can be field changed and then repaired at a more convenient time. Appurtenances required on the mainline pressure sewer are flushing cleanout connections and air relief valves at pipeline high points.

One major cost advantage of pressure sewers is that the pipe need not be laid to line or grade and can be placed to avoid obstacles. Installing a tracer line is recommended when pipe location is field determined. Because pipeline materials are usually of nonconductive materials, a tracer wire is an inexpensive solution for line relocation. Waste production from pressure systems is normally less than for conventional systems—75 gpcd vs 100 gpcd,* and there may be significant treatment cost savings if the lower value is allowed by regulatory agencies.

There are considerations common to both system types. Easements to provide access for maintenance must be obtained by the managing entity

*Estimates vary with source from <50–>100 gpcd.

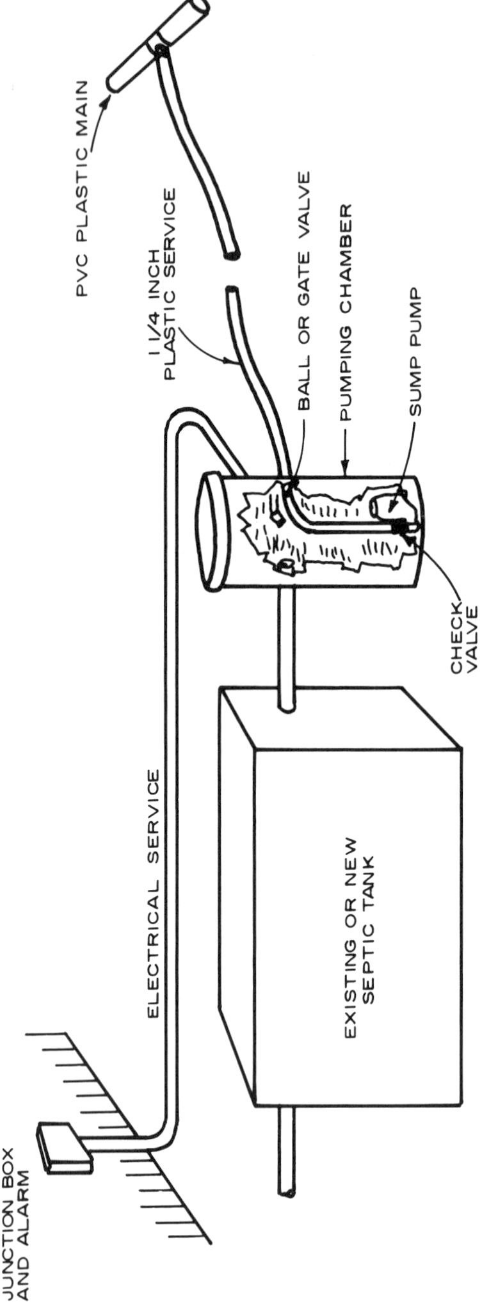

Figure 4. Typical STEP system (courtesy of U.S. EPA).

from all affected property owners. Careful public relations is required during design and construction, as many homeowners are sensitive to the location and appearance of the pumping unit. In some cases it may be necessary to camouflage the installation by means of landscaping. An extensive program for homeowner awareness must be maintained in a successful system; homeowners have been known to turn off alarms rather than notify maintenance personnel.

Grinder Pump Units

The two types of grinder pumps in general use today are the submersible centrifugal type (Hydro-Matic, F. E. Myers, Toran, Peabody Barnes and others) and the progressing cavity, positive displacement type (Environment/One). The centrifugal type will deliver a wide range of varying flows, depending on the number of units connected to the mainlines. The positive displacement type delivers a rather constant flowrate (approximately 11 gpm) against a wide range of discharge heads.

Careful consideration must be given to the mainline hydraulic gradient when selecting centrifugal pumping units for pressure sewer systems because the pumping rate of an individual unit will vary significantly with line pressure, depending on the number of other units operating simultaneously.

Solid materials are frequently found in normal wastewaters. Dry hard objects may enter and stop a centrifugal pump (until the object is removed) without causing any damage. On the other hand, a stone or similar object is likely to pass through a progressing cavity type, but, in so doing, may cause permanent rotor damage.

Because grinder pumps receive direct household wastes, some grease-related problems may be expected, especially where the household has a garbage grinder. There have been station malfunctions where grease accumulation on control floats was excessive; periodic washdown of floats may be required. Examination of pressure lines at one operational system has reportedly revealed a noticeable reduction of pipeline diameter, resulting in reduced carrying capacity attributable to grease buildup.

STEP Units

As noted earlier, the STEP unit is the pressurization unit receiving waste after it has passed through a standard septic tank. The basic overall advantage to this system is the treatment accomplished in the septic tank. Waste characteristics of typical septic tank, household waste and municipal waste are generally as follows:

Parameter	Septic Tank Effluent [1-3]	Household Waste Without Grinder	Household Waste With Grinder [4]	Medium Municipal [5]
BOD_5	100-180	415	465	200
SS	50-75	296	394	200
Grease	10-20	123	129	100

Specific advantages for this type of system are as follows:

1. The pressurizing pump can be an inexpensive submersible sump pump capable of handling 0.5- to 1-inch solids, as larger solids are settled out in the septic tank; high-horsepower pumps are not required for solids shredding.
2. The 1.5- to 2-foot clear space at the tank top can be utilized for storage of approximately a 24-hour flow during power outages.
3. Grease-related problems previously described are eliminated, as grease is trapped in the septic tank.

Septage can be disposed of in a variety of ways, depending on the facilities available. The following are a few that may be considered:

1. Land Disposal. This is perhaps the most frequently used method of septage disposal (spreading with a truck). The main restrictions are any heavy metals present (although not likely in rural systems) and nitrogen loading. Soil bacteria will transform the rich septage ammonia nitrogen to nitrate nitrogen, which may be leached below the plant root zone. Storage facilities will be needed to hold septage during precipitation to prevent runoff and to allow for bacteria dieoff.
2. Composting. This would require ample availability of a mixing agent (wood chips, etc.) and heavy equipment, and an end use for the product.
3. Transport to Treatment Facilities. Nearby sewage treatment plants are also a frequent acceptor of septage. Septage has been disposed of by adding it to the liquid stream or the sludge stream. In any case, the effect of adding septage must be studied for its effect on the treatment process. A properly designed septage handling facility should be provided that incorporates unloading, screening, degritting, equalization and controlled addition facilities, as sludge dumping of septage may upset treatment systems. The unloading station should be hard surfaced with washdown facilities.

EXISTING PROJECT EXPERIENCE

Willliams & Works has been, and is currently, involved in the design of numerous wastewater collection systems that incorporate hundreds of grinder pump stations. As examples, two systems completed by the firm are discussed below. The first was designed in 1972 and completed in 1974, so several years of operational experience are available; the other was completed in 1979.

The Harbor Springs area wastewater facility serves the city of Harbor Springs, Michigan, as well as inland lakeshore areas in Little Traverse and Littlefield Townships, plus the village of Alanson and unincorporated community of Conway (Figure 5). The collection system is basically a gravity and pumped sewer system constructed in 1972-74, but has 50 individual grinder pumps. There are two small localized pressure systems, with a total of 17 individual residential grinder pump units discharging to a gravity line at two locations. The majority of the remaining grinder units serve individual low-lying homes, where it was more cost-effective to install a grinder pump discharging to a gravity line than to lower several thousand feet of gravity line in areas of high groundwater tables.

Average costs at that time for 27 single grinder pump units were $2431/unit. The cost for a 1.25-inch polyethylene pressure service line averaged $5.90/ft. Thus, the total cost for serving an individual low-lying home was

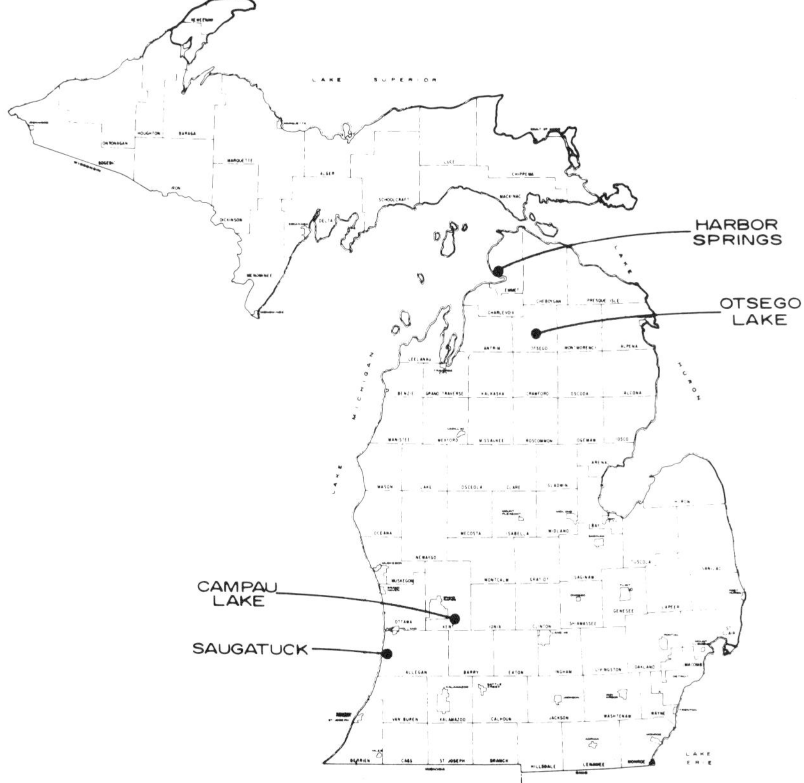

Figure 5. Location map.

approximately $2950 (with curb stop and an average of 75 feet of 1.25-inch service). Disadvantages associated with this system are as follows:

1. A large percentage of septic tanks will be found inadequate and will need to be replaced during construction.
2. Odors can be expected where a pressure system discharges to a gravity manhole because of anaerobic conditions.
3. The waste pumped is more corrosive; plastic pump impellers are preferred.
4. The septic tanks must be pumped every three to five years to retain the effectiveness of the system.
5. The septage must be disposed of suitably.

STEP systems have been constructed in Idaho and Oregon. The consultant on the Oregon project indicates that service call frequency has been approximately 18 months per unit, and pump replacement appears to be required about every five years. In areas where many tanks need to be replaced, it may be advantageous to install a complete prefabricated FRP combination septic tank and pumping chamber for uniformity.

Typical septage characteristics as published by EPA [6] are as follows:

Parameter	Mean Concentration[a]	Minimum Reported	Maximum Reported	Variability[b]
Total Solids (TS)	40,000	1,132	130,475	115
Total Volatile Solids (VS)	26,000	4,500	71,402	16
Total Suspended Solids (SS)	15,000	310	93,378	301
Volatile Suspended Solids (VSS)	18,100	3,660	51,500	14
Five-Day Biochemical Oxygen Demand (BOD_5)	5,000	440	78,600	179
Chemical Oxygen Demand (COD)	45,000	500	703,000	469
Total Organic Carbon (TOC)	15,000	316	96,000	73
Total Kjeldahl Nitrogen (TKN)	600	66	1,900	29
NH_3(N)	150	6	380	63
NO_2	0.7	0.1	1.3	13
NO_3	3	0.1	11	110
Total P	150	20	760	38
PO_4	64	10	170	17
Alkalinity	1,020	522	4,190	8
Grease	9,561	604	23,368	39
pH (units)	6 to 9	1.5	12.6	8
LAS	150	110	200	2

[a]Values represent ratio of maximum to minimum values.
[b]All values in mg/l, except where noted.

Assuming a community of 1000 people with 285 homes, nearly 50,000 gallons per year of septage would have to be disposed of at 600 gallons/tank, and tanks would have to be pumped at 3 1/2-year intervals.

There were two instances in this project where alternative construction bids were received for pressure vs gravity systems. The locations were in the villages of Alanson and Conway. The following is a comparison of the two alternatives:

	Conway	Alanson
A		
6-inch house service	400 ft[a]	500 ft
8-inch gravity line	740 ft	846 ft
Forceline	–	410 ft
Lift stations	–	1
Cost	$65,542	$66,766
B		
Single grinder pump station	8	10
1.25- to 3-inch forceline	1470 ft	2520 ft
Cost	$73,010	$49,100

[a]Estimated.

Obviously the pressure sewer alternative proved costly in Conway, while the opposite was true in Alanson.

In previously mentioned areas where pressure systems were installed, the main pressure line in the streets ranged in size from 1.5–3 inches. The cost of the main pressure line serving 17 homes averaged $1150 per home plus $2950 for pump and service line, for a total of $4100 per home for a small pressure system.

The Harbor Springs Area Sewage Disposal Authority began keeping records of the time required for maintenance of grinder pump units. Records for 1978 indicate a total of 328.5 hours, including 43 hours for callouts for the 50 units. This would indicate approximately one callout per unit per year, assuming one hour per callout; regular preventive maintenance required an average of 5.7 hours per year. The preceding would indicate a monthly maintenance cost of $3.90 per unit, assuming employee wages of $1200 per month. Pump replacement costs would need to be included in an overall O&M budget, with a 10-year pump life being reasonable for budgeting.

All grinder pumps in the Harbor Springs system are Hydro-Matic units. The client reports that most problems encountered are related to grease accumulation on pumps and controls. The grease interferes with the action of float-activated mechanical switches, causing the control float switch to "stick" in the open or closed position. Over the life of the system, three pump motors have burned out when the control float switch has become "stuck" in the open position. Present design utilizes suspended mercury float switches, which are expected to reduce or eliminate this problem.

The other significant problem has been the winter freezing of individual discharge lines where the pipe is installed at an insufficient depth. Lines would be especially susceptible where residents are seasonal, as is typical of Harbor Springs. Operating personnel indicate that they are able to thaw a frozen section within 200 feet of the pumping unit by removing the pump and feeding hot water into the discharge line. Operators in other areas indicate that a sodium chloride salt solution placed in discharge lines is effective where there are no winter inhabitants.

The second installation is a wastewater collection and treatment project to serve the villages of Saugatuck and Douglas, Michigan. This project was bid in early 1978 and is now operational. Fifty-three single and double grinder pump units were bid at unit costs of $6766 and $9750, respectively. In one particular area within the village of Douglas there was a concentrated area of 38 low-lying homes and cottages along the Lake Michigan shoreline. A gravity sewer was constructed along Lakeshore Drive, considerably above typical house elevations. All residents were served by single grinder pump units, with the exception of a double grinder pump unit where a home and adjacent cottage were owned by a single property owner. Except for five units that discharged directly into the gravity system, the remainder were served by small pressure systems with groups of four to seven grinder pump units connected to a main pressure line with discharge to the gravity sewer line.

The cost of 29 single grinder pump units, 4 double grinder pump units and pressure line averaged approximately $7800 per property owner. The equipment installed is manufactured by F. E. Myers Company; and the collection system is operational, with grinder pumping units operating satisfactorily.

Planned Projects

Caledonia Township in Kent County, Michigan and Otsego Lake in Otsego County, Michigan are among a number of projects in the planning stage where alternative systems are being evaluated. The Caledonia Township project consists basically of serving the Campau Lake area. In accordance with the requirements of PRM 78-9, alternatives under consideration are as follows:

I. Conventional gravity sewer system with land application treatment.

II. Rehabilitation of individual septic tanks, small-diameter gravity sewer system with two community drainfields, and subsurface land application of septage.

III. Pressure sewer system with grinder pumps, and community septic tank and drainfield with subsurface land application of septage (excluding from the collection and treatment system a small area on the southeast where the groundwater table, soils, topography and lot size are conducive to septic tank and tile field systems). Onsite systems in this area would be upgraded to meet current county regulations.

IV. Rehabilitation of individual onsite septic tanks with pressure sewer system, consisting of septic tank effluent pumps (STEP), septic tank pumpout and land application of effluent at a central treatment facility (12 acres of lagoons and 27 acres of irrigation). Septage would be periodically pumped and injected into the soil at the treatment facility.

Cost-effective analysis showed alternative II to be the most cost-effective, with alternative I only slightly more; alternative IV was the least cost-effective. The estimated local cost for alternative II was significantly lower than alternative I because a larger portion of cost was eligible for grant funding. The following is a display of the costs:

	Alternative I	Alternative II	Alternative III	Alternative IV
Total Net Present Worth	$3,740,000	$3,478,000	$4,535,000	$4,932,000
Total Local Cost	$1,009,000	$ 592,000	$ 577,000	$ 942,000

The present recommendation to the community is to select alternative II for Step 2 design but with parallel design and bidding of both I and II, with the final selection based on actual bids received.

The proposed wastewater project for the Otsego Lake Area consists principally of serving 10–11 miles of the Otsego Lake shoreline. A feasibility study conducted earlier this year to evaluate a completely pressurized STEP system in comparison with a conventional system (with land treatment) found, as in the Campau Lake project, that the STEP pressure system was not cost-effective. Currently, various combinations of individual onsite treatment, community septic tank and drainfields, and reduced central treatment are being evaluated.

SUMMARY AND CONCLUSIONS

The overall goal of wastewater projects is pollution abatement at the least cost to the individual community. Past and present experience has shown that alternative pressure systems are a reliable and often less costly means of wastewater transport and may become even more appealing as experience is gained and technologies improve. However, the choice of system must depend on the system or the combination of system types that will best serve the needs of the community.

REFERENCES

1. Weibel, S. R., C. P. Straub and J. R. Thoman. *Studies on Household Sewage Disposal Systems–Part 1*, U.S. Public Health Service Publication (1949).
2. Bendixen, T. W., M. Berk, I. P. Sheehy and S. R. Weibel. *Studies on Household Sewage Disposal Systems–Part 2*, U. S. Public Health Service Publication (1950).
3. Weibel, S. R., T. W. Bendixen and J. B. Coulter. *Studies on Household Sewage Disposal Systems–Part 3*, U. S. Public Health Service Publication No. 397 (1954).
4. Witt, M., R. Siegrist and W. C. Boyle. "Rural Household Wastewater Characterization," in *Home Sewage Disposal, Proc. Am. Soc. Ag. Eng.* (1975).
5. Metcalf and Eddy, Inc. *Wastewater Engineering* (New York: McGraw-Hill Book Co., 1972).
6. Kreissl, J. F. Memo on Septage Analysis, U.S. Environmental Protection Agency, Cincinnati, OH (February 2, 1976).

21

PRESSURIZED SUBSURFACE EFFLUENT DOSING–THE TEXAS EXPERIENCE

Sherman W. Hart
Chief, Division of Wastewater Technology
Texas Department of Health
Austin, Texas 78756

INTRODUCTION

A somewhat unique method for disposing of domestic wastewater effluent was introduced in Texas several years ago by Z Industries, Friendswood, Texas, manufacturers of the Nutt-Shell sewage treatment system. This disposal method, identified as Pressurized Subsurface Effluent Dosing (PSED), has proved to be an effective, efficient method of onsite wastewater disposal, particularly in soils that are marginally suited for conventional septic tank-absorption field systems. This chapter focuses on the evolution of PSED; current empirical design criteria; descriptions of process variations; and problems encountered with the system.

DESCRIPTION OF THE PROCESS

The PSED process consists of pumping treated effluent through small-diameter perforated pipe into an enclosed (covered) trench (Figures 1-4). The effluent is either absorbed into the surrounding soil or rises to the surface and is dissipated to the atmosphere by evapotranspiration. A low-pressure pump is utilized for this process, with controls provided to turn the pump on and off and for an alarm in case of system malfunction. Dosing is accomplished by pumping the effluent from a separate compartment (pump well) and establishing a fixed quantity of effluent to be pumped when the pump is activated.

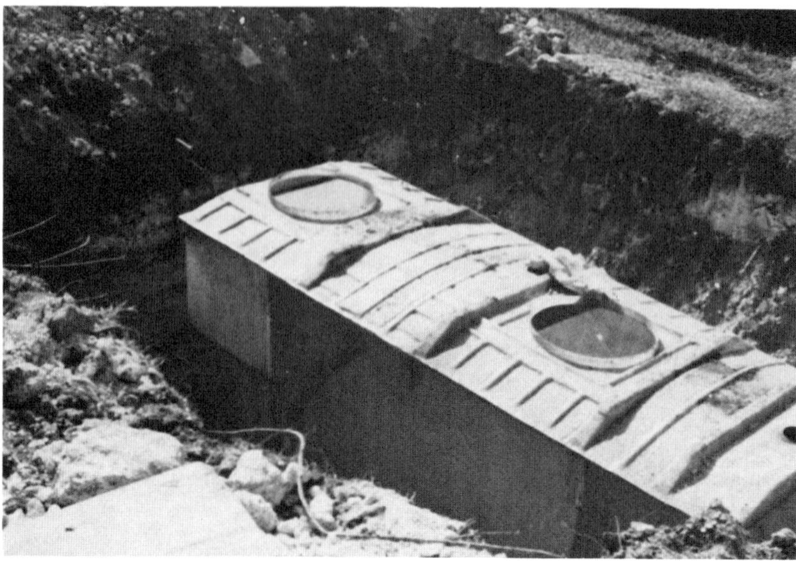

Figure 1. Installation of a typical Nutt-Shell aerobic treatment unit with self-contained pump well.

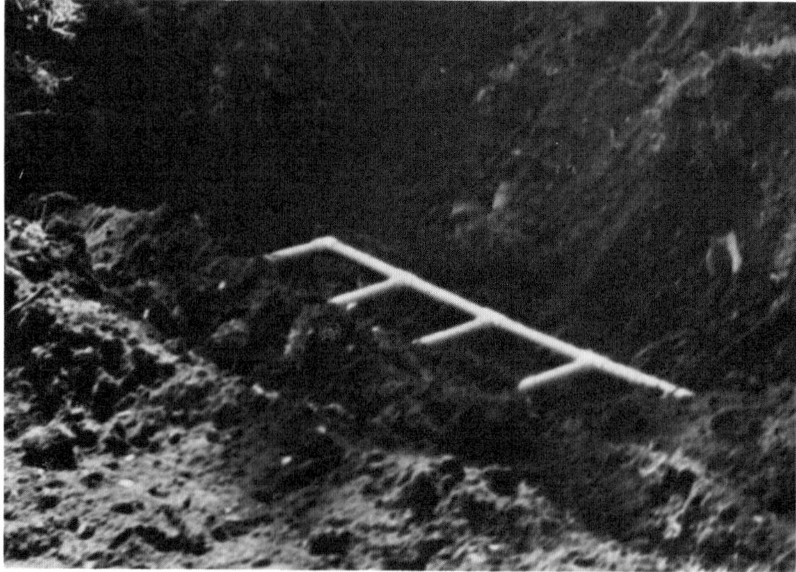

Figure 2. Typical bed installation for combining soil absorption with evapotranspiration for effluent disposal.

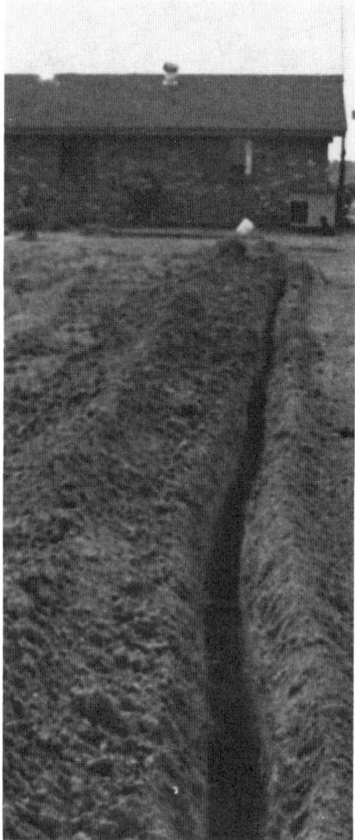

Figure 3. Typical narrow trench dosing installation with one trench uncovered.

EVOLUTION OF THE PROCESS IN TEXAS

The initial systems utilizing pressure dosing were installed in Montgomery County, Texas (near Houston) which is experiencing an extremely high growth rate. Subdivisions were constructed on soils totally unsuited for conventional septic tank systems prior to the adoption of county septic tank regulations. Many of these subdivisions experienced almost complete septic tank system failure at each dwelling in the subdivision. Partially treated effluent was surfacing in the backyards of the dwellings and flowing into barrow ditches. Public health nuisance conditions abounded, and the local health department was concerned about the possibility of disease transmission.

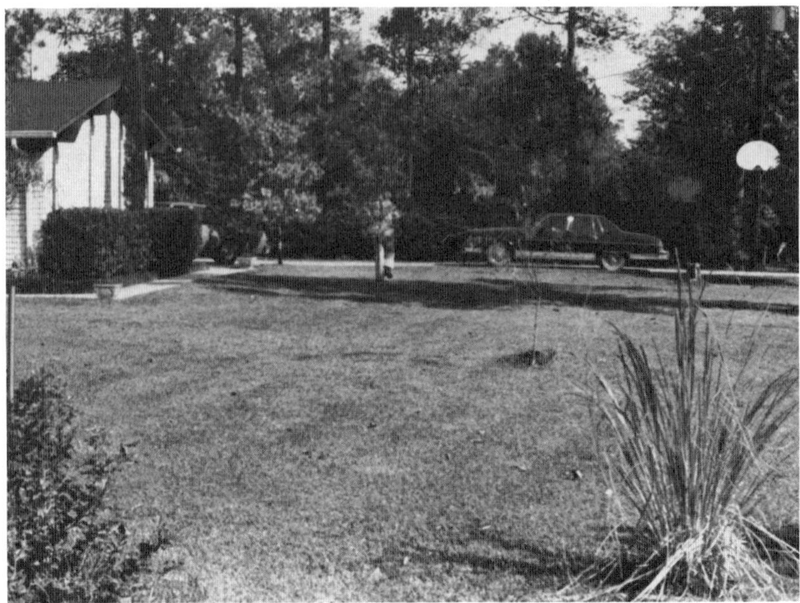

Figure 4. PSED system operating properly. Note striations in grass locating covered dosing pipe.

Montgomery County officials were approached by the manufacturers of the Nutt-Shell aerobic treatment system, who were granted permission to install some of these systems on an experimental basis in the abovementioned subdivisions. It was concluded that any improvement over the existing situation would be helpful. A considerable decrease in surfacing effluent was observed after the systems were installed. The system has been refined during the last five years and has evolved into an excellent method of subsurface effluent disposal.

ADVANTAGES AND DISADVANTAGES OF THE PSED PROCESS

The greatest advantage of the PSED process over a conventional septic tank drainfield is the cost of materials and installation. Because treated effluent is pumped through small-diameter perforated pipe, the cost per lineal foot is much less than that of conventional drainfield pipe (Figure 5). This small-diameter pipe is buried directly in trenches without gravel bedding,

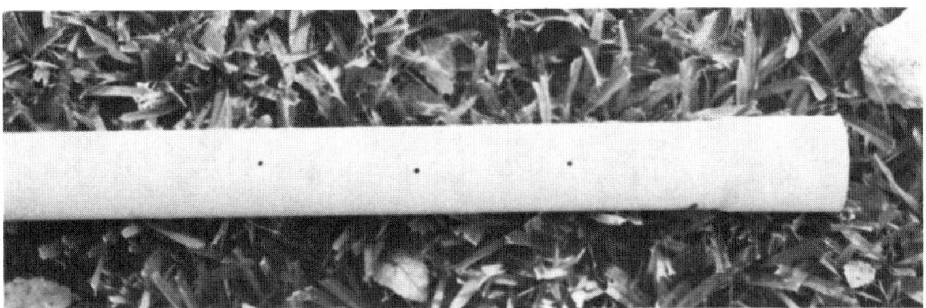

Figure 5. Typical pipe used in the PSED systems. The above illustration is 1 1/4-inch-diameter pipe with 1/8-inch-diameter holes drilled on approximately 3-inch centers.

which eliminates the cost for the gravel and associated transportation costs. Moreover, narrow trenches are utilized, reducing excavation cost. Compaction and smearing of trench walls are less than would occur if the system were installed by a backhoe, as is generally the case with conventional trenches. The overall cost reduction makes it economically feasible to literally install thousands of feet of drainfield to obtain large soil–effluent contact areas. The extensive soil–effluent contact areas receiving periodic dosing of the effluent permit subsurface disposal of wastewaters in tight soils.

The major disadvantages of the PSED process are the operation and maintenance (O&M) costs associated with the mechanical equipment. A positive-pressure pump is required along with some method to control the pressure in the drainfield. On–off and alarm switches are also required to control the pump. In most cases the pumping system is preceded by some type of aerobic treatment unit, which contains a mechanical aerator. All these items will require periodic maintenance and replacement at the homeowner's expense. For this reason, PSED systems that minimize mechanical components are desirable.

PSED EMPIRICAL DESIGN CRITERIA

Through cooperation with the Nutt-Shell company, various local health departments and the Texas Department of Health, general design criteria have evolved for a typical PSED installation (Figure 6). These criteria are empirical in nature and based on observations and modifications of existing PSED systems currently in use in Texas. To date, more than 300 of these systems have been installed in all areas of the state except in far West Texas.

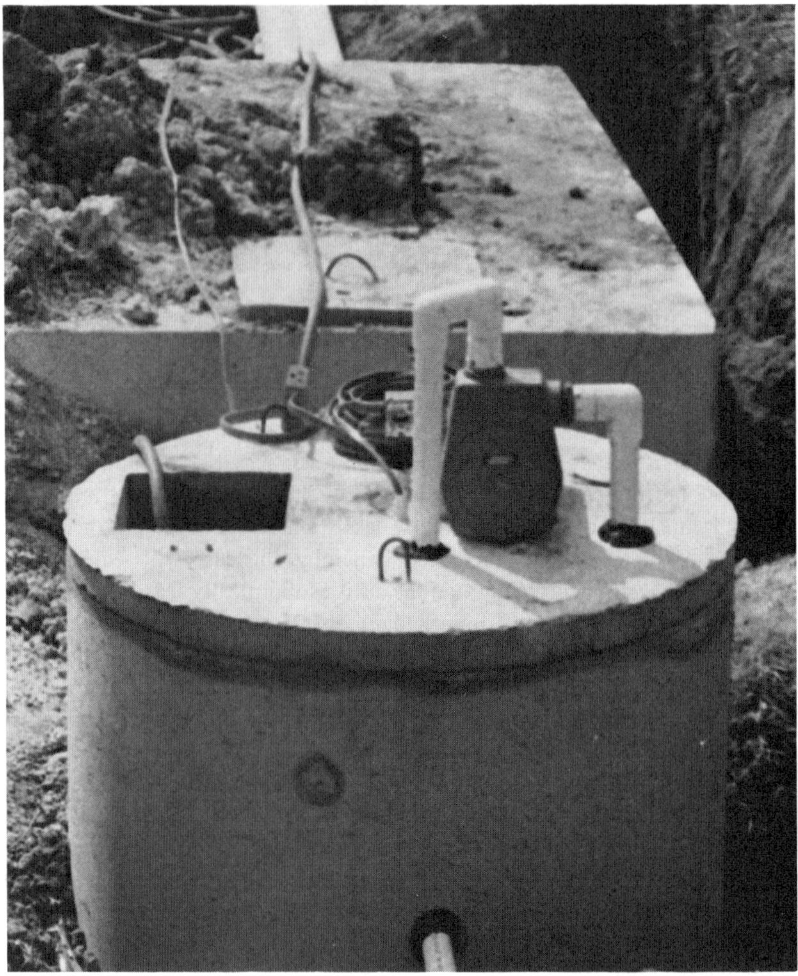

Figure 6. Unique design currently under study that uses a PSED system following a two-stage (baffled) septic tank. Pump well with pump on top is in foreground.

Pipe Specifications

The perforated pipe used to distribute the effluent is constructed of polyvinylchloride (PVC), polyethylene (PE) or similar materials, and ranges in diameter from 1–2 inches. Holes of $\frac{1}{8}$-inch diameter are drilled through the pipe inline on approximately 3-inch centers. Standard tees, elbows and other fittings are used to construct a gridded distribution system (Figure 7).

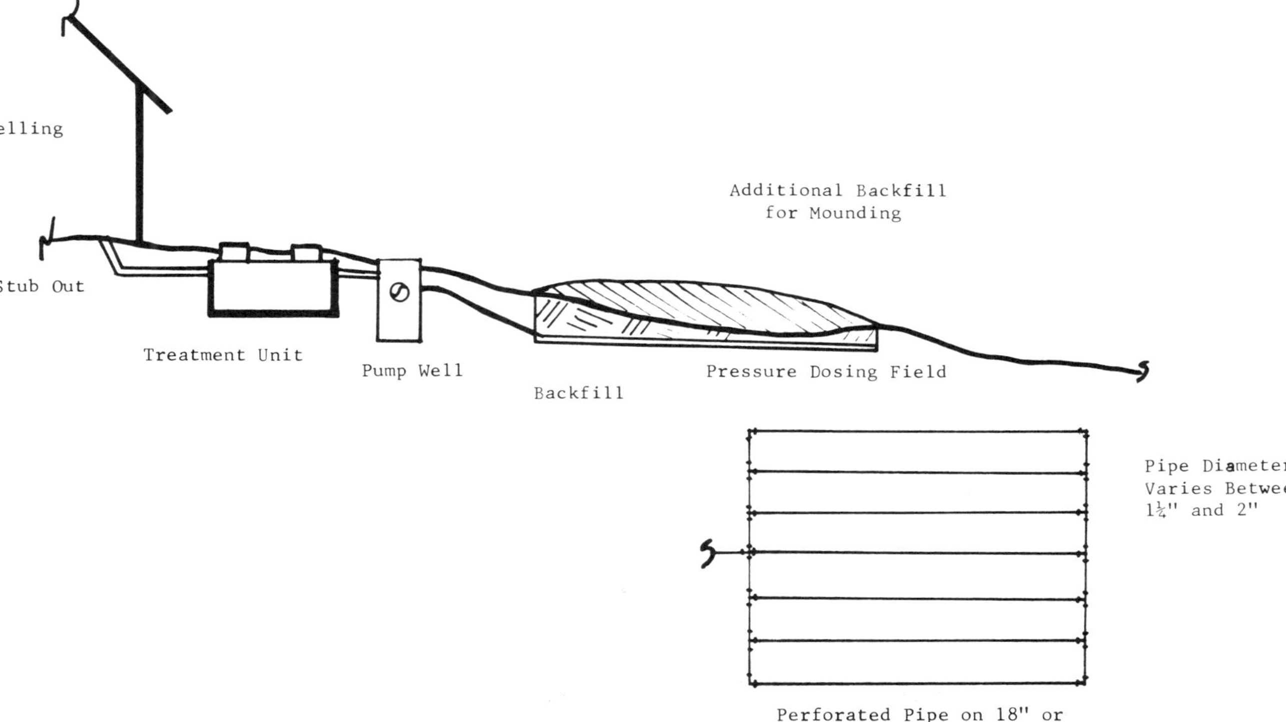

Figure 7. Typical pressure dosing system.

Trench Construction and Sizing

Trenches are excavated to a depth that varies from 18 to 30 inches, depending on soil conditions (Figure 8). In very tight clay soils the trenches are shallow (18 inches), while deep trenches (30 inches) are used in sandy soils. Trench width is not important; however, trench widths are usually held to a minimum of 6 inches to minimize excavated material. The pipe is placed in the trench with the perforations toward the trench bottom. It is very important that all the trench bottom in the overall drainfield locations be level and on the same elevation for equal effluent distribution.

The trenches are sized according to the specifications in Figure 9, which was derived from the state of Texas septic tank standards and is based on the assumption that each lineal foot of pressure line is equivalent to one square foot of conventional absorption trench area [1]. The number of feet of pressure pipe per gallon of effluent per day varies from approximately 9 inches at percolation rates of 5 minutes per inch to 10 feet at rates approaching 140 minutes per inch. The trenches should be spaced no closer than 18 inches and line lengths restricted to 100 feet or less to minimize pressure loss in the pipe.

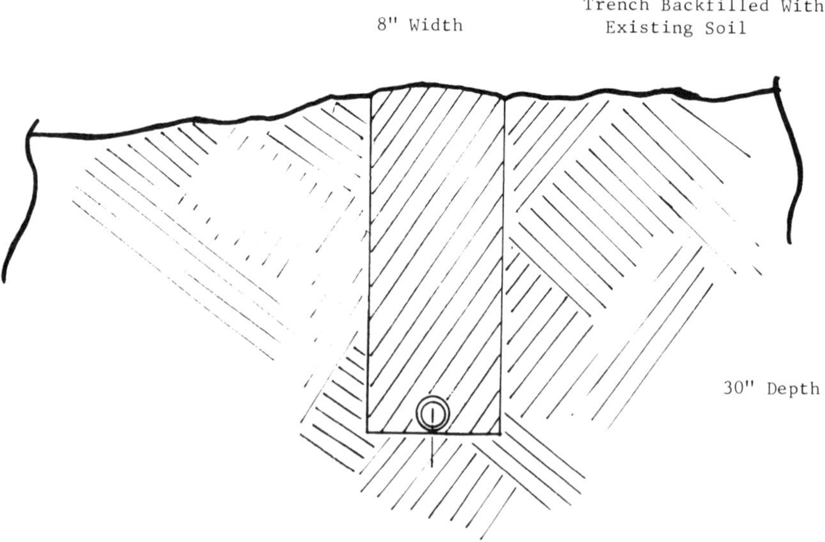

Figure 8. Typical cross section of a PSED trench in soil with medium-to-low permeability.

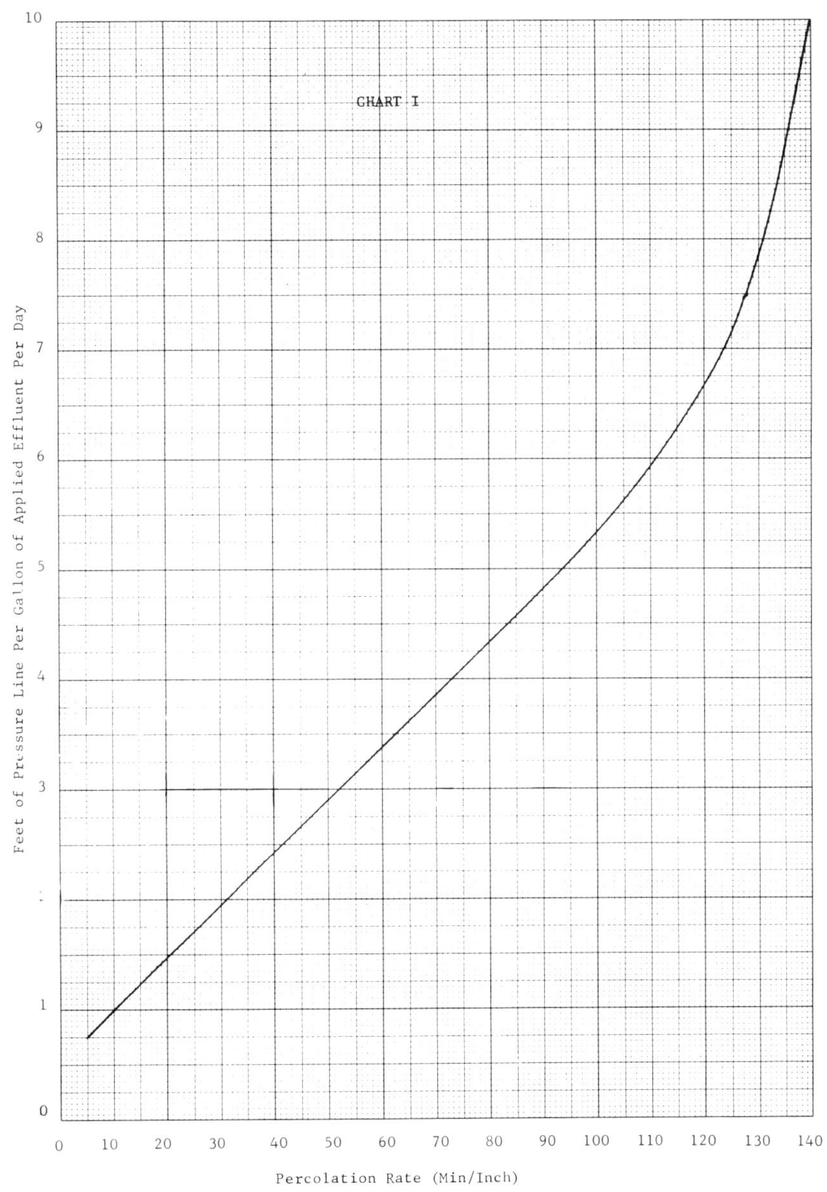

Figure 9. Specifications for sizing the trenches for a PSED system.

Soil percolation should be evaluated very carefully utilizing a good percolation test procedure, such as the one described by Dr. Timothy Winneberger [2]. The soil structure should also be investigated to determine the ultimate trench depth. Experience in installing pressure dosing systems is invaluable in arriving at the proper depth of trench (based on the above considerations). If the soil is layered, for example, it may be possible to construct a trench so that the sidewalls are in contact with a permeable soil layer, although the topsoil may be a heavy clay. In this case deep trenches should be employed, even though the topsoil type would indicate the use of shallow trenches. The recommended procedure for trench evaluation is as follows:

1. Remove a core sample of soil to a depth of at least 36 inches.
2. Identify soil type of dominant structure (clay, clay loam, silt, sand, etc.).
3. Determine whether any soil stratification is present.
4. If no stratification is present, conduct at least four percolation tests at four separate locations.
5. If stratification is present, conduct a percolation test in the soil layer(s) that appear to be the most permeable.
6. Size pressure distribution system accordingly.

In cases where the topsoil is permeable and subsoil consists of clay, the trenches may be constructed in the clay but a permeable soil cover used to permit the effluent to move up into the topsoil (Figure 10). Obviously, the primary design consideration is to introduce the effluent directly into the most permeable soil layer or to provide a path for the effluent to reach a permeable soil layer.

Pump Design and Pumping Specifications

The pump, pump well and controls used in a PSED system must be designed to provide proper pressure and flowrate so that a dosing cycle compatible with the subsurface field can be maintained. Under normal conditions for single-family dwellings, three to four dosing cycles per day are required, with approximately 100 gallons of effluent discharged to the dosing field per cycle. Large dosing fields in very tight soils require larger quantities of effluent dosed per cycle and fewer cycles per day. Maximum dosing pressure at the pump should not exceed 3 psi. Pressure loss through the dosing field will reduce this pressure to approximately 1.5–2.0 psi. If the pump will supply a higher pressure than 3 psi at the desired flowrate, some provision must be built into the system to control pressure. The simplest type of flow control consists of a valved bypass line, which will return some of the effluent back to the pump well.

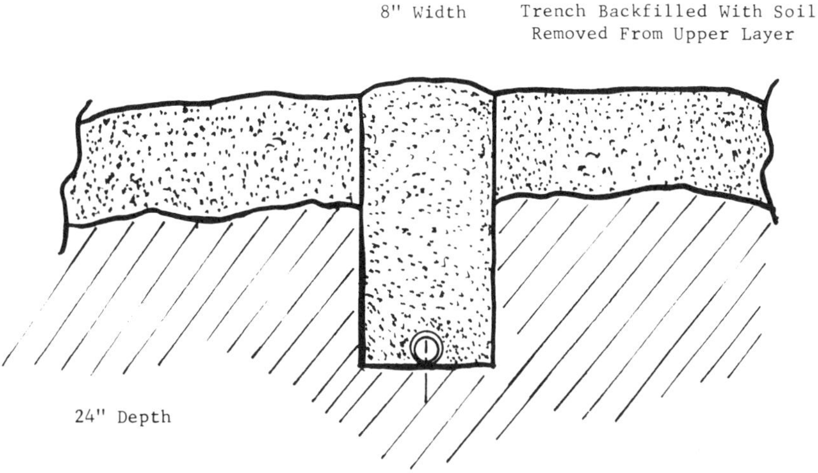

Figure 10. Typical trench cross section in layer soil with the upper soil layer having good absorptive characteristics.

The pumps must be constructed to operate in an anaerobic environment and should be capable of pumping small solids. Several reasonably priced satisfactory pumps are currently being marketed. Mercury float switches should be used to turn pumps off and on and to provide a high water alarm should difficulty arise.

Pump wells must be sized to hold at least one dosing cycle of effluent (approximately 100 gallons) plus additional storage in case of pump failure. The optimum size for pump wells is considered to be 150- to 300-gallon capacity. Concrete or fiberglass tanks may be purchased in this size range and are often utilized as pump wells. Pump wells are an integral part of the Nutt-Shell systems, thus eliminating the cost for an extra tank.

PSED PROCESS VARIATIONS

Another advantage of the PSED system over gravity systems is evident when one considers alternate methods of effluent disposal, such as evapotranspiration beds and mound construction. As long as sufficient surface area is available, the configuration or elevation of the effluent disposal area is not critical because the effluent is pumped into the area and the pump can be adjusted to compensate for rather large changes in elevation.

Evapotranspiration beds are used to a considerable extent in Texas, especially in the more arid parts of the state. A rather simple pressure-dosed system can be constructed by excavating a large area (2000 square feet or more) to a depth of 2 feet and filling the area with sand after installing a gridded pressure piping system. The top of this excavation is then mounded with topsoil, and plants and grasses with good transpiration qualities are planted. This type of construction eliminates the need for conventional gravel bedding and sand wicks normally required in evapotranspiration system design.

By eliminating the excavation and building the system above the ground, a mound design is created and can be used in areas with high groundwater tables. Mound systems used in conjunction with PSED have been installed on the coastal plains of Texas with good results.

PSED PROBLEMS

There is virtually no onsite system that is totally free of operating problems or periodic failure. PSED is certainly no exception, and a brief discussion of the major system pitfalls is in order here.

It is imperative that PSED systems be maintained properly because they utilize several mechanical components. Most homeowners will not provide adequate maintenance and often it is difficult to find someone to repair the systems. Plumbers and septic tank installers are not familiar with the process. Therefore, if many of these systems are to be installed in a subdivision, some type of maintenance contract should be established between the homeowners and a service company familiar with the process. In the long run, the money invested in this type of service contract will be worthwhile.

PSED systems will fail under one or more of the following conditions:

1. too much pressure applied by the pump;
2. soil structure with permeability so low that the effluent will not be absorbed;
3. PSED system designed too small for soil conditions and effluent load; and
4. soil saturated by long periods of heavy rains.

In all of these cases the failure occurred by effluent breaking through the surface of the dosing field (Figure 11), usually at a low point in the field. Such breakouts are not obvious during wet weather conditions; however, they will be observed after drying has taken place because the breakout point will continue to discharge effluent.

The first corrective procedure when a breakout occurs is to try to place additional topsoil over the dosing field. If the dosing field was adequately sized, the addition of topsoil will cure the problem. Should this not prove successful, a reevaluation of the field sizing may be required and the field

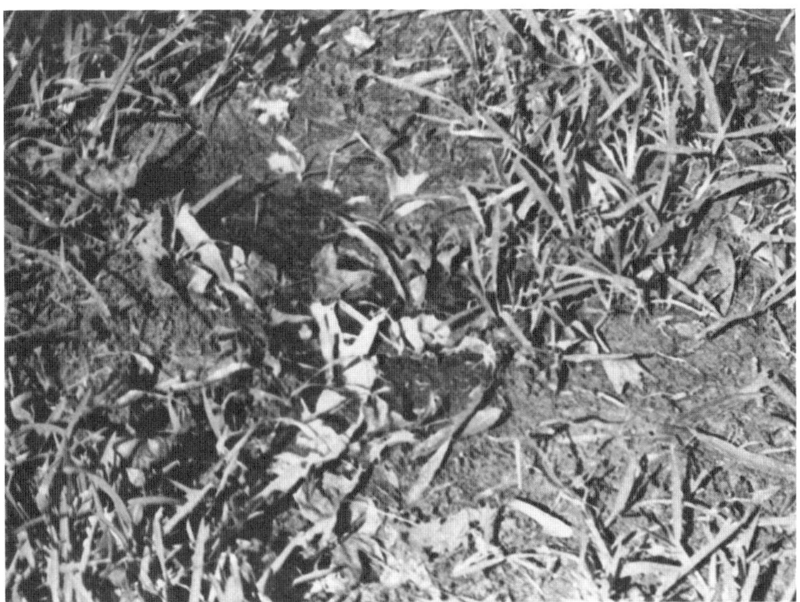

Figure 11. System malfunction caused by improper effluent distribution. Dosing pipe was not placed in a level trench. Note localized breakout of effluent.

expanded accordingly. Field expansion may also be required if family water usage increases. This situation has been observed on several occasions but is offset to some extent by the fact that the systems are simple to expand if land is available. Additional trenches can be provided and additional dosing pipe can be manifolded and connected into the existing system without concern about interfering with the existing drainfield or maintaining proper gravity flow and equalization in the system.

REFERENCES

1. Texas Department of Health. "Construction Standards for Private Sewage Facilities," Texas Department of Health, Austin, TX (1977).
2. Winneberger, J. T. "Correlation of Three Techniques for Determining Soil Permeability," in *On-Site Waste Management, Volume III*, Hancor, Ohio: Hancor, Inc., pp. 26, 29.

22

MANAGEMENT OF ALTERNATIVE SYSTEMS: ISSUES, PROBLEMS, CONSTRAINTS AND OPPORTUNITIES

Kenneth C. Wiswall, P.E., Senior Project Engineer
Peter A. Ciotoli, AICP, Senior Project Planner
Weston Environmental Consultants
West Chester, Pennsylvania 19380

INTRODUCTION

The management of onsite and small community wastewater systems is a topic that has been receiving increasing attention over the past several years. As more and more small communities attempt to apply this kind of technology, it has become apparent that these systems have unique administrative and operational needs that must be provided for to ensure successful implementation. It has also been recognized that providing for these needs requires special institutional arrangements. This presentation will attempt to illustrate different approaches to the development of appropriate management programs in these situations.

MANAGEMENT ISSUES

The design of an alternative wastewater system management program will reflect the type of technology applied, the institutional options available, and various financial, legal and political issues that may apply in a particular case. These factors represent constraints that determine the feasibility of different management approaches. Each community will face a different set of constraints, so will require a custom-designed management program. Nonetheless, certain basic and common issues will apply in any case in which onsite and small community systems are considered.

CASE STUDIES

A study of "Institutional Arrangements for the Management of On-Site and Alternative Wastewater Systems," sponsored by the U.S. Environmental Protection Agency (EPA) Municipal Environmental Research Laboratory under the Small Flows Program is currently investigating experiences of communities that have established management programs for alternative systems. As part of this study, nine communities were selected as case studies representing different forms of management programs. These communities are listed in Table I, together with a brief description of the management program. Of the nine case studies, six involve the management of individual systems, including standard septic tank–drainfield systems, as well as alternative onlot systems (e.g., aerobic plants, sand mound drainage areas, etc.). The other three are examples of community systems involving low-pressure sewer collection systems and clustered treatment systems. In each case the choice of technology and management approach applied was the result of a set of circumstances unique to the particular community. Nonetheless, the experience of these communities demonstrates how various problems and constraints can be overcome through the design of an appropriate management program.

CHOICE OF TECHNOLOGY

The design of a management program usually follows the design of the wastewater systems utilized. In most cases the type of system is selected to suit the physical site conditions, with little consideration of management needs. In fact, most of the factors affecting the choice of collection and treatment alternatives are related to site characteristics and treatment level requirements. However, certain basic management issues should be considered in the technical evaluation of alternatives. These relate to the financial capacity and operational capability of existing or proposed management agencies. The financial and manpower resources necessary to support a proposed wastewater system should not place an undue burden on the community.

Table I. Case Study Communities

Community	Management/Agency	Program Description
Acton, Massachusetts	Municipality	Community septage management program using private haulers with publicly owned and operated treatment facility.
Fairfax County, Virginia	County Health Dept.	County onsite system permitting program that applies comprehensive site evaluation, system design and installation criteria.
Marin County, California	County Health Dept.	County onsite management program, where periodic inspections of septic tank systems are made to check performance.
Rural Towns, Vermont	Soil and Water Conservation Districts	Cooperative effort between state, municipality and conservation districts in Vermont to provide site evaluation and system design services to homeowners.
Auburn Lake Trails Georgetown, California	Public Utility District	District manages onsite and alternative systems at one large subdivision through performing site evaluations, design systems, system inspection and water quality monitoring.
Stinson Beach, California	Water District	District manages both new and old onsite and alternative systems for small community.
Lake Meade, Pennsylvania	Municipal Authority	Authority designs, installs, owns and operates grinder pump-pressure sewer system around the lake.
Port Charlotte, Florida	Private Utility Co.	A publicly regulated private utility owns, designs, installs and maintains septic tank-effluent pump systems at two major developments.
Otter Tail County, Minnesota	Homeowners' Association	Lake homeowners' association manages septic tank-effluent pump system around lakes.

Individual vs Small Community Systems

Whether to use individual systems or small community systems will depend primarily on soil conditions and the density of the units. When suitable soils prevail and average lot size is greater than half an acre, onsite systems will generally be the most cost-effective and least maintenance-intensive solution. In the case of existing developments where onsite systems are presently in use, the actual performance of those systems should be assessed to determine the feasibility of preventing or correcting operational problems. Whenever onsite systems are proposed, the long-term impact on local groundwater supplies should be a major consideration. Even properly functioning septic tank systems discharge nitrates that potentially can accumulate in groundwater to levels exceeding U.S. Public Health Service standards.

When individual systems are not applicable, some form of centralized collection of wastewater will be required. In small community situations, nonconventional methods such as low-pressure sewer systems often offer considerable capital cost savings over gravity sewer systems. These alternative collection methods are also more flexible in their ability to serve isolated clusters of development in a more cost-effective way. The choice between different collection alternatives will be based on relative cost-effectiveness, performance reliability and operational demands.

Treatment options will be influenced by regulatory requirements and land availability. The use of treatment facilities with surface discharge is often limited in small community situations where receiving streams are typically small and very sensitive to wastewater effluent discharges. In such cases, subsurface disposal or land application are often proposed. Land availability (i.e., sites with suitable soil characteristics) and impact on groundwater are the major considerations when evaluating these options.

The following case study examples illustrate how these technical evaluations and other nontechnical issues influence the choice of technology in actual situations.

MANAGEMENT APPROACH

The scope and effectiveness of a management program are a function of the services the agency or combination of agencies provide. The functions or services to be provided should be determined by the nature of the wastewater problem, the types of systems utilized, and the economic and manpower resources of the management agency(ies).

The nature of the wastewater problem (i.e., the extent and seriousness of failing existing systems) and the local site constraints will determine the minimum functional requirements necessary to provide a service equivalent to that provided by conventional sewerage systems. The more restrictive the site constraints, the more involved will be the necessary management functions.

Management Functions

The major management functions include the following:

- Planning
- Site Evaluation
- System Design
- Installation Supervision
- Operation and Maintenance (O & M)
- Financing
- Water Quality Monitoring
- Systems Inspection
- Public Education
- Program Coordination

When individual systems are considered, the site evaluation and system design functions are particularly important to avoid improper applications of onlot systems. Installation supervision and operation and maintenance are also important for assuring proper construction and continued operation of the system. The latter two services inherently involve greater administrative and operating staff requirements.

With the centralized community systems (i.e., collection and treatment), the operation and maintenance function is the most critical. However, installation supervision is also very important and may contribute to significant reductions in startup problems when a system first comes online.

The other functions listed also apply, regardless of the type of systems being used. Most of these relate to the day-to-day administration of a program dealing with budgetary matters, regulatory requirements and public relations. From our experience, the function of public relations is very often the key to the success of a program. In dealing with nonconventional approaches to wastewater management it is very important to educate the public about the service being provided. In most cases it is necessary to convince the people that they need the proposed system in the first place.

Institutional Arrangements

There are many options when it comes to defining management responsibilities. One or several existing or newly created agencies can serve to carry out different functions. The choice will depend on the scope of management functions to be provided and the capability of existing agencies to fulfill them.

A management program can be administered by any one or a combination of the following three agencies:

1. *Public agencies*. These include municipal governments or counties, as well as other government agencies, such as regional planning agencies, boards of health and conservation districts.
2. *Special service agencies*. These include special districts or public authorities created for a special purpose, such as a water and sewer district or a sanitary district.
3. *Private sector entities*. These include private contractors (e.g., land developers), private utility companies, rural cooperatives and property owner associations.

Financial, Legal and Political Issues

State enabling legislation and local government charters will determine the legality of different types of institutional forms in a particular area. The following considerations should be taken into account when evaluating institutional options.

1. The *legal authority* to tax, collect revenues, secure financing, gain access to private property and enforce regulations should be provided either through enabling legislation, governmental charter or by service agreement.
2. Any designated management agency should be *financially stable* in terms of revenue base (taxes, user charges, grants, etc.) and bond rating.
3. *Administrative and operating* staff needs should be realistically assessed. The ability to satisfy these needs through existing agency staff and the local availability of qualified people should be carefully evaluated.
4. The management agency should have *public obligation* in the sense of having long-term responsibility to serve the public. Third-party agreements involving a local government, performance bonds and public utility commission regulation are possible means of gaining this assurance.

In any case, when alternative systems are proposed, regardless of the reliability of the technology, the long-term performance of such systems cannot be assured without addressing the adequacy of the management program in terms of these considerations.

CASE STUDIES

The following discussion of case study experiences presents the factors and circumstances that led to the development of the respective management programs.

Acton

Seven major studies concerning wastewater management in Acton have been prepared since 1965. The first two studies, completed in 1966 and 1972, recommended sewer construction (estimated to cost $10 million in the 1966 study) largely because the town was experiencing a rapid rate of growth, and soils were considered unsuitable for onsite systems. Only 15% of the town's land is considered suitable for onsite systems. These recommendations were rejected by the town's residents as being too costly and unnecessary, given the perceived adequacy of existing onsite systems.

Three subsequent studies, prepared in 1975 and 1976, questioned the need for sewers in the town and recommended that the use of onsite systems be continued. Onsite disposal appeared in these studies to be satisfactory from the viewpoint of public health, costs, density of development and environmental impact.

To resolve the conflicts of previous studies, a 201 (Step 1 planning) study is being prepared. The plan, which is expected to support the use of individual subsurface disposal systems on a townwide basis, recommends:

1. continued reliance on onsite disposal as the most cost-effective alternative in view of the town's present stands and surveillance program; and
2. an educational campaign to encourage homeowners to maintain their systems properly.

An integral part of Acton's current reliance on subsurface disposal is its program for handling septic wastes. Since the early 1960s the town has provided a site for the disposal of septage. The present lagoon facilities (costing approximately $47,000 for materials) were financed completely by the town. Labor and equipment were supplied by the town's highway department, which is responsible for maintaining the septage disposal facility, while the health department reviews and issues permits for onsite system construction and replacement.

Acton maintains strict local regulations regarding design, installation and operation of private subsurface disposal systems. These regulations are complemented by an active inspection and surveillance program, reinforced by careful recordkeeping, so that subsurface systems are constructed according to approved designs. Each new septic tank system or system repair must have a construction permit and operational approval from the Board of Health.

Acton is able to administer this management program principally because of the professional and technical staff employed by the town. The town residents are highly educated, and public involvement in the onsite wastewater management program is facilitated by the town meeting form of government, which encourages active citizen participation in community programs. The common goal in this case is to avoid the cost and associated impacts of proposed sewer systems by demonstrating that onsite systems can be managed effectively.

Fairfax County

The Fairfax County Health Department began a comprehensive onsite system regulatory program in 1954 in response to politically unpopular capital expenses required for sewering areas with failing septic tanks. In the early 1950s the County experienced many septic tank failures attributable to inadequate planning, design and construction. After issuing bonds to support the needed sewer extension, the Board of Supervisors directed the Health Department to develop a program that would prevent future failures. The Health Department (EHD) decided that soil suitability would be the basis of a prevention program. The soils extension service of Virginia Polytechnic Institute (VPI) mapped all of Fairfax County for soils at 400 ft/in. to establish an information base. The EHD drafted legislation, which the Board of Supervisors enacted, to require a set of permits for a developer to install a septic tank. To verify soils data, site testing (supervised by Health Department staff) is required for any proposed subdivision of land.

Fairfax County's program is aimed at preventing problems through construction of adequate onsite wastewater disposal facilities. The result is a failure rate that has dropped from 6-8% during the early 1950s, to zero since the mid 1960s. The emphasis of the program is regulation of system design and installation. The EHD believes that a county-operated/sponsored O&M program would be beneficial, but the atmosphere for expanding local programs is not strong. Also, difficulties are foreseen in managing a program with more than 20,000 component systems. The county feels that program objectives are accomplished by rigorously regulating planning, design and construction by the private sector.

Marin County

In 1967 Marin County retained the services of a consultant to study the problem of individual disposal systems and identify future sewerage facility needs. That study showed that in the preceding 40-year period, Marin County had experienced a growth in population from about 40,000 persons in 1930 to more than 200,000 persons in 1970.

As of 1967, about 70% of the county's residents were served by public sewers maintained by numerous special districts throughout the county.

The continued use of onsite systems outside of these districts seemed to pose a threat to public health, most particularly in areas near existing or proposed water supply reservoirs. In 1963 the county upgraded its rules and regulations governing onsite systems to conform with the U.S. Public Health Service and Federal Housing Authority standards. Adoption of these criteria strengthened county control over the design and installation of onsite systems. In 1971 the passage of County Code 18.06 considerably expanded the approach to onsite system management in Marin County because it not only further upgraded the standards for onsite system design and construction, but incorporated a periodic inspection program to monitor system performance.

The Marin County experience with onsite management has shown that it is possible to incorporate an inspection program within an existing government framework. The relatively small number of households in the program, the restriction of the inspection program to only new systems, and the nominal publicity given to the program have helped it evolve into a well-operating program. The future exercise of the right-of-entry and inspection capabilities of the county's Health Department, along with the extension of the inspection program to preexisting systems by the county's supervisors, are believed to have strengthened the program.

Vermont Onsite Specialist Program

The onsite specialist program was promoted primarily by members of the Vermont Association of Conservation Districts (VACD) program in the state (i.e., farmers, concerned citizens, and Cooperative Extension Service (CES) and Soil Conservation Service (SCS) personnel) in response to the problem of malfunctioning onsite systems in scattered rural areas. Because of the lack of technical assistance and other reasons, local health officers had paid insufficient attention to administering these regulations. Therefore, it was felt by the conservation district representatives that local health officers needed assistance in administering state health regulations governing individual sewage systems.

As state legislation does *not* mandate adoption of local ordinances governing onsite systems, few towns had ordinances. Those that did found them difficult to enforce without technical support. The SCS and CES helped develop and implement this program through the conservation districts using SCS soil survey data as the technical basis for reviewing onsite system designs. To help implement the program on a statewide scale, a uniform onsite ordinance contract form was prepared, and the primary focus for program administration shifted to the Vermont Association of Conservation Districts (VACD). The VACD is currently lobbying to achieve complete statewide implementation of the onsite specialist program and attempting to become more involved in planning and design of alternative wastewater systems for small communities (e.g., through the 201 facilities grants program).

The program is politically acceptable to local governments because it is sponsored by the soil and water conservation districts (an existing agency), rather than a government unit. Further, local control and enforcement of onsite system regulations have been maintained. The onsite specialist serves only in a technical advisory role. Despite the apparent success of the program, the onsite specialist program has not been accepted statewide. Many towns are unwilling to participate voluntarily, and as long as the state does not require local health ordinances governing individual sewage systems, this is likely to continue. Objections have been raised by professional engineers and system installers who feel that the onsite specialists encroach on their work. On the other hand, many installers and individual homeowners greatly appreciate the advice of the specialists. Other concerns relate to the adequacy of the specialists' background and training and the potential conflict of interest that exists because the specialists are involved in designing individual sewage systems, as well as in administering local health regulations governing these systems.

Auburn Lake Trails

Trans America Development Co., the original developer of Auburn Lake Trails, had prepared a series of site plans and detailed feasibility studies for the development (November 1969–May 1971). The initial plan called for installation of a centralized water supply system with onsite septic tank systems for wastewater treatment and disposal. In late 1970 the California Water Resources Control Board (WRCB), Central Valley Region, raised concern over soil depths, slopes, high water tables, etc. in the area being developed and issued an order prohibiting onsite systems. Instead, it recommended central services. Estimated costs for installing a sanitary sewer system in the development were $3.6 million, or nearly $2000 per lot for collector sewers and wastewater treatment facilities. The initial high capital cost, coupled with the anticipated low buildout rate for the subdivision (approximately 3% annually), made it economically unfeasible to sewer the development at that time. Based on data cited in several feasibility studies prepared by the developer's consultant, it was argued by the county's health department representative and the developer's consultant that the proper performance of onsite systems could be ensured through a management program. The WRCB subsequently issued an order allowing the use of onsite systems on most lots, with the requirement for a management program through the existing Georgetown Divide Public Utility District (GDPUD) to "assume responsibilities for the design, installation, maintenance and repair of any sewage disposal system constructed within the subdivision" (Waste Discharge Requirements-WRCB 72-2).

As a result, a special sewer improvement district was created by resolution of the GDPUD Board of Directors in June 1971 (Ordinance 71-3), and a full-time wastewater program manager was hired by the GDPUD in the fall of 1971 to develop and administer the program. The onsite management program has evolved through the mutual efforts of the GDPUD wastewater manager, the developer's sanitation (assistant general manager) and El Dorado County Health Department personnel. The result is a coordinated program where the GDPUD, the developers and the county's health department share onsite management responsibilities.

Stinson Beach

In 1961 the Marin County Health Department conducted a survey to determine the adequacy of wastewater disposal in the Stinson Beach area. The results of the survey showed that the use of onsite systems for wastewater disposal constituted a public hazard, and that a public district should be formed to deal with the problem. The following year the Stinson Beach County Water District was formed to act as the wastewater planning agency and to provide sewerage services for the coastal community.

Subsequent water quality sampling of the community's water resources between 1961 and 1972 by the county and state health departments indicated that coliform counts exceeded the water quality standards established by the state WRCB. These findings led the San Francisco Regional Water Quality Control Board to adopt Resolutions 73-13 and 73-18 (September 1973), which required phasing out all onsite wastewater systems in Stinson Beach by October 1977. The resolutions also placed a ban on new buildings with onsite wastewater systems.

Several wastewater management plans and feasibility studies were prepared, all of which proposed a centralized sewage collection and treatment system for the entire community. These recommendations were rejected by the residents because of high user costs and the contention that alternative solutions had not been adequately considered.

Prompted by these objections and the recognized need to investigate alternative solutions, the district and the state WRCB initiated another feasibility study in 1975 (through the 201 Program—Step 1 planning grant) to survey existing onsite systems and document the extent of the problems associated with these systems. After evaluating a wide range of alternative solutions, the onsite alternative program was recommended as the "best" alternative. It was further recommended that the selected program be administered by an onsite system wastewater management district and that a sampling and inspection program be instituted to monitor onsite system performance. Special state enabling legislation (SB 1902) was prepared and adopted (in 1976) that essentially gave the Stinson Beach County Water District the explicit authority to manage privately owned onsite wastewater systems. This legislation was subsequently expanded to allow the creation of onsite wastewater management districts statewide.

Although the onsite wastewater management program at Stinson Beach has been operating only since January 1978, it has already done much to demonstrate the viability of onsite systems serving the wastewater management needs of an existing community. The District, in its efforts to provide sewerage services for the community resident, has become a respected, visible and active local service agency. It has established itself as a service organization by emphasizing public awareness and education regarding onsite system practices. The Water District's Board of Directors has been very supportive of the onsite management program thus far, and has been willing to exercise enforcement authority in several cases to ensure compliance with program regulations.

Lake Meade

In the early 1970s septic tank systems around Lake Meade began to fail. The lake had shown early signs of eutrophication, necessitating a chemical treatment program for weed control. The community continued to develop, using holding tanks as an emergency method of wastewater management. New septic tank systems were not permitted by Pennsylvania regulations in soil conditions like those found near the lake. Eventually the sewage treatment plant near Gettysburg, where the pumpage from Lake Meade holding tanks was disposed of, refused to accept any more of Lake Meade's wastewater, and the Department of Environmental Resources (DER) subsequently issued a moratorium on new construction in the community until the wastewater problem was resolved.

The Lake Meade Municipal Authority (LMMA) then initiated meetings to discuss alternative methods for resolving the lake's water quality problems from malfunctioning septic tank systems. The LMMA was originally created by the developer (in 1969) to plan for, own and maintain sewerage services for the community. It was not until 1976, however, that the LMMA was legally activated to provide wastewater disposal services (by resolution of Reading and Latimore Townships). Based on engineering studies, a plan was selected that called for a low-pressure sewer collection system utilizing individual grinder pumps and a fairly sophisticated treatment plant.

Preliminary investigations into financing alternatives for the LMMA indicated that the community was probably not likely to receive a 75% grant under the Federal Water Pollution Control Act Amendments of 1972 (PL 92-500) because of the community's low position on the state priority list. As a result, attention was directed to local financing and grants and loans from other federal and state agencies. In 1976 the Authority received funds from the Farmer's Home Administration (FmHA) and a grant from the Department of Commerce, State of Pennsylvania. More than $1 million in grants and $528,000 in low-interest loans were secured by the LMMA.

To be eligible for these funds the community had to provide a portion of the funds necessary to construct and acquire its proposed sewage collection, transportation and treatment system. Funding for the community's share was arranged by the Authority's bond counsel with a local bank.

The process of developing the institutional framework and developing the powers of the Authority to provide sewerage services was carried out primarily through the active involvement of the Lake Meade Property Owners' Association. Because of the private nature of the lake community and the Property Owners' Association's responsibilities for providing municipal services to the community (including security, ambulance and fire service, trash removal and road repairs), the early LMMA members were motivated to find an acceptable wastewater management solution.

Port Charlotte

During the 1960s, the General Development Utility Company (GDU) was faced with a problem familiar to many land developers. Because of poor soil conditions, seasonal high water tables, and faulty installation by independent contractors, many difficulties were being encountered with conventional septic tank-drainfield systems. GDU, through economic analysis and financial feasibility studies, realized that the cost of providing conventional gravity sewers to many sparsely populated, widely scattered communities was prohibitive. This scattered type of land development is typically associated with "homesite developments," where lots are sold in a parcel of land without immediate plans for building on those lots.

The environmental and economic impacts of serving this type of development with conventional onsite systems or gravity collection systems led GDU to design and install a septic tank effluent pumping (STEP) pressure sewer system in a section of Port Charlotte in 1970. In 1972 the system was extended to the Gulf Cove area in Port Charlotte, which became the official test area for expansion of the Suburbanaer pressure sewer system via a state demonstration project. GDU's Suburbanaer system has received "conditional" approval from the Florida DER, with final approval dependent on the completion of the current demonstration program. Suburbanaer systems maintenance personnel are drawn from existing utilities, operations staff and generally perform work for both Suburbanaer and conventional sewer systems.

The future of the Suburbanaer project remains somewhat tentative at this point. The Florida Department of Environmental Regulation has been less than enthusiastic about the project, even though pressure sewer systems have been installed elsewhere in the state. Perhaps a primary reason for DER's reluctant attitude toward the GDU project and the STEP system is the initial lack of cooperation between GDU, the county health department and the Florida DER in applying the new technology. The initial STEP systems were installed with approval by county and state agencies without prior submission of design specifications, projected number of units to be installed, maintenance requirements, etc. This lack of supporting information at the early stages of the project eventually led the Florida DER to establish the demonstration project. Through this demonstration project, it is felt that a better understanding and improved communication between GDU and the Florida DER can be achieved. Indications are that the two parties are moving in that direction.

Otter Tail County

With the adoption of the Shoreline Management Ordinance in October 1971, Otter Tail County became one of the first counties in the state of Minnesota to establish and adopt an administrative and regulatory program governing the use of onsite wastewater systems in lake communities. The statewide shoreline management program was established to: (1) provide a comprehensive review of onsite systems located within sensitive shoreline areas; and (2) establish the regulatory framework for upgrading and/or rehabilitating failing systems and address noncompliance within these shoreline areas.

The county has been innovative in finding collective solutions to existing failing or nonconforming onsite systems that must be remedied under the state act and county ordinance.

In a desire to conform to the county's Shoreline Management Ordinance, and with persuasion by the county's Department of Land and Resource Management, the Rothsay Camp Property Owners Association decided to construct a small community (i.e., cluster) wastewater system to meet its wastewater needs. The only legal agreement signed by the members was a Deed of Easement to permit construction, operation and maintenance of a system that would cross the property of each member. The deed further stated that when a property was sold, the new owners would be obligated to comply with its requirements. The system consists of individual septic tanks discharging to a common subsurface drainage field located a sufficient distance from the lake.

A key to this program's success has been that the wastewater systems are affordable (and less expensive than individual solutions) and can be easily managed and maintained by local residents. The successful implementation of this program is the product of the willingness of the individual homeowners to cooperate, and the ability of the County Department of Land and Resource Management (particularly its executive director) to provide an effective liaison between state agencies, county elected officials, and local permanent and seasonal residents. Most important, the Rothsay Camp Association's wastewater management program is typical of the voluntary participation style utilized throughout the state, particularly in its rural recreation-oriented areas, and stems from a desire on the part of local residents to seek preventive solutions to wastewater disposal problems.

CONCLUSIONS

These nine examples do not begin to represent all the possible approaches to managing individual and small community wastewater systems. However, they do illustrate a range of institutional arrangements that can be applied to suit different management needs. It should be apparent that the design of a management program should reflect the level of technology being applied, as well as the management capability of the community. Each program we have observed is a product of individual efforts in response to a unique wastewater problem that makes the best use of the resources available to the community. The nine case studies presented all represent successful management programs and demonstrate the viability of nonconventional approaches to wastewater management.

23

DESIGN AND INSTALLATION SUPERVISION BY AN ONSITE MANAGEMENT DISTRICT

Richard N. Prince, R.S., M.P.H., Water Quality Superintendent
Marie Eisen Davis, C.P.S.S., M.S., Geologist
Georgetown Divide Public Utility District
Georgetown, California 95634
Kent B. Seitzinger, R.S., Assistant Project Manager
Transamerica Development Company
Cool, California 95614

INTRODUCTION

Since the inception of the program in 1971, the Georgetown Divide Public Utility District (GDPUD) has tried to incorporate the best available technology for its onsite waste management activities. As previously reported by other authors [1-3], the District operates a management program for the Auburn Lake Trails Subdivision in Cool, California.

Some of the services provided under the public management concept are: (1) site evaluation, (2) system design, (3) construction management, (4) construction inspection, and (5) operational management.

In view of these mandated activities [4] and the uniqueness of the concept, GDPUD has enlisted the advice and talent of numerous consultants and agencies to achieve these ends. The result of that research has been the formation of a program that provides the required services while offering a means of using the feedback to modify future designs.

SITE EVALUATION

To borrow from a recent U.S. Environmental Protection Agency (EPA) publication on alternatives for small wastewater treatment systems, " . . . the first step in designing community wastewater facilities is to characterize the local environment" [5]. This statement can be no less true for the design of an individual onsite system.

In Auburn Lake Trails, the site evaluation process (Figure 1) is initiated by the request of the prospective home builder. Once alerted, a District representative commences the initial evaluation equipped with a topographical map, a plot plan drawn to scale showing the proposed homesite (the latter is provided by the prospective builder), a magnetic compass and a clinometer, used to measure slope.

The initial survey provides a general analysis of the surface features of the parcel, including:

1. Topography (lay of the land)
   - a. Slope
   - b. Contour
2. Physical Features,
   - a. Rock outcroppings
   - b. Surface water
   - c. Floodplains
   - d. Vegetation
   - e. Road cuts
   - f. Available area

Essentially, this step ascertains whether there are limiting factors to be dealt with.

Provided that the findings support the installation of an onsite system, a series of color-coded stakes are placed in the selected disposal area. These markers serve as a guide to the backhoe operator, now scheduled to excavate stair-stepped pits to predetermined depths (shown by the color-coded stakes).

On completion of the excavating phase, percolation tests are conducted at selected levels in the pits by technicians trained in multiple facets of onsite disposal practice.

When these tests have been completed, a second site evaluation is conducted by a technologist armed with the results, the previously mentioned maps, as well as Soil Conservation Service (SCS) maps. The preliminary design hinges on this intensive analysis and a thorough understanding of the newly exposed soil profiles. The visual inspection is based on a series of keys, which identify a soil's ability or inability to handle the application of wastewater.

Several excellent sources detail many of the basic ingredients or characteristics present in a soil column, which impart information regarding the ability of that profile to accept the application of wastewater [6-10].

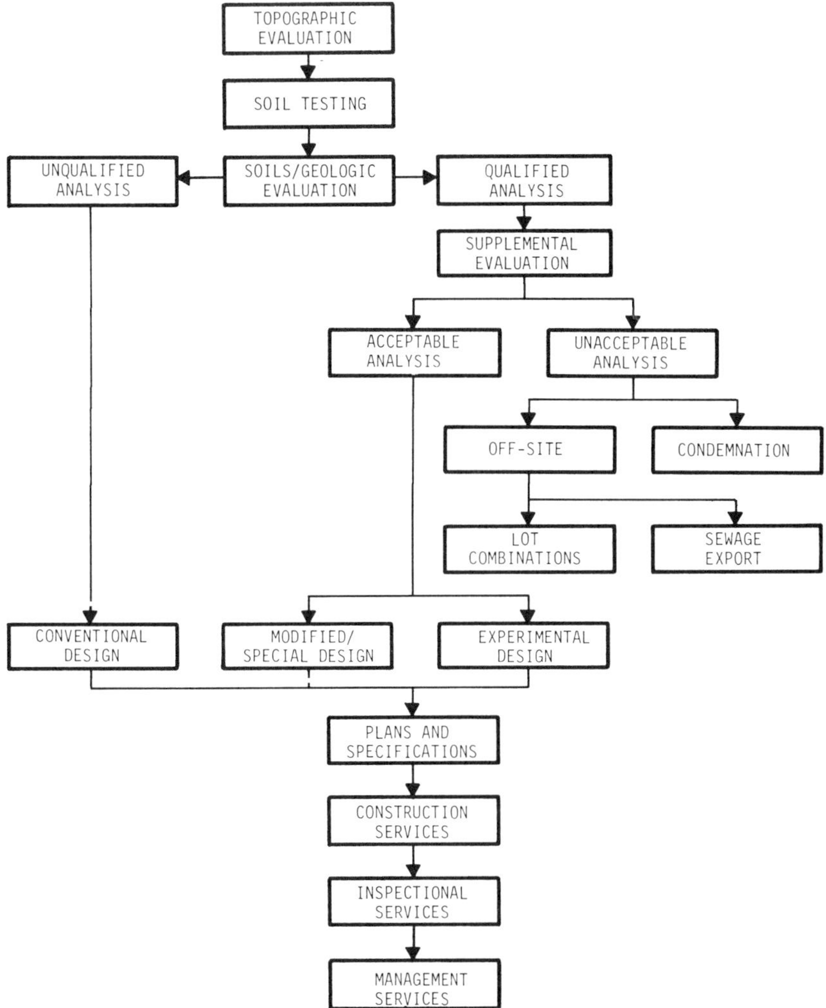

Figure 1. Auburn Lake Trails procedural scheme for onsite evaluation.

The relatively detailed investigation includes identifying and locating the following:

- soil type and depth of each horizon
- soil colors
- soil textures
- soil drainage

- smear potential
- the presence/absence of gleying or mottling
- the presence/absence of groundwater
- the presence/absence of restricting layers
- the condition and depth of the parent material
- the depth and relative density of vegetative root systems

Some aspects of the inquiry will have to be qualitatively judged, while factors such as soil color and texture may be quantitatively measured by color charts (Munsell), or hydrometer testing [11,12].

Should unusual or extraordinary findings be noted, photographs of the profile or feature are taken; the information then becomes a part of the permanent record, maintained for that site.

SYSTEM DESIGN

Once the data are correlated, it is then possible to select pertinent parameters for the design phase. The criteria chosen are based on:

1. the specific site characteristics noted;
2. the demands of the home environment (i.e., structure configuration, the presence of driveways, outbuildings, etc.)
3. the anticipated loading rate of the dwelling;
4. the pretreatment indicated; and
5. the maintenance and surveillance program.

In general, with the use of conventional soil absorption systems, the District subscribes to the principle of dosing and resting [13]; consequently, each such design includes two equivalent fields separated by a diversion valve. Additionally, each line within a field incorporates a 4-inch capped riser by which the District can make liquid level measurements and/or collect effluent samples.

A system constructed under controlled circumstances, where there is (1) an in-depth soils analysis, (2) the ability to measure water consumption, and (3) known storage capacity, provides a wealth of information concerning how such a system will function under field conditions. This system becomes an in situ percolation test, automatically compensating for sewage effluent, the presence of clogging mats or the phenomenon of hydraulic head. On a long-term basis, this type of controlled and monitored installation seems to be the best source of future design information.

A further advantage to this monitored installation, but one that is not generally lauded, is that surveillance can detect problems and anticipate failure if conditions remain unchecked. In theory, corrective action can be taken prior to the actual daylighting of effluent.

If the inquiry suggests that conventional means of onsite disposal are unacceptable, District evaluation shifts to other options that may lend themselves to the parcel (Figure 2). Each alternative is weighed according to: (1) the specific site conditions, (2) the ability of that system to achieve the objectives required, (3) the cost of installation, and (4) the projected depreciation and operating expenses. In effect, the cost/benefit ratio is a prime consideration in the case of alternative designs.

Experience in Auburn Lake Trails indicates that invariably there are instances where no combination of efforts will effectively and economically solve onsite problems. In such circumstances, the remaining available options are: (1) the combination of two or more parcels to reduce restrictions to a tolerable level; (2) provision for offsite disposal in an area with acceptable site conditions; and (3) condemnation—the parcel may be recommended for incorporation into the subdivision's scenic greenbelt system as a last resort.

When a design has been finalized, plans and specifications are drawn and sent to the El Dorado County Health Department for review, approval and permit issuance.

CONSTRUCTION MANAGEMENT

After many frustrating experiences, it is apparent that a system designer cannot always expect construction to proceed smoothly according to an approved set of plans. Not infrequently, major modifications in site conditions, having profound if not lethal effects on the adequacy of an onsite system, appear to be necessary. Additionally, arbitrary changes in trench depth or location, effluent distribution or just poor construction techniques yield equally unacceptable results [14]. In some cases, little can be done after-the-fact to obviate the damage. The District's approach to this problem has been to offer preconstruction services to eliminate or reduce the frequency of such occurrences.

By request, GDPUD employees locate and stake a disposal system as it appears on approved plans. This service requires dispatching a crew of two equipped with transit and rod; contours are determined and lines are laid out and flagged accordingly.

For contractors new to Auburn Lake Trails, District policy dictates that a staff member confer with them to ensure their familiarity with design requirements and construction practices necessary to achieve an acceptable installation. Because of the fragile environment, they are made to understand

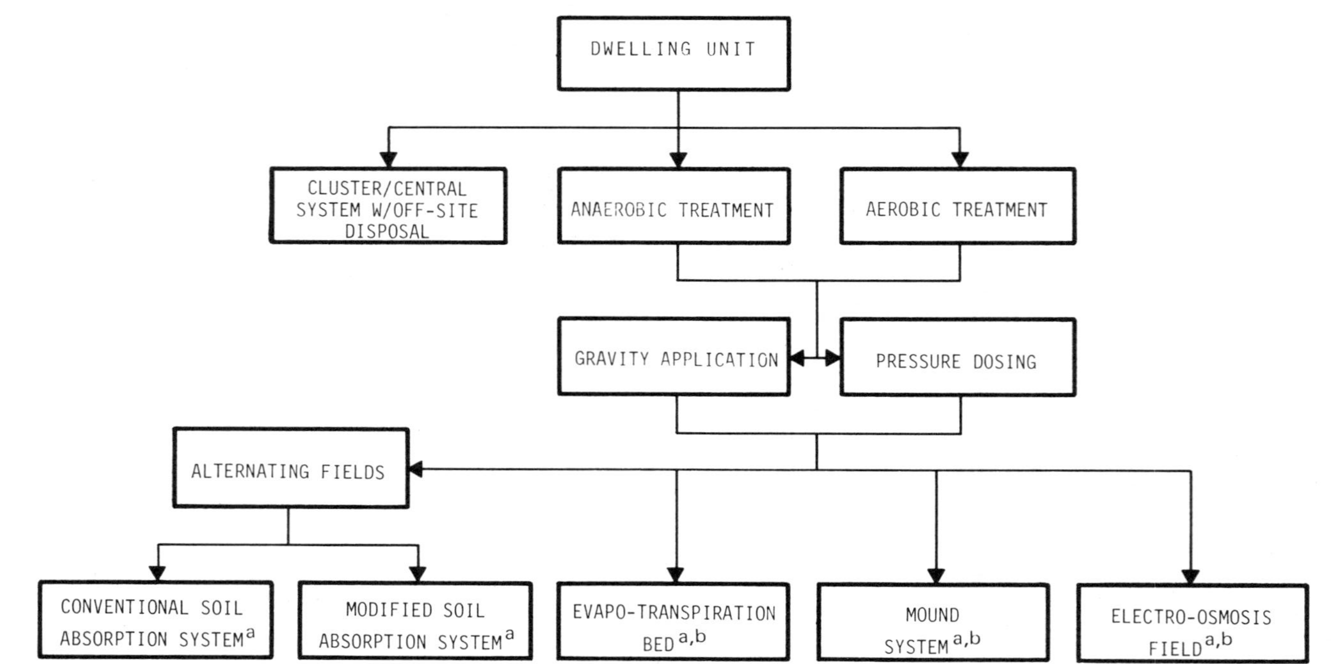

Figure 2. Auburn Lake Trails alternative approaches to onsite disposal: (a) reduced flow features and/or advanced treatment may allow a modification in system sizing; (b) this unit is currently classified as experimental in El Dorado County, California.

that District control must be maintained in all aspects of design and construction. The system layout service is still in its infancy, having been implemented approximately one year ago. Therefore, its effectiveness cannot yet be evaluated realistically.

INSPECTION SERVICES

This facet of the program dovetails with construction management aspects in that multiple inspections are made during the course of construction. The exact number will vary with: (1) the intricacy of design, (2) the complexity of the site, and (3) the competence of the contractor.

The inspector has been trained to recognize characteristic soil conditions, in addition to being familiar with standard construction practices [15,16]. His observations will then have greater meaning in the overall performance of the system. If conditions are significantly different than those found in the testing program, steps can be initiated to overcome the problem prior to the unit's being placed into service.

Once the system has been finished to the District's satisfaction, an accurate plot plan, showing exact dimensions, is prepared to simplify future maintenance activities.

An inventory card is prepared when the home is occupied, and the system becomes a part of the surveillance and maintenance program. Semiannual inspections determine the condition of the system. Effluent depths are measured, valves are alternated and other steps are taken as required. Recently, the District added the requirement that capped risers (8-inch well casing) be provided on the septic tanks [16] to allow for more frequent and economical inspection of the scum and sludge levels; semiannual inspection now appears realistic.

CONCLUSIONS

Georgetown Divide Public Utility District's experience over the past eight years indicates that public management of onsite wastewater disposal systems can be an appropriate function of government.

An integrated program involving onsite evaluation, system design, construction management, inspection services and operational management provides mandatory safeguards for maintaining the public's health and environmental quality while reducing economic and energy demands commonly associated with more conventional means of disposal.

As this field receives increased emphasis, the additional sophistication that will follow can only expand the benefits derived.

REFERENCES

1. United States General Accounting Office. "Community-Managed Septic Systems-A Viable Alternative To Sewage Treatment Plants," Controller General's Report to the Congress, Report No. CED-78-168, U.S. Government Printing Office, Washington, DC (1973), p. 25.
2. Roy F. Weston, Inc. "Management of On-Site and Alternative Wastewater Systems," paper presented at the Technology Transfer Seminar, Wastewater Treatment Facilities For Small Communities, United States Environmental Protection Agency, 1979.
3. Wheeler, G., and J. Bennett. "On-Site Wastewater Management Districts in California," paper presented at the Alternative Wastewater Treatment Systems Workshop, Champaign, IL, June, 1979.
4. California Regional Water Quality Control Board, Central Valley Region. "Waste Discharge Requirements for Auburn Lake Trails Subdivision," Order 72-2, Exhibit B (1971).
5. United States Environmental Protection Agency. "Alternatives for Small Wastewater Treatment Systems, On-Site Disposal/Septage Treatment and Disposal," EPA-625/4-77-011 (1977).
6. Born, S. M., and D. A. Stephenson. "Hydrogeologic Considerations in Liquid Waste Disposal," *J. Soil Water Cons.* 24 (2): 426-431 (1969).
7. Franks, A. L. "Geology for Individual Sewage Disposal Systems," *Calif. Geol.* 195-203 (September 1972).
8. Birkeland, P. W. *Pedology, Weathering, and Geomorphological Research* (New York: Oxford University Press, Inc., 1974), pp. 269-273.
9. Parker, D. E. "Soil Evaluation of Sites for Soil Absorption Systems," *Proc. Third Nat. Conf.* (Ann Arbor, MI: Ann Arbor Science Publishers, Inc., 1976), p. 139.
10. United States Department of Agriculture, Soil Conservation Service. *Soil Survey Manual*, Handbook No. 18, U.S. Government Printing Office, Washington, DC (1962), pp. 173-188.
11. Day, P. R. "Report to the Committee on Physical Analyses, 1954-55, Soil Science Society of America," *Soil Sci. Soc. Am. Proc.* 20 (2): 167-169 (1956).
12. Bouyoucos, G. J. "Hydrometer Method Improved for Making Particle Size Analyses of Soils," *Agron. J.* 54: 464-465 (1962).
13. McGauhey, P. H., and J. H. Winneberger. "A Study of Methods of Preventing Failure of Septic Tank Percolation Systems," Federal Housing Administration, U.S. Government Printing Office, Washington, DC (October 1967), pp. 6-11.
14. Otis, R. J., W. C. Boyle, J. C. Converse and E. J. Tyler. "On-Site Disposal of Small Wastewater Flows," Small Scale Waste Management Project, University of Wisconsin, Madison, WI (1977), p. 42.
15. Commonwealth of Pennsylvania, Department of Environmental Resources. "Technical Manual for Sewage Enforcement Officers," Harrisburg, PA (1975).
16. Davis, M. L. "System Inspectors Manual," unpublished report, Georgetown Divide Public Utility District, Georgetown, CA (1978).

24

OPERATION AND MAINTENANCE FUNCTION OF AN ONSITE WASTEWATER MANAGEMENT DISTRICT

Michael R. Batz
Wastewater Technician
Stinson Beach County Water District
Stinson Beach, California 94970

INTRODUCTION

On January 17, 1978, the San Francisco Bay Area Regional Water Quality Control Board (RWQCB) passed a resolution allowing for the continued use of onsite systems for the disposal of wastewater in the community of Stinson Beach under the management of the Stinson Beach County Water District (SBCWD). If, after a three-year test program, the RWQCB is satisfied with the performance of the onsite systems with respect to water quality and the management program conducted by SBCWD, the RWQCB will consider amending the Basin Plan to allow for the continued long-term use of onsite systems.

In formulating a management program that would meet with the RWQCB's approval, the SBCWD developed a detailed set of rules and regulations to govern the use of onsite systems and the management of the program. In addition, the SBCWD agreed to file with the RWQCB monthly self-monitoring reports, as well as an annual report. It was agreed that the annual report should contain (1) both tabular and graphic summaries of the monitoring data obtained during the previous year; (2) a comprehensive discussion of the compliance record; and (3) the corrective actions taken or planned that may be needed to bring the onsite systems into full compliance with the requirements of the RWQCB and SBCWD.

BACKGROUND

Development of Onsite Management District: An Overview

Onsite systems of various types have been used for the disposal of liquid wastes in Stinson Beach since its inception as a summer community in the late 1800s. In 1961 a survey was conducted by Marin County to determine the adequacy of wastewater disposal in the Stinson Beach area. Based on the results of the survey, it was concluded that the existing disposal method involving the use of septic tanks constituted a public health hazard and that a public district should be formed to deal with the problem. The Stinson Beach County Water District (SBCWD) was formed in 1962 to provide sewerage services to Stinson Beach and those surrounding areas not already within the Bolinas Public Utility District.

Between 1961 and 1972 the Marin County Health Services and the state health departments continued to collect water samples from Easkoot Creek for bacterial analysis. The principal finding derived from those tests was that the coliform counts usually exceeded the water quality standards established by the State Water Resources Control Board (SWRCB). These findings led the San Francisco Regional Water Quality Control Board (RWQCB) to adopt Resolutions 73-13 and 73-18 in September of 1973. The resolutions required that all onsite septic tank systems within the Stinson Beach area be eliminated by October 1977. In addition, a ban on new buildings with onsite disposal systems was included.

During this same period (1961-1972), nine engineering studies were conducted to determine what should be done to correct the situation. These reports are summarized in the literature [1]. In each case the proposed plans were rejected because of local opposition or failure of the plans to meet county or state water quality regulations.

The SBCWD, serving as the wastewater planning agency for the community, responded to the Regional Board resolutions (adopted in 1973) by hiring an engineering firm to investigate the problem and arrive at a solution. The consulting engineers selected proposed a central treatment system for Stinson Beach [2] that eventually was rejected by the community in a special election on March 5, 1974. The local residents had a variety of reasons for rejecting a central treatment system, the strongest being the high costs associated with the construction of a treatment plant for a population of fewer than 1000. The residents also contended that alternative solutions were not investigated thoroughly.

Prompted by the residents' objections and a recognized need for further study, the SBCWD, in conjunction with the SWRCB, decided to initiate an objective investigation of the engineering and environmental factors associated with all alternatives. In July 1975, Eutek, Inc. was selected as the engineering consultant to perform field and preliminary engineering work to evaluate the efficiency of existing onsite septic tank systems and to develop other possible waste treatment alternatives. In September 1975, the URS Research Company was selected as the environmental consultant to perform an environmental assessment and prepare the necessary Environmental Impact Report (EIR) based on the alternative concepts developed by Eutek, Inc.

After a number of trials and tribulations, the third draft of the engineering report was completed in April 1977 [3] and the final one in October 1977 [4]. The principal finding documented in these two reports was that of all the alternatives evaluated, the continued use of onsite systems was the most cost-effective and environmentally acceptable. The recommended program for the continued use of onsite systems involved (1) the establishment of an onsite wastewater management program, and (2) the establishment of a sampling and inspection program to monitor onsite system performance.

Even before the engineering study was approved in July 1975, it was apparent that special legislation would be required if the continued use of onsite systems was to be a viable alternative. As conceived at that time, the legislation would make it possible under California law to form a management division for onsite systems within the SBCWD. The SBCWD would then be empowered legally to deal with the RWQCB. Thus, in November 1975, some four months after the initiation of the engineering study, preliminary contact was made with Senator Peter Behr's office. He agreed to sponsor legislation that would make it possible to form a management division for the operation and maintenance (O&M) of onsite systems. On March 18, 1976, Senator Behr introduced Senate Bill 1902 to administer onsite systems. After committee hearings, it was passed by the legislature on September 13, 1976.

Starting on September 27, 1976, dialogue was initiated between the SBCWD and the RWQCB concerning the implementation of an onsite wastewater management program for the community of Stinson Beach. Working together with the Board and staff of the RWQCB, the staff of the SBCWD began compiling a set of rules and regulations that could be used as a basis for managing the proposed program. It took until December 10, 1977 to develop an acceptable set of rules and regulations [5] and to work out the administrative details between the agencies. Based on the availability of an acceptable set of rules and regulations and the enabling legislation that made the District a legal entity with which the RWQCB could deal, the staff of the RWQCB recommended that the implementation of the program be approved on a trial basis. On January 17, 1978, the RWQCB passed a resolution allowing for the continued use of the onsite systems for the disposal of wastewater in the community of Stinson Beach under the management of the SBCWD. If, after a three-year test program, the RWQCB is satisfied with the performance of the onsite systems with respect to water quality and the management program conducted by the District, the RWQCB will consider amending the Basin Plan to allow for the continued long-term use of onsite systems.

Condition of Onsite Systems

Based on the house-to-house onsite survey conducted in 1975-76 [3], some 75 onsite systems were found, or were assumed, to be failing. The number and distribution of the failing systems by geographic area is summarized in Table I. The observed causes of these failures are summarized in Table II. Most of the failed systems had received little or no maintenance, had been installed improperly, poorly constructed or overused. Also, many people were hesitant to spend money to maintain or repair/replace their systems with the possibility of a proposed sewer. An analysis of the results of the survey showed that the average age of the working systems was about 14 years. The average age of the failed systems was estimated to be 20 years.

Objective of the Wastewater Management Program

The principal objective of the Onsite Wastewater Management Program undertaken by the SBCWD is to ensure that the quality of the waters in the community of Stinson Beach is maintained through the effective control and management of the onsite systems used for the disposal of wastewater.

Table I. Observed Onsite System Failure by Community Area [3]

Area	Surveyed Systems[a]	Failing Septic Tank Systems
Seadrift	139	1
Patios	51	1
Calles	85	18
Old Town	122	21
Highlands	48	3
Panoramic	11	2
Stinson Beach Total	456[b]	46[c]

[a]As of April 1976.
[b]Excludes 29 cesspools identified throughout the community.
[c]Includes 7 systems assumed failing because of refusal of residents to allow system to be surveyed.

Table II. Observed Causes of Onsite System Failures [3]

Cause	Number Observed	Percent of Total
Septic Tank/Leach Field (presumably clogged leach field)	17	44
Poor Leach Field Design	10	26
Inadequate Septic Tank Maintenance	6	15
High Groundwater/Poor Drainage	4	10
Undersized Septic Tank	2	5
Totals	39[a]	100

[a]Excludes 7 systems assumed failing because of refusal of residents to allow system to be surveyed.

OPERATIONS

Implementation of the Onsite Wastewater Management District (OSWMD) and its program by the SBCWD involved: (1) the development of office procedures; (2) the issuance of permits and citations; (3) the initiation of the monitoring program; (4) the continuation of the water quality monitoring program; and (5) the submission of monthly reports to the RWQCB.

Development of Office Procedures

Development of specific office procedures to handle the paperwork associated with the OSWMD was a significant part of the program implementation. Although this work had, in part, begun with the preparation of the District's "rules and regulations," in which various reporting forms had been developed, a separate bookkeeping and accounting system had to be established for the OSWMD. In addition, files had to be set up for the vast amount of paperwork involved, even for such a small district. Files that are maintained include: (1) card files to record when each inspection is completed and when the next is due; (2) a system folder for each home; (3) mailing lists; (4) correspondence; and (5) lists of systems in need of repair.

Issuance of Permits and Citations

On January 19, 1978, 60 Failing System Citations were issued; on January 24, 1978, 434 Interim Permits to Operate were mailed to the residents of Stinson Beach.

Citations

Citations were issued to homes with failing systems based on information obtained during the house-to-house onsite survey conducted during 1975-76 [3]. Included in this category are homes with cesspools, deteriorated septic tanks and/or drainfields, and clogged drainfields. Systems where the homeowner refused to respond either to the initial survey or to a wet weather resurvey were also included in this category. Forty-two additional citations have been issued to homes with systems that were found to be failing between January 17, 1978 and October 1, 1979.

Permits to Operate

Interim Permits to Operate were issued to homes where the onsite systems were found to be operating satisfactorily during the onsite survey conducted during 1975-76 [3]. Failing systems that had been corrected since the onsite survey was completed were also issued Interim Permits to Operate; they are included in the total count of permits (434). In addition, 20 Permits to Operate have been issued to new systems.

Interim Permits are issued for one year, at which time each system is to be inspected. If the system passes the inspection or has been repaired, a two-year Permit to Operate is issued. If a system is found to be operating only marginally, it may require special monitoring to determine whether it should be cited as a failed system. If a failing system is found, a Failing System Citation Report is issued. Along with the Citation, a timetable for correction of violations is presented to the homeowner.

Inspection and Monitoring Program

The inspection and monitoring program was initiated in January 1978 for systems constructed under Marin County Code 18.06, for systems that have been repaired and for those requiring two-year inspection. It should be noted that the SBCWD has assumed the two-year inspection responsibility for systems designed and constructed under the Marin County septic system ordinance No. 18.06.

Inspection Program

With notification of a scheduled inspection appointment, a drawing and explanation of the need to provide permanent access to the septic tank is included. Each homeowner is required to provide such access for inspection purposes. The inspection includes documenting the following information for each onsite system:

- age of the septic tank system components
- past maintenance
- number of residents
- number of bedrooms and bathrooms
- tank dimensions and volume
- sludge and scum thicknesses
- tank construction and condition.

After noting these details, water is run into the tank at a rate of 30 gallons per person or 60 gallons per bedroom, whichever is greater. The outlet to the drainfield is observed to record any increase in the liquid level as the tank is being surcharged. The drainfield absorption rate is also measured. Recommendations are made to the homeowner based on the levels of material in the septic tank and absorption rate versus measured water usage.

Monitoring Program

Those systems found to be operating marginally (requiring minor alterations, maintenance or water conservation) during the onsite survey conducted in 1975-76 [3] were placed in the special monitoring category. Also placed in this category were high groundwater demonstration systems, alternative waste disposal systems and separate greywater systems.

Forty-six systems were included in this category in January 1978. Each was inspected during 1978, some up to three times to ensure their proper operation. Of these, approximately 80% have been placed on the regular two-year inspection schedule.

Water Quality Monitoring Program

The full-scale water quality monitoring program was initiated in January, 1978. Seven surface water and six groundwater sampling stations are involved. Surface water sampling is conducted on a weekly basis; groundwater sampling is done every two weeks. Samples are collected and sent to a private laboratory for bacteriological analysis. In addition, chemical determinations are conducted in the field for surface waters every two weeks and quarterly by a laboratory. It should be noted that some limited water quality monitoring had been conducted by the SBCWD since the completion of the onsite system study in 1976.

Stations S5 and S6 are affected by tidal waters from the Bolinas Lagoon. The high coliform counts obtained at these stations are partially attributable to large wildlife populations in the lagoon.

Submission of Monthly Reports to RWQCB

As agreed with the RWQCB, the SBCWD is to submit monthly Self-monitoring Reports in which the results of the water quality sampling program are presented and discussed. In addition, Failed System Status Reports, in which the status of the failed systems is delineated, are submitted every two months. The first Self-Monitoring Report (for January 1978) was submitted on February 17, 1978; the first Failed System Report on March 15, 1978; and the First Annual Report in July 1979.

MAINTENANCE

The average age of septic tank systems in Stinson Beach is approximately 18 years, while the average age of systems found to be failing is close to 25 years. With regular inspections, routine maintenance and proper design and installation, the working life of each system is expected to increase.

History

In reviewing the history of the development of Stinson Beach, several points should be noted:

1. Many of the homes were built as second homes.
2. Many homes were used only during the summer months and occasionally on weekends.
3. Families would gather in groups for their vacations at the beach.
4. There was little or no supervision over the design, materials of construction and installation of the onsite disposal systems for these homes.

In many cases, maintenance was conducted only after a problem existed and usually only temporary repairs were made. Most homes are now occupied on a full-time basis.

Using the District's rules and regulations, many of the improperly designed and installed systems are being replaced with systems designed to operate properly under current conditions.

Routine Maintenance

Each homeowner is responsible for providing access, doing routine maintenance, and for the repair or replacement of his septic tank system.

Prior to an inspection by the District, it is the homeowner's responsibility to provide access ports at both the inlet and outlet ends of the septic tank. The ports must have inside dimensions of at least 12–20 inches and must extend to, or above, the ground surface. After the inspection, the homeowner is advised of necessary maintenance or repairs. If repairs are required, the District will withhold the operating permit until the work has been completed and inspected.

Costs for any maintenance are borne by the homeowner. Costs incurred include those for septic tank pumping, derooting, installing outlet baffles or tees, and installing greywater sumps.

The District maintains a list of local, willing workers–people with experience in locating, providing access to and doing minor maintenance to the septic tank.

Repair or Replacement of Onsite Systems

Under the SBCWD's rules and regulations, once a Failing Onsite Disposal System Citation Report (citation) has been issued, the homeowner is required to repair or replace the cited components. A failed system would include one that surfaced effluent, was a cesspool, was deteriorated, was improperly designed or installed, or one that was undersized. Guidelines outlining the process for replacing or repairing an onsite system are set forth in the rules and regulations.

The homeowner is required to submit an engineered proposal to the District. Criteria from ordinances in the rules and regulations for drainfield design, location and setback requirements must be incorporated in the engineer's design. In his design, the engineer must consider the geology, hydrology and topography; if possible, user attitudes should also be reflected in the design. Special system designs using greywater and/or alternative systems must be approved by the SBCWD and the RWQCB.

Once plans have been approved, the homeowner must hire a contractor to install the system component(s). After installation, the District must inspect the work prior to any backfilling. Once the system passes the final inspection, a two-year operating permit is issued.

Enforcement

If a homeowner refuses to repair a cited system after repeated notices, the District has several enforcement action options. Termination of water service, termination of occupancy or contracting with an engineer and contractor to design and install a replacement system are among the options.

Costs for the engineer and contractor would be billed to the homeowner or placed as a lien against the property.

If the homeowner does not provide access for inspection after three notices, the system is classified as failing and abatement proceedings are initiated. The process is terminated if the system is inspected and found to be working properly.

Funding

Operating funds for the onsite program are obtained from permit fees billed to the homeowner. These fees are set during the annual budget preparation to cover expected operating costs for the next fiscal year. A two-year Demonstration Grant was received this year from the California State Water Resources Control Board. The grant funds will be used to cover a portion of the salaries and to provide low-interest loans for homeowners who are required to repair or replace their systems and can show financial need.

The District is also in the process of completing the Step 1 Facilities Planning Study. On the successful completion of the Step I plan, the District will seek to obtain funding for the design and construction of failing onsite systems. This will require the completion of Step II and III reports.

Public Relations

The establishment of good public relations has been extremely important in the successful implementation of the onsite program. Every home in the community was studied during the 1976 onsite survey, and user attitudes and feelings about centralized wastewater treatment versus retaining and upgrading the existing onsite systems were recorded. A majority of the people favored and supported retaining onsite treatment.

Since the program was implemented in 1978, the District has provided a variety of educational materials to the residents of Stinson Beach. These have been in the form of newsletters and a Homeowners and Users Guide for Onsite Wastewater Disposal Systems. This information provided a list of maintenance tips along with some do's and don't's for operating the systems, and answered questions about the use of onsite wastewater disposal systems.

Having a local, centralized office where records of each onsite system are maintained, old as well as new residents have access to the history of their systems. Many questions are answered by means of telephone conversations, office visits and visits to peoples' homes.

This public relations program has contributed to the development of an informed public that supports the efforts of the District in the establishment of a responsible and effective long-term onsite system management program.

REFERENCES

1. Tchobanoglous, G., R. C. MacArthur and D. K. Wood. "Review of Wastewater Management Problems in Stinson Beach, California," report prepared for BASSA, Davis, CA (October 1974).
2. Brown and Caldwell Consulting Engineers. "Wastewater Collection, Treatment and Disposal," report prepared for Stinson Beach County Water District, San Francisco, CA (January 1974).
3. Eutek, Inc. "Stinson Beach Wastewater Facilities Planning Study Project Report," revised third draft, Sacramento, CA (April 1977).
4. URS Company. "Final EIR, Stinson Beach Wastewater Management Plan," San Mateo, CA (October 1977).
5. Stinson Beach County Water District. "Wastewater Management Program Rules and Regulations," Stinson Beach, CA (December 1977).

25

DESIGN AND INSTALLATION OF SMALL COMMUNITY SYSTEMS

Malcolm K. Lee
Administrator of Land and Resource Management
Otter Tail County
Fergus Falls, Minnesota 59537

INTRODUCTION

Otter Tail County is located in West Central Minnesota approximately 60 miles southeast of Moorhead, Minnesota and Fargo, North Dakota. The landscape is extremely scenic, with rolling hills of cultivated farmland dotted with numerous marshes and lakes. In geographic area, Otter Tail County is the sixth largest county in Minnesota and ranks eleventh in population, with a normal or fixed population of approximately 46,000. The lake area includes approximately 174,000 acres. About 25% of the county's population is located in the county seat city of Fergus Falls, which has a population of 13,000. About 90% of the remaining population is located in or on lakeshore. The county, which contains 10% of Minnesota's 12,000 classified lakes, has been estimated to have a summer population of 250,000.

The scenic beauty of the land and the excellent lakes attract both seasonal and year-round residents from the Minneapolis-St. Paul and Fargo-Moorhead areas, among others. Even though tourism is a significant part of the local economy, the county's primary base remains agriculture. The average annual precipitation is 20 inches and the temperature range is from a low of −35°F in winter to above 90°F in summer.

The lakes of Otter Tail County are important for many reasons, a primary one being the taxes derived from lakeshore owners, both seasonal and year-round residents. These taxes are a vital source of income for supporting local units of government and school systems. In one township alone 96% of tax revenues generated comes from lakeshore residents.

Prior to 1971 there were no controls to guide the development and integration of shoreland into the unincorporated shoreland areas of Minnesota. Likewise, there were no sewage system requirements. Many small lakeshore lots were platted without regard for the crowding potential of the lake and the inherent problems associated with sewage being generated from these small communities.

In many instances lots were platted in areas subject to seasonal flooding and with very high groundwater tables. In some areas the soils were absolutely unsuitable for a soil absorption sewage system. The results were contaminated wells, and rapid eutrophication of the lakes was visible.

THE SHORELAND MANAGEMENT ACT

In 1969, because of pressure from lakeshore owners, local units of government and the general public, the Minnesota legislature enacted "Statewide Standards and Criteria for Management of Shoreland Areas." This is legally referred to as Minnesota Statute 1969, Chapter 777, commonly referred to as the Shoreland Management Act.

Basically, the pressure came from landowners who did not want to see their lakes polluted and their possible investment of $300/foot of water frontage become worthless. Secondly, the local units of government and schools knew that lakeshore was a valuable source of tax revenue. In addition, there was a mass desire by the general public to preserve an important natural resource.

The Shoreland Management Act dictates minimum lot size, sewage regulations, land elevation above the high water table for both building and sewage purposes, grading and filling in shoreland areas, and numerous other requirements. To be more explicit, the Shoreland Management Act classifies lakes into three categories:

1. Natural Environment Lakes
   Minimum lot size is 200 feet of lake frontage and 80,000 square feet of lot area (almost an acre). Sewage system setback from the high water mark is 150 feet.

2. Recreational Development Lakes
   Minimum lot size is 150 feet of lake frontage and 40,000 square feet of lot area. Sewage system setback from the high water mark is 75 feet.

3. General Development Lakes
   Minimum lot size is 100 feet of lake frontage and 20,000 square feet of lot area. Sewage system setback from the high water mark is 50 feet.

There is also a fourth classification, called Rivers and Streams; however, the isolation requirements are the same as for a General Development Lake.

In addition, a standard isolation distance for all classes of lakes is required for isolation of the well from the sewage system. This distance varies, depending on whether the well is less or more than 50 feet deep. The isolation distance ranges from 50 to 100 feet.

Meeting the Requirements

The deadline for local units of government to enact and enforce the regulation was July 1, 1972. The Shoreland Management Act did not "grandfather" in existing sewage systems. Lots platted prior to October 15, 1971 were "grandfathered" in for dwelling purposes only. Many of the small lots platted and "grandfathered" could not meet the minimum sewage isolation distance requirements established by the Shoreland Management Act. For example, no septic tank was to be closer than 50 feet from a well, yet there are numerous platted lots that are only 50 feet in width and 100 feet in depth. The Act also set a minimum sewage setback from the lake high water mark, a dwelling, the side lot lines, etc. There were, and are, many lots in Otter Tail County that could not comply with these minimum requirements.

In most cases, the substandard lots can accommodate only a septic tank or a holding tank. To avoid any misunderstanding, a septic tank may be defined as a watertight tank of sound and durable material not subject to excessive corrosion or decay.

CONCEPT OF A COMMON DRAINFIELD

In anticipation of eliminating noncomplying existing illegal sewage systems, a solution to the problem had to be found. In September of 1971 a Home Sewage Treatment Workshop was sponsored by the University of Minnesota and conducted by Professor Roger Machmeier. Professor Machmeier recommended that perhaps a common drainfield established at a remote area would meet the elevation and setback requirements. To his knowledge this was a new and untried concept. With this suggestion in mind, numerous onsite evaluations of existing sewage systems were made with horrifying results. Wells had been installed adjacent to cesspools; in many cases cesspools and septic tanks overflowed directly to the lake; numerous cesspools were in the groundwater table; and in some instances sewage was piped directly into the lake. The following recommendations were made to solve these problems:

1. Each dwelling would have a properly sized septic tank.
2. The outlet of each septic tank would discharge to a common trunk line.
3. The trunk line would be so installed that by gravity flow the effluent liquid would flow to a miniature pump station, such as a 500-gallon or larger septic tank.
4. In the pump station, a pump capable of pumping liquid to a common drainfield some distance away would be installed where proper distance from the lake could be achieved and the land elevation was proper.
5. The common drainfield area would need to be owned in common by all users or they would need to obtain an easement from the property owner.

Selection of a Community

An area for such a system had to be selected and most importantly, the residents had to be convinced of this idea. The opportunity came in the spring of 1974 for a small community of 12 dwellings on Lake Lida known as the Rothsay Camp (Figure 1), which was incorporated in 1915. In addition to the lake frontage, the Rothsay Camp property owners own in common a 24-acre parcel of land directly across the township road from their lake lots and also a pie-shaped acre parcel of land directly adjacent to an end lot.

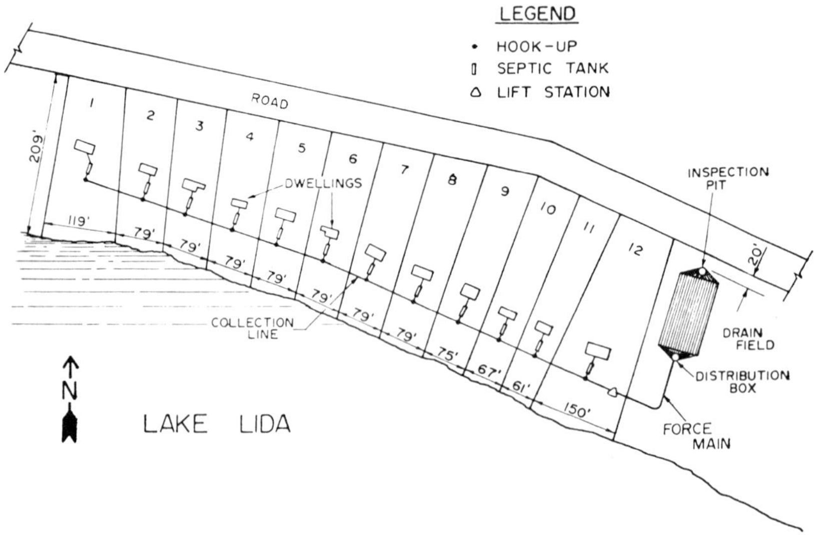

Figure 1. The Rothsay Camp.

Both parcels had an elevation of approximately 18 feet above the high water mark and could meet the drainfield setback requirement.

The collector system concept at first seemed to them to be a favorable solution until it became known that their system would be an experiment. The property owners also felt that the estimated cost fell far short of those of municipal systems they were familiar with. In fact, some even said that the engineering costs alone would be more than what was quoted for the entire system. A total figure for the collector system, drainfield, pump station, labor and materials of $14,400 (or $1200 per dwelling) had been given. It was suggested to them that if the final bids were too high they could be rejected and costly holding tank systems installed to solve their sewage problem. They accepted the offer.

Procedure

The following is what was needed to be done:

1. The system was to be sized using the number of bedrooms—each bedroom generates 70 gpd of liquid. Therefore, an inventory of the total number of bedrooms in Rothsay Camp was needed, to which was added a 25% expansion factor.
2. Percolation tests needed to be taken in the proposed common drainfield area. Each perc rate carries a soil absorption square footage space requirement. The total number of bedrooms and the percolation rate were computed to give the total drainfield size requirement.
3. The grade elevation needed to be taken for the trunk line to obtain the proper grade for gravity flow.
4. The pump station needed to be sized.
5. The type of pump needed to be selected and a dual pumping system was recommended. If one pump failed the other one was to "kick in" automatically and a signal light was to come on.
6. An overflow tank next to the pump station was also anticipated for use in case of a power outage. This overflow tank would equal the total gallons of the combined residential water pressure system tanks. If the power went off, the pumps would not operate, so no sewage would be discharged to the system other than what was in the individual pressure tanks.

Modification of the System

This was all documented and bids were requested. The problem became more complex at this time because no one had installed such a system locally. Only one installer expressed an interest, but fortunately it was a very reliable local firm. In consultation with him, the following changes were made.

1. The overflow tank next to the pump station would be eliminated. Consultation with the local power company representatives revealed that in 20 years the longest power outage had been 2½ hours and that it was a controlled outage during a transformer changeover, which occurred at 2:00 A.M. All residents had had prior knowledge of when the outage would take place.

2. The dual pump concept was removed because the installers always had at least one pump on hand for emergency purposes. In addition, the installer was located less than eight miles from the Rothsay Camp area.

The installer's bid for the trunk line, drainfield, material and labor was $834.00 per dwelling. Work commenced within four weeks and the system was in operation on Labor Day of the same year (Figure 2). New septic tanks were installed at each residence that needed a septic tank of greater capacity. This additional expense to each affected resident cost no more than $600.00. Some of the lots had properly sized tanks in their old system and these were utilized with the collector system. These residences had no additional cost other than connecting to the trunk line. The following are some points of interest on this collector system:

1. The trunk line is down only 4 feet and, in some instances, is in the groundwater table.
2. At no time is there standing water in the trunk line.
3. Biological heat generated from bacterial action in the septic tanks apparently helps to avoid line freezing.
4. The pump in the pump station operates only when the tank is 60% full. A float regulates this action. Thus a dosing system is achieved which is a desired drainfield concept.
5. The pump station annual estimated power consumption would not meet the minimum annual electric company charge. Therefore, it was wired directly to the nearest dwelling and each year the other parties included in the system pay their share of $3.00 for a total estimated annual electric cost of $36.00.
6. Every septic tank is pumped annually to remove the sludge and ensure water clarity.
7. The pump manufacturer did the friction loss computation at no charge.
8. The system has been in operation for five years.
9. Last, but not least, the system meets all Shoreland Management Act requirements, without pollution of wells or natural resources.

Now there are more than 30 collector systems in operation in the U.S., ranging in size from 3 dwellings to 28 dwellings.

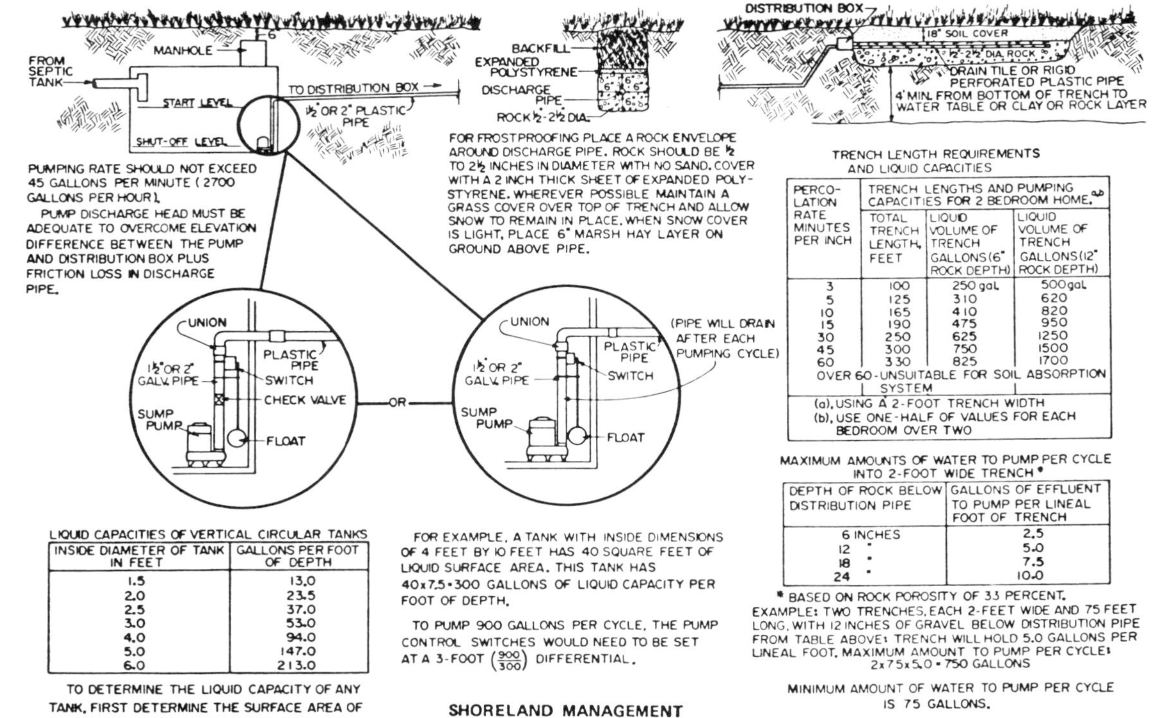

LIQUID CAPACITIES OF VERTICAL CIRCULAR TANKS

INSIDE DIAMETER OF TANK IN FEET	GALLONS PER FOOT OF DEPTH
1.5	13.0
2.0	23.5
2.5	37.0
3.0	53.0
4.0	94.0
5.0	147.0
6.0	213.0

TRENCH LENGTH REQUIREMENTS AND LIQUID CAPACITIES

PERCOLATION RATE MINUTES PER INCH	TRENCH LENGTHS AND PUMPING CAPACITIES FOR 2 BEDROOM HOME.[a,b]		
	TOTAL TRENCH LENGTH, FEET	LIQUID VOLUME OF TRENCH GALLONS (6" ROCK DEPTH)	LIQUID VOLUME OF TRENCH GALLONS (12" ROCK DEPTH)
3	100	250 gal.	500 gal.
5	125	310	620
10	165	410	820
15	190	475	950
30	250	625	1250
45	300	750	1500
60	330	825	1700
OVER 60-UNSUITABLE FOR SOIL ABSORPTION SYSTEM			

(a). USING A 2-FOOT TRENCH WIDTH
(b). USE ONE-HALF OF VALUES FOR EACH BEDROOM OVER TWO

MAXIMUM AMOUNTS OF WATER TO PUMP PER CYCLE INTO 2-FOOT WIDE TRENCH*

DEPTH OF ROCK BELOW DISTRIBUTION PIPE	GALLONS OF EFFLUENT TO PUMP PER LINEAL FOOT OF TRENCH
6 INCHES	2.5
12 "	5.0
18 "	7.5
24 "	10.0

Figure 2. Pumping station.

RESULTS

To recap a few collector system strong points:

1. Professional engineering service may not be required for small collector systems. Most installers can use a transit proficiently.
2. There is much free, reliable advice about pumps and pump stations available from the pump manufacturers and their field representatives.
3. All necessary materials are readily available, and even the septic tanks are manufactured locally.
4. Electrical requirements are not complex.
5. Control is local and there is no need to involve more than the local permitting unit of government, i.e., no need to deal with Washington or state bureaucracy.
6. Finally, the cost saving compared with a normal municipal professionally engineered and designed sewage system is approximately 4 to 1.

The costs quoted thus far have been for the Rothsay Camp system installed in 1974. Costs have gone up somewhat in the interim, but some have remained the same.

In 1979 a collector system was installed on another lake for an area called Dunnvilla. The groundwater table is approximately 3 feet below the ground surface, which drives up the installation costs because of the necessity of dewatering the area. While not completed as of this date because of a high water problem, this system will include 28 dwellings, plus a large nightclub, golf course club house and pro-shop. The drainfield, pump station and septic tanks have been installed and the nightclub is hooked up to the system. This system includes dual pumps with signal lights. The central drainfield is more than 900 feet from the pump station. The estimated cost of the completed system is approximately \$70,000. Included in this figure is \$3000 for dewatering the area for installation of the septic tanks at the pump station, \$4500 for driving an encased sewage line under a state highway, and \$3000 for costs associated with crossing the Pelican River. It is estimated that the nightclub costs alone are about \$20,000, so the cost per dwelling unit is estimated to be approximately \$1800. This figure is still about a 4 to 1 savings over a municipal system being planned in another of the lakeshore areas.

CONCLUSIONS

Small collector systems are an effective means of solving sewage problems on substandard lots and lots that cannot meet the requirements of a combination septic tank–drainfield system because of isolation distances, soil limitations, etc. The costs are reasonable, especially when compared with a "municipal type" system. Valuable water resources are protected, the collector systems do work, and the owners are satisfied.

26

THE OPERATION AND MAINTENANCE OF THE SUBURBANAER (STEP) SYSTEM

Paul C. Kloser, Manager, Product Development
Harold E. Schmidt, President
General Development Utilities, Inc.
Miami, Florida 33131

INTRODUCTION

General Development Corporation (GDC) is one of Florida's oldest, largest and most respected developers of planned communities. GDC has seven major communities in Florida comprising a land area of some 273,000 acres.

General Development Utilities, Inc. (GDU) is a subsidiary of GDC and is one of the largest private utilities in the state, providing water, sewer and gas services to more than 28,000 customers in all seven GDC communities. Approximately a decade ago, GDU became interested in developing an alternative to conventional gravity sewers because of (1) their high cost, (2) failures of septic tank–drainfield systems within their communities, and (3) the possibility that these systems might be outlawed at some future date. The prohibitive front-end cost of developing new slow growth areas by means of the conventional gravity sewer was also a major consideration.

THE SUBURBANAER STEP SYSTEM

After considerable study, the President of GDU, decided on a septic tank effluent pressure system (STEP) as an alternative method. The first units were installed in Port Charlotte in 1970 and were so successful that today there are several hundred units in operation in both Port St. Lucie and Port Charlotte communities.

The interceptor tank presently being used in the Suburbanaer System is a 1050-gallon fiberglass tank, the pump chamber being an integral part located in the upper section at the discharged end. A neck extension is added to bring the pump section to grade, and a decorative patio stone is placed over the lightweight, fiberglass wide lip cover. The original units consisted of a concrete tank followed by a Flextran pipe chamber. A reinforced flat concrete cover was caulked and sat on the lip of the chamber. This caused some odor complaints, especially if care wasn't taken during the caulking process. The fiberglass wide lip cover has eliminated any odor emanating from the pump units.

The pump presently used in the Suburbanaer is a Hydromatic one-third-horsepower submersible pump, Model #OSP 33A. Most pumps are cast iron, but because of the scale buildup that takes place around the intake area if the pump is not serviced annually, new pumps are provided with bronze foot and baffle plates, bottom plates and diaphragm guard. The remainder of the pump is coated with selected coal tar epoxy, resulting in a pump that remains clean after years of service. Bronze pumps likewise show little deterioration even after six years of service. On the bronze and epoxy-coated pumps there is little or no scale buildup, but rather a slime buildup on the top and sides of the pumps, with the intake areas remaining relatively clean. When the system was first put into operation it was anticipated that pump life and pump-related problems would be the main failures encountered. As it turned out, hardware problems and faulty installation techniques were the chief culprits.

On most of the original units a cast iron swing check valve was used, with hose connectors and steel clamps. The cast iron valve did not hold up well and the steel clamps rusted through after a year or two of service, causing the hoses to blow off. This accounted for most of the service calls during the first two years of operation of the Suburbanaer System. Brass Camlock disconnects likewise proved to be generally unsatisfactory, as were recent attempts to use nylon clamps. Bronze swing checks and gate valves have proved themselves with up to nine years of service to date, as have PVC valves. The handles on the gate valves rust and are now either treated or removed, but the remainder of the valve shows little deterioration after years of service.

Air-locking of the pumps resulted in many service calls, with fifteen recorded in 1977. This problem was eliminated by drilling a small 1/8-inch hole in the nipple between the pump and swing check valve. One service call this year resulted because the air relief hole was made with a nail set instead of a drill, causing rough edges on the inside of the nipple and eventually a lint accumulation, which clogged the hole.

The hardware presently being used in the pump chamber includes polyvinylchloride (PVC) threaded fittings, bronze valves, PVC hose inserts, radiator hose and 300 series stainless steel clamps. These have all been time proven and offer an indefinite service life.

One of the advantages of the fiberglass tank is that one can drill and tap holes for the PVC fittings. Pipe joint compound is used, and the adaptors are threaded through the pump chamber wall to make a watertight seal. A 4-inch PVC pipe is inserted through the bottom of the chamber into the tank, serving both as a pump-out port and a ready access to check tank sludge depth. In 1976 GDU carried out a small sludge accumulation study [1]. The results compared favorably with a large study conducted in 1949 by the U.S. Public Health Service [2], which indicated an average accumulation of approximately 10 gpy per person. The federal study also showed that after six years solids accumulation increased at a decreasing rate. The Suburbanaer units had not been in operation long enough in 1976 to verify this point. In practice, however, after nine years of service it has never been necessary to pump out *any* Suburbanaer tanks because of sludge accumulation. Two tanks have been pumped because of a scum blanket clogging the tank inlet tee. In both instances, the housewife admitted to regularly disposing of grease and cooking oils down the sink drain. This practice was discontinued and a recent check showed little or no scum on these tanks. During the solids study only a very small percentage of tanks were observed to have any scum accumulation.

COMPLIANCE WITH GOVERNMENT STANDARDS

To determine compliance with applicable tensile and flectural ASTM standards, a strength of materials expert at the Engineering Department of the University of Miami was commissioned to study the material properties of the Suburbanaer interceptor tank. It was found that with a thickness of less than 3/16 inch, the strength and elastic modulus properties exceeded applicable ASTM standards by a comfortable margin. To comply with Florida statutes, the Suburbanaer tank is a minimum of 1/4-inch thick. In addition, prior to use water is added to the tank to check for leaky seams. The tank is then filled completely and allowed to stand for a minimum of 24 hours.

The tank is set with a backhoe, the neck of the pump chamber set at final grade elevation. The service line from the tank to the main line is a 1.5-inch (PR160) PVC pipe, as is the line that serves as a conduit for the pump and mercoid float cords. A PVC ball check valve is installed upstream from the line tap. The tap is made, the valve checked for leaks and the service line connected to the pump chamber. Ring and bell joints or solvent weld joints are equally acceptable. The pump is discharged and the system checked for leaks prior to backfilling.

Hand backfilling to protect the service line is recommended before completion by the backhoe. The PVC line tap has a brass cutting head, which can also serve as a shutoff valve. Carelessness during installation of earlier units resulted in the cutter not being backed off all the way, partially blocking the service line, and a subsequent slow discharge rate. This has been overcome first by being careful, and also by timing the discharge rate as part of the installation procedure.

SAFETY FEATURES

The original Suburbanaer units used a standard electrical plug with a waterproof receptacle. New units utilize a twist lock arrangement to prevent its being used for other purposes. This has resulted in the pump being left unplugged and a service call being required.

Each unit is supplied with a high water level warning system generally consisting of a mercoid float switch and a buzzer/light alarm. When the first units were installed in the early 1970s, it was anticipated that if there were to be problems they would probably be related to pump failure. These units were provided with a warning light activated by pump burnout or power failure. As pump failure has not been a major problem, high-level alarm systems are now being installed on these early units.

New homes in areas served by the Suburbanaer System are specially prewired to provide both for the pump and the warning alarm by running two wires from the electrical panel box to the outside wall receptacle. This outside receptacle should be located within several feet of the plumber's stub-out pipe to allow for standard pump cord length. For existing homes not prewired for the alarm, alternate alarm systems are available. One of these, called a "mini-trol," requires only one 115-V lead. The pump and the mercoid float switch are wired directly into the unit, which has a built-in horn and light. This unit can also be locked to prevent tampering. Another unit in use utilizes a 9-V battery as a power source. The mercoid float is wired into the transmitter located at the outside receptacle. The receiver with a buzzer and light is plugged in at some convenient location in the house, normally the garage or utility room. The unit has advantages at commercial locations in that the receiver can be located some distance away. A unit has been installed at a country club, and the receiver has been located in the pro-shop, which is always manned if the club is open.

When the high-level alarm is triggered on GDU's new units, a reserve capacity of 150 gallons is provided in the pump chamber and the tank freeboard. With an average water consumption of less than 200 gpd for an average family in GDC's communities, this allows 18 hours to service the unit before the homeowner is inconvenienced.

CUSTOMER SERVICE FEATURES

New Suburbanaer customers are provided with an information packet that describes basically how the system works. Included in the packet are a wall plaque with appropriate service call phone numbers, which is mounted at the location of the buzzer, and a self-addressed, stamped postcard to the State Environmental Regulatory Agency, which can be used if the customer has any complaints regarding the system.

The Suburbanaer mainlines to date are PVC (PR160) 3-, 4- and 6-inch-diameter new pipe, brown in color. On a good day, a three-man crew with a trencher can lay up to a mile of pipe at a 36- to 42-inch depth. This in contrast to installing gravity lines, where a 12-man crew with a large backhoe, a loader, expensive surveys, laser gun, etc., can lay up to 300 feet at a 15- to 20-foot depth. Infiltration into the system is virtually eliminated, of course, with the pressure system considerably reducing plant construction, operation and maintenance (O&M) costs. Moreover, no line accumulations have ever been observed and *no* line maintenance has ever been required.

The effluent from the system is discharged either to the conventional sewer or, in Gulf Cove area of Port Charlotte, to the Suburbanaer Waste Treatment Facility. In Port St. Lucie, effluent discharge to the conventional treatment facility constitutes approximately 20% of total plant flow. The Suburbanaer Treatment Facility presently receives waste from 37 homes with a recorded flow of approximately 8000 gpd. The plant is a modified extended aeration facility with an aerator capacity of 15,000 gallons. Aeration time is presently set at 15 minutes on and 30 minutes off, effluent BODs and total suspended solids (TSS) are consistently averaging 2-3 ppm. Corrosion is negligible, and odors are probably less than experienced at a conventional facility.

ADVANTAGES OF THE SYSTEM

A number of advantages for pressure sewers have been cited [3-8], some of which are as follows:

1. Pressure sewer systems are feasible in lieu of conventional gravity sewers in outlying urban areas utilizing septic tank–soil absorption systems.

2. Pressure sewer systems offer the best alternative available in servicing suburban areas, sparsely populated rural areas, seasonal communities, rocky and hilly areas and waterfront property, among others, where the cost of conventional gravity sewers is prohibitive.
3. Pressure sewer systems allow a designer freedom in the site layout of new developments.
4. The cost of the pressure system in new developments is spread over the years as development and construction progress, instead of the heavy initial capital outlays required with gravity sewers.
5. Small PVC system lines and pressure lines may be installed quickly just below the frost line in narrow trenches, with the only equipment needed being a small trencher and/or a backhoe.
6. The need for overflow manholes and lift stations is reduced or eliminated.
7. Lines may be laid along the roadway or in existing utility easements, eliminating the need for obtaining rights-of-way.
8. Infiltration is eliminated. In most cases, this will reduce plant sizing requirements by half.
9. Community disturbance and environmental damage are minimized.

Additional advantages of the Suburbanaer System, which utilizes an interceptor tank as an integral part of the system, are as follows:

1. Significant treatment occurs in an interceptor tank [2,9,10]:
   a. 65–80% of the BOD is removed.
   b. 70–90% of the suspended solids are removed.
   c. 70–90% of the hexane extractables (grease) are removed.
2. The conversion of the remaining BOD within the tank to a soluble BOD, coupled with the low suspended solids, allows treatment by a simple oxidation process, such as extended air, resulting in considerable savings in both plant construction, and operation and maintenance.
3. The soluble organic matter discharged from the tank can be further reduced within the system by various oxidizing agents, filter media and other chemicals.
4. The cost of organic removal is considerably less when anaerobic treatment is employed.
5. Less sludge (approximately 1/4) is accumulated by anaerobic as compared with aerobic treatment.
6. Less costly treatment plants are required because wastes are treated at the point of origin.
7. Maintenance costs are extremely low.
8. The interceptor tank and effluent holding chamber provide adequate emergency storage capacity in the event of a mechanical or electrical power failure [11].

CONCLUSIONS

Pressure sewers may not be the best alternative in every situation, and the system today is certainly not the ultimate. However, the Suburbanaer System offers a simple, practical, common sense alternative, and GDC is committed to its use in its communities in those areas where gravity sewers are financially prohibitive. When one consider's that neither hardware nor pumps have yet been designed specifically for STEP systems, and that general interest in developing such hardware and pumps has been minimal or nonexistent, the Suburbanaer has established an excellent track record.

A point has been reached where annual maintenance, if desired, serves more as a customer public relations project than a system necessity. As effluent systems increase in popularity and specific hardware and pumps become available, one can anticipate that "package" STEP systems will be commonplace in the relatively near future.

REFERENCES

1. General Development Utilities, Inc. "Sludge Accumulation Study," Miami, FL (1976).
2. Weibel, S. R., C. P. Straub and J. R. Thoman. "Studies on Household Sewage Disposal Systems-Part I, U.S. Public Health Service Publication (1949).
3. Carcich, I. G., L. J. Hetling and R. P. Farrell. "A Pressure Sewer Demonstration," USEPA Report No. R2-72-091 (1972).
4. Carcich, I. G., L. J. Hetling and R. P. Farrell. "The Pressure Sewer: A New Alternative to Gravity Sewers," *Civil Eng.* 44 (5): 50-53 (1974).
5. Mekosh, G., and D. Ramos. "Pressure Sewer Demonstration at the Borough of Phoenixville, Pennsylvania," USEPA Report No. R2-73-270 (1973).
6. Clift, M. A. "Experience with Pressure Sewerage," *J. San. Eng. Div.*, ASCE 94 (5): 849-865 (1968).
7. Hendricks, G. F. "Pressure Sewage System and Treatment at Grandview Lake, Indiana," paper presented to ASAE Convention, Pullman, Washington, 1971.
8. Rose, C. W. "Rural Wastes: Ideas Needed," *Water Wastes Eng.* 9 (2): 46-47 (1972).
9. Bendixen, T. W., M. Berk, J. P. Sheehy and S. R. Weibel. "Studies on Household Sewage Disposal Systems-Part II," U. S. Public Health Service Publication (1950).
10. Weibel, S. R., T. W. Bendixen and J. B. Coulter. "Studies on Household Sewage Disposal Systems-Part III," U. S. Public Health Service Publication No. 397 (1954).
11. Environment One Corporation. *Design Handbook for Low Pressure Sewer Systems* (1973).

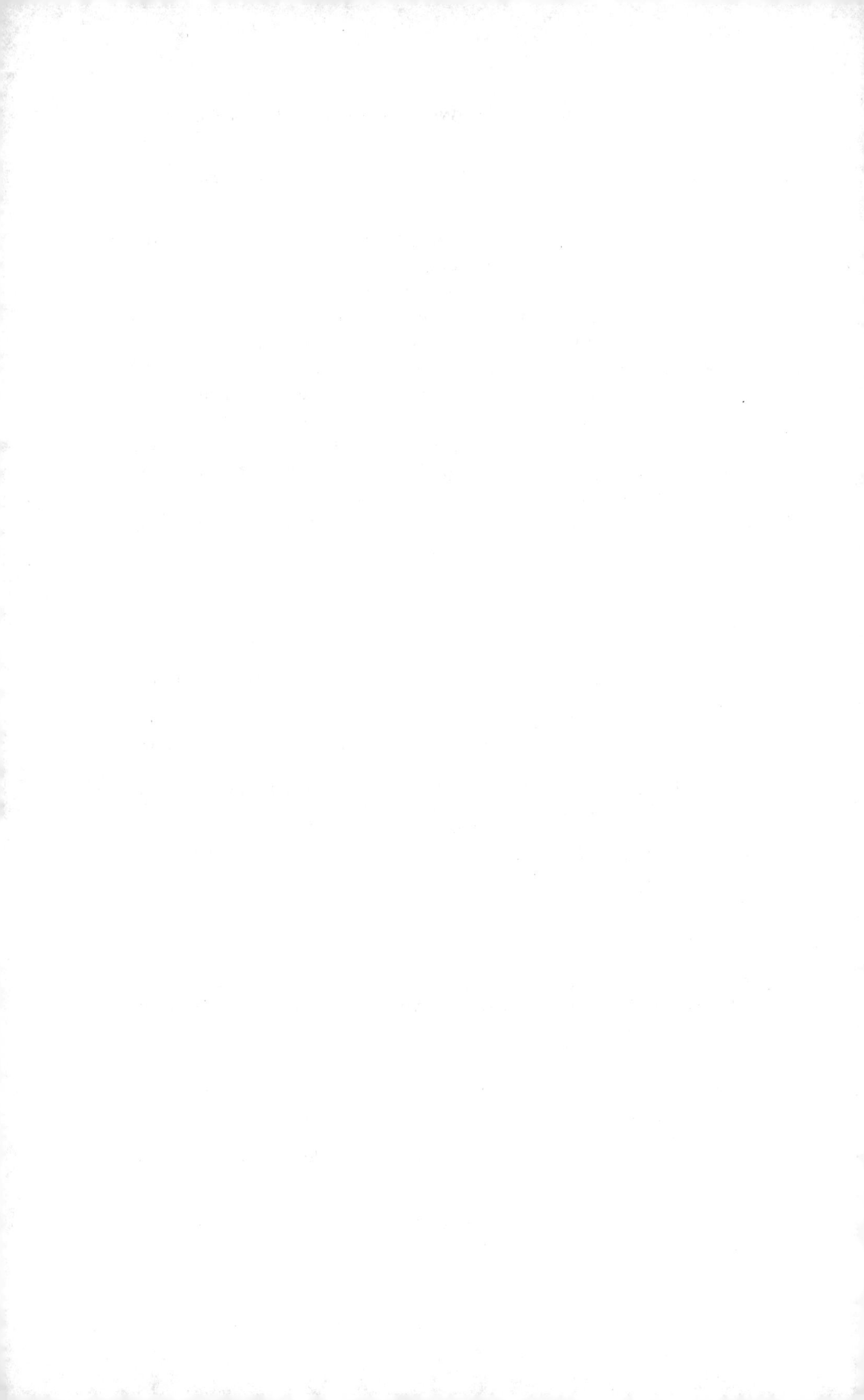

27

ONSITE SYSTEMS FOR DEVELOPING AREAS

Witold Rybczynski
Associate Professor
School of Architecture
McGill University
Montreal, Quebec, Canada H3A 2A7

INTRODUCTION

A discussion of onsite wastewater technologies for developing countries in the 1970s must be prefaced by three important provisos. First, as far as rural sanitation is concerned, and here onsite systems are the exclusive solution for developing countries, very little new technology has been developed that is not already described in the classic World Health Organization (WHO) monograph by Wagner and Lanoix [1]. If there has been less than total success in rural sanitation, and indeed this is the general opinion, then it is not because of a lack of appropriate technologies, but rather because of failures in application, and perhaps failures in properly understanding the social and cultural parameters of improving and changing defecation habits.

Second, although the technological options with regard to onsite waste disposal have remained largely unchanged, the situation in the urban and semiurban areas of the developing countries has changed drastically in the last decade. It was generally assumed in the 1950s that the traditional waste disposal solution, underground sewers, would be applicable to the cities of what was to be called the Third World. This has not proved to be the case. Recent figures released by WHO reveal that whereas in 1970 27% of the urban population in developing countries had sewerage connections, in 1975 this figure had actually declined to 25%. To make matters worse, another

25% had no access to any sanitary system at all [2]. The problem of urban sanitation has not been ignored; on the contrary, all the best efforts to implement conventional sewerage solutions have not been able to keep up with the problem. However, there are indications that now, other lower cost options are finally being considered. Hence, although onsite waste disposal systems have not changed, the context for their application has. Onsite systems, which were previously considered to be exclusively rural in character, must now be reexamined as possible urban solutions.

Third, although there has been a shift to recognizing onsite systems as potential urban technologies, it is probably a mistake to consider them as "alternatives" to offsite disposal, as some have recently done [3,4]. Although this paper focuses exclusively on onsite systems, there are a variety of offsite systems, particularly cartage and vacuum truck systems, but also modified waterborne systems, which are also appropriate solutions. It is likely that, in many cases, the onsite solution will be a first step in an upgrading process that may well lead to some form of offsite system.

CLASSIFICATION OF ONSITE SYSTEMS

There are many ways in which waste disposal systems have been classified: wet or dry, privy or waterborne, according to biological process (infiltration, decomposition, etc.) or according to technological sophistication. A useful practice with respect to low-cost technologies is to differentiate between onsite (or household) and offsite (or community) systems. The former implies small, individual systems; the latter implies systems that require organization and action at the scale of the community. Of course, onsite systems may serve the entire community through a process of agglomeration.

The focus here will be on the onsite technologies, which may be classified according to five general categories, as has been done in a recent World Bank report [5]. The usefulness of these categories is that they represent the current state-of-the-art:

1. Pit latrines (Figure 1)
2. Pour-flush toilets (Figure 2)
3. Composting toilets (Figure 3)
4. Aquaprivies (Figure 4)
5. Septic tanks (Figure 5)

The basic characteristics of these systems are well known, having been described by Wagner and Lanoix [1] and in more recent publications [6].

A literature search carried out in 1977 for the International Development Research Centre in Ottawa turned up more than 500 documents dealing with low-cost sanitation technologies, many of them onsite systems [7]. A brief description of the five classes of onsite systems follows:

Pit Latrines

This is traditional "hole-in-the-ground" solution, which also includes improvements such as vent pipes and offset pits to facilitate emptying. Pits are used until full. Then they are either relocated or emptied and reused.

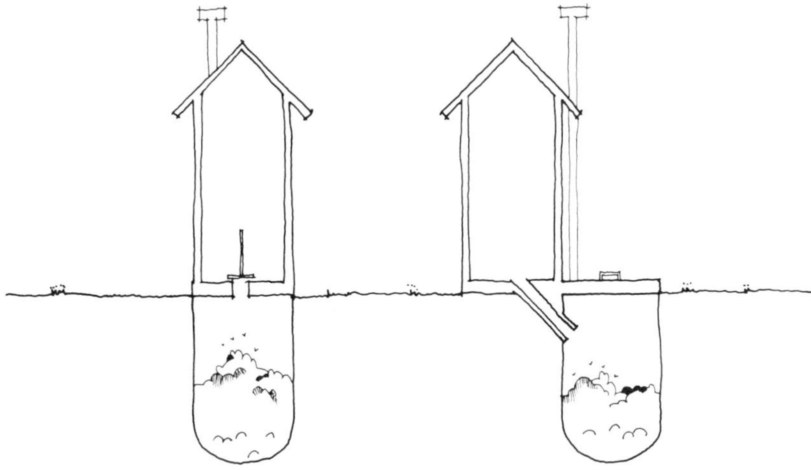

Figure 1. Pit latrines–simple and offset.

Pour-Flush Toilets

This is a modified pit latrine. A manually flushed water seal prevents flies and odors from escaping the pit. This permits the squatting plate to be located inside the house if required. A variety of pour-flush fixtures have been designed (ceramic, concrete, plastic), both for sitting and squatting.

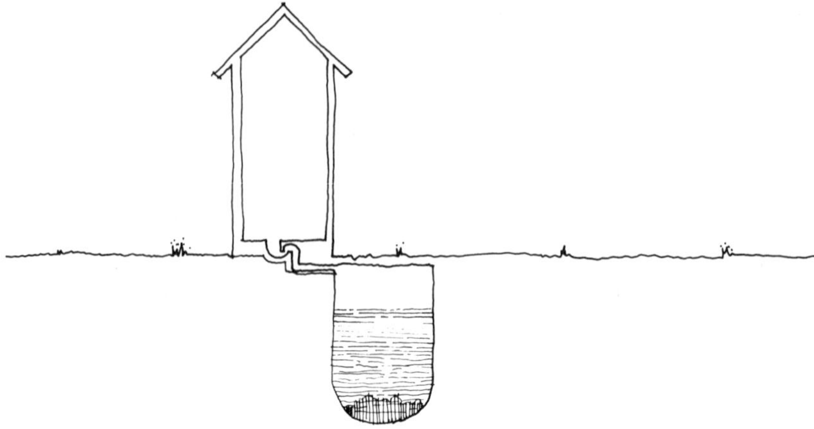

Figure 2. The pour-flush toilet.

Composting Toilets

Composting toilets are containers within which human excreta is collected and undergoes biological decomposition, either aerobic or anaerobic. A variety of composting toilets exist, generally either a continuously used single compartment or alternatively used twin compartments. The product is a nutrient-rich humus.

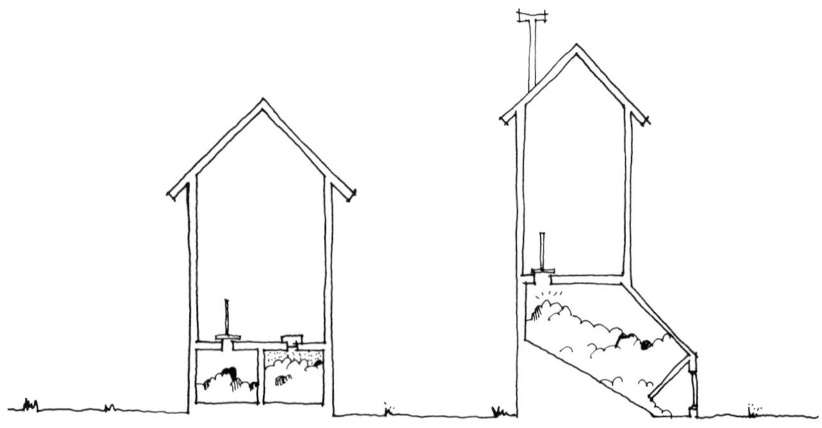

Figure 3. Composting toilets–twin compartment and continuous types.

Aquaprivies

The aquaprivy resembles the septic tank in some ways, except that the water seal is effected by a drop pipe that is submerged below the water level in the tank. Like the pour-flush toilet, a small amount of water is required to operate an aquaprivy. The overflow from the tank is displaced into an adjacent soakage pit. Aquaprivies require periodic desludging.

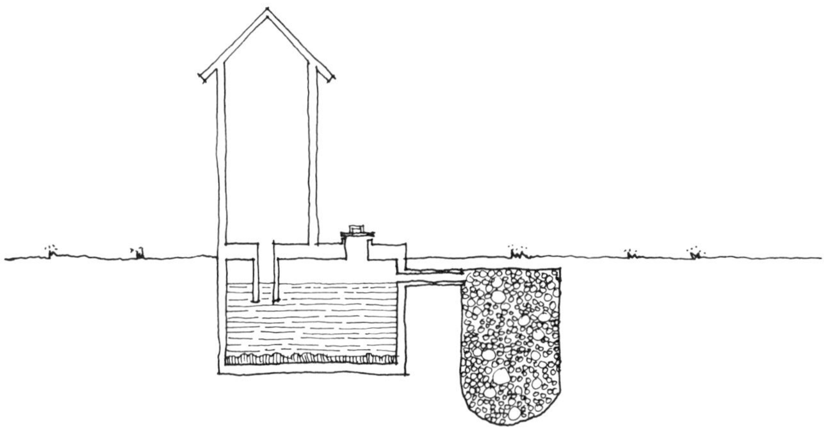

Figure 4. The aquaprivy.

Septic Tanks

The septic tank consists of a retention settling tank and a soakage pit or infiltration field. The septic tank is normally connected to a water flush toilet and can accommodate large amounts of wastewater. Like the aquaprivy, the septic tank requires periodic desludging.

FACTORS AFFECTING THE CHOICE OF A SYSTEM

Although the five classes of onsite systems are generally well understood in a rural context, their application to urban situations requires that a number of factors be taken into consideration. Some of these relate to rural installations as well; other are unique to the urban setting.

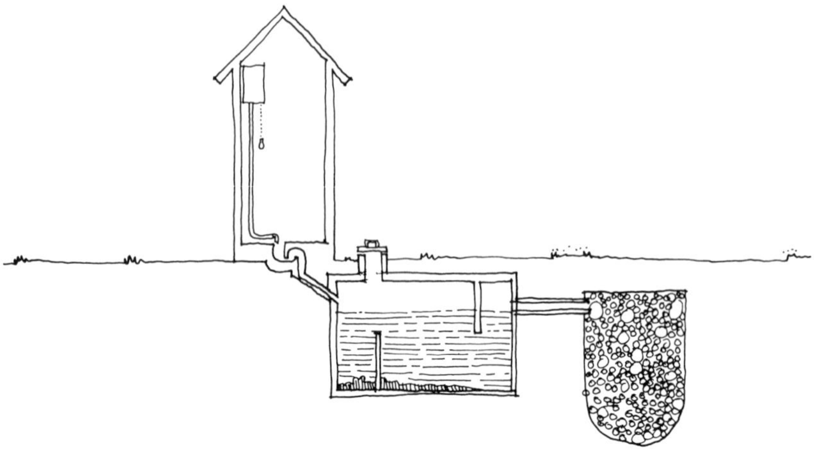

Figure 5. The septic tank.

Water Supply

The availability of water is a major factor in choosing an onsite system. The pit latrine and composting toilet require no water at all to operate. Small amounts of water are used for pour-flush toilets and relatively larger amounts for aquaprivies and septic tanks. Because most urban inhabitants in the developing countries do not have piped water house connections, their problem of sanitation is primarily that of excreta disposal, not, as in American cities, wastewater disposal. This is a crucial difference in choosing an appropriate waste disposal system.

Soil Conditions

The composting toilet is the only onsite system that is entirely above-ground and does not depend on favorable soil conditions. All other systems depend to a greater or lesser extent on sufficient soil porosity for infiltration. Relatively dry systems, such as the pit latrine, can be installed in more impermeable soils than the pour-flush toilet. Aquaprivies and septic tanks require high-porosity soils to function successfully.

Settlement Density

It is likely that composting toilets could be introduced at relatively high densities, although this has not been recorded to date. Pit latrines and pour-flush toilets may function at densities up to 200–300 persons per hectare, although in hot dry climates this has been recorded to be two or even three times higher. Aquaprivies and septic tanks can be installed at a maximum density of about 100–150 persons per hectare, assuming ideal soil conditions. The main limitation of onsite systems is that in all cases they are ground related; that is, they are suited to one- or two-level houses with ground access, but *not* suited to multilevel housing.

Self-Help

The use of self-help in implementing servicing systems is just as important in the urban areas as in the rural village. And the onsite systems, originating as they do in the village, all have some potential for user construction. This potential may be a bit greater with pit latrines, pour-flush toilets and composting toilets than with aquaprivies and septic tanks.

Cultural Adaptability

Onsite systems such as septic tanks, aquaprivies and pour-flush toilets are suitable in regions where religion or tradition prescribe anal cleansing with water (e.g., Muslim areas and in most parts of India). Dry onsite systems may be unsuitable here. On the other hand, in areas where solid materials are used for cleansing (e.g., parts of Africa), experience has shown that pour-flush toilets tend to become clogged. Finally, in cultures with no tradition of excreta reuse, the introduction of composting toilets may be problematic.

UPGRADING ONSITE SYSTEMS

The point has already been made that it is probably a mistake to consider onsite sanitation systems as "alternatives" to offsite technologies. The choice of an onsite system in an urban area should take into account future upgrading. The urban environment is a dynamic one and as water consumption grows, or density increases, or as expectations rise with growing prosperity, it is likely that the "appropriateness" of a particular solution will also change.

There are a number of ways in which onsite systems can be upgraded. Pit latrines can be fitted with liners and turned into parts of a cartage system. Composting toilets could likewise become part of a municipal cleanout system. Aquaprivies can become wet vaults in a vacuum truck system. Both pour-flush toilets and aquaprivies could be ultimately connected to a small-diameter sewer.

Onsite systems can provide high levels of service in terms of hygiene and convenience at significantly reduced cost and, in most cases, without depending on increased water consumption. At the same time they do not preclude future improvements and upgrading. The World Bank research study estimated that over a 30-year period the upgrading that finally would result in pour-flush toilets that overflow into a small-diameter sewer will cost about one-half the present cost of conventional sewerage [5].

The 75% of the urban population in the developing countries presently not served by sewers have had few options. A reexamination of onsite systems for urban application is now in order.

REFERENCES

1. Wagner, E. G., and J. N. Lanoix. "Excreta Disposal for Rural Areas and Small Communities," WHO Monograph No. 39, Geneva (1958).
2. World Health Organization. "Community Water Supply and Excreta Disposal in Developing Countries: Review of Progress," *WHO Stat. Rep.* 29 (No. 10) (1976).
3. Stoner, C. H., Ed. *Goodbye to the Flush Toilet* (Emmaus, PA: Rodale Press, 1977).
4. Van der Ryn, S. *The Toilet Papers* (Santa Barbara, CA: Capra Press, 1978).
5. Kalbermatten, J. M., et al. "Appropriate Sanitation Alternatives: A Technical and Economic Appraisal "Summary Report," P.U. Report No. RES20, unpublished report of the World Bank, Washington, D.C. (1979).
6. Pacey, A., Ed. *Sanitation in Developing Countries* (New York: John Wiley & Sons, Inc., 1978).
7. Rybczynski, W., et al. *Low Cost Technology Options for Sanitation: A State of the Art Review and Annotated Bibliography* (Ottawa: International Development Research Centre, 1978).

28

INNOVATION IN ONSITE TREATMENT SYSTEMS

George W. Reid
Regents Professor and Director
Bureau of Environmental and Water Resources Research
University of Oklahoma
Norman, Oklahoma 73069

INTRODUCTION

Sewage treatment can be classified as conventional or onsite. Onsite sewage treatment can be further classified as hydraulic, biological and/or thermochemical. So communities have a choice between conventional treatment and one of the three general classifications of onsite techniques. The selection should be made according to which provides the best service at the least cost for construction and operation and maintenance (O&M). Finally, the selection of one technique does not preclude the simultaneous use of one or more. To be able to make these choices one must develop a model(s) of the systems and have available the necessary technology and technical coefficients. That is, one must know processes, efficiencies and costs. There exists abundant information on conventional systems.

COST OF ONSITE TREATMENT

A considerable body of technology has also been amassed on onsite treatment, that is, technology on hydraulics, biological and thermochemical treatment techniques: however, there is very little known about onsite costs of the thermochemical alternative under mass production and distribution; however, the information is particularly abundant on hydraulic and biological

Table I. Collection Systems–Population and Density Versus Energy Requirements and Annual Costs (1976) [1]

Population of Agencies	Miles of Sewer	Population per Mile	Annual Sewer Line Cost ($/mi)	Number of Lift Stations	Installed Pump Horsepower	Energy Consumed (millions kWh)
10,000	29	345	185	5	52	0.0239
36,685	128	287	297	5	220	0.120
43,000	153	281	910	22	1390	0.608
84,700	337	251	521	5	16	0.006
89,200	360	248	839	26	565	NA[a]
309,000	1211	255	469	48	3112	4.0
383,000	1600	239	2444	57	1997	1.93
557,000	1450	385	674	13	NA	NA
728,400	1355	538	1370	5	855	0.491
			Range of Values			
10,000–728,400	29–1600	239–538	185–2444	5–57	16–3112	0.006–4.0

[a]NA = not available.

methods, including lagoons, septic tanks, etc. Onsite treatment technology has developed for application to rural or dispersed sites. Recently, however, it is becoming apparent that onsite treatment is perhaps the only viable alternative to conventional systems in urban sites. In rural areas, where the combination of sewers and a central plant is not economically feasible, the septic tank, lagoon, etc. are methods of choice. On shipboard, offshore oil rigs, toll bridges and in suburban and recreation areas of unsuitable soil conditions, the thermal toilet is used. Because of the recycle potential, thermochemical onsite technology is appropriate for water-short areas, as well as where water is conserved or sewers are underused or pressurized.

An intriguing potential for onsite–thermal methods is found in the lesser developed countries. Obviously there are places that really require no supporting evidence where onsite technology applies. However, what about the onsite alternative in American cities? The proposed comparison is onsite versus conventional sewerage systems, and the bottom line is cost.

The conventional system has progressed from storm drainage to combination storm and sanitary sewers, and finally to separate sewers with sewage treatment. The sewerage system lost some of its economy when separate sewers became necessary. Sewage treatment is amenable to considerable

Table II. Cost per Household per Year for Wastewater Services in Communities with Populations of Less than 50,000 [2]

Cost/Household/Year ($U.S.)	258 Facilities (%)	83 New Facilities (%)
100–200	40	75
200–300	10	20
>300	>0	>0
<100	50	5

Table III. User Charges per Month for Wastewater Services in Communities with a Population of Less than 50,000 [2]

User Charge/Month ($U.S.)	Community Size
<12	All other communities
12–20	10,000 or smaller
20–30	Some communities

Table IV. Comparison

Method	Name	Country	Unit Cost $0–100	Unit Cost $100–500	Unit Cost $500–1000	Unit Cost Over $1000
Incinerating	Destroilet	USA			*	
	Ecett	Sweden			*	
	Electro Standard	Sweden			*	
	Elonette	Sweden		*		
	Incinolet	USA			*	
	Toarett	Sweden		*		
	Xpurgator	USA				*
Composting	Clivus Multrum	Sweden				*
	(Same Name)	(USA)				*
	Mull-Toa	Norway		*		
	(Biu-Let)	(USA)			*	
	Saniterm	Sweden			*	
	Toa-Throne	USA			*	
	Farallones Privy	USA	*			
		Denmark	*			
	Kern Compost Privy	USA		*		
	Mulbank	Sweden		*		
	(Ecolet)	(USA)			*	
	Humumat	Canada				
	Kombio	Norway			*	
	Mull-Toa Jumbo	Norway			*	
	KPS Miljoklosett	Norway		*		
	Tropic	Norway		*		
Biological	Cycle-Let	USA				
	Bio-Flo	USA			*	
	Jet Flush	UK		*		
	Monomatic	USA		*		
	Potpourri	Canada	*			
	Craft Toilet	USA		*		
Vacuum	Vacu-Flush	USA			*	
	Electrolux Vacuum Sewage System	Sweden				*
	Airvac	USA				
	Envirovac	USA			*	
	Lectra/San	USA				
Aerobic	Digestomatic	USA				
	Aerobic Home System	USA				
	Sewerless Toilet	USA				*
	Waste Tamer	USA				
	Microx	USA				

of Devices and Systems

		Requirements				
Operating Costs	Capacity (persons)	Water	Power	Chemicals	Effluent	Primary Application
3–5¢/u[a]	4–16		*		A[b]	Second home
6¢/u	4–6		*		A	Second home
5¢/u	4–6		*		A	Second home
4¢/u			*		A	Second home
5¢/u	4–12		*		A	Industry
8¢/u			*		A	Second home
	4–20		*		A	Developmental
	4–40				S[c]	Home
	4–40				S	Home
	3–4		*		S	Second home
	3–4		*		S	Second home
24¢/day			*		S	
	4–6		*		S	Second home
	4–6				S	Rural
	4–6				S	
	4–6				S	
6¢/day	2–4		*		S	Second home
6¢/day	2–4		*		S	Second home
			*		S	
					S	
			*		S	
			*		S	
			*		S	
		*	*	*	L[d]	
4¢/day	1–12			*	L	Second home
	100/u		*	*	L	Portable
	100/u		*	*	L	Airlines
	50/u			*	L	Portable
	200/u		*	*	L	Marine
	4+		*		L	Marine
	4+		*		L	Recreation area
			*		L	Community
			*		L	Community
	3–5		*		L	Marine
		*	*		L	
		*	*	*	L	
		*	*		L	
		*	*		L	
		*	*		L	

Table IV,

Method	Name	Country	Unit Cost $0–100	$100–500	$500–1000	Over $1000
Aerobic (continued)	Cromaglass	USA			*	
	Flo-Thru	USA				*
	Bio Disc	Canada				*
	Aquarobic	Canada				*
Oil Flush	Magic Flush	USA				*
	Aqua Sans	USA				*
	Sarmax	USA				

[a]u = use.
[b]A = ash.
[c]S = solid.
[d]L = liquid.

economies of scale; that is, one can treat larger amounts of waste at increasingly lower per capita costs (Figure 1), but the cost of conveying sewage to the plant increases with size. For example, at a population level of 10,000, sewers would cost $185–200 per mile per year. At a population level of 100,000, the cost would be $800 per mile per year, or four times as much. For 500,000 people, the cost reduces to $700 per mile per year (Table I) [1]. Sewerage system charges generally range from $1500 to $2000 per household, with a hypothetical monthly cost of $23–30 per month (Tables II and III) [2]. (This is estimated at 8% for 20 years financing charges.)

The cost of conventional systems includes both conveyance and treatment, with conveyance charged separately from treatment. Also included are the cost of financing and debt retirement, usually equal to capital cost. Each additional increment to the system costs more, due to upstream location and inflation.

In addition to conveyance and treatment cost, there are also environmental costs entailed in large or metropolitan treatment plants, and these are inescapable. For example, a small town of 10,000 will discharge to a water course, at 90% treatment efficiency, a population equivalent to 1000 people. A city of 100,000 discharges at a 10,000 population equivalent. So size and central plants create concentration discharge problems. One could suggest increasing the treatment level by 10–99% and reducing the discharge level to a population equivalent of 1000, but at what cost? Because the costs are a function of what is yet to be removed, the last 10%, will probably cost as much as the first 90%. And this says nothing about nutritional pollution.

continued

Operating Costs	Capacity (persons)	Requirements			Effluent	Primary Application
		Water	Power	Chemicals		
	4–25	*	*		L	Home/industry
	6	*	*		L	Home
	5–500	*	*		L	Home/industry
	8	*	*		L	Home
	4+		*		L	Second home
	4+		*		L	Recreation area
	4–6		*		L	Home/recreation area

COMPARISON OF FINANCING ARRANGEMENTS FOR CONVENTIONAL AND ONSITE SYSTEMS

The other issue is one of financing. Central systems usually require 20 to 40-year loans, with aggregate carrying charges equal to or in excess of, capital costs. Finally, because of federal assistance (PL 660 and others), many of the costs are passed to Washington then back to the citizen, with at least a 20% loss.

Onsite systems are dispersed, and are generally "pay-as-you-go," increasing with inflation and finance charges. If all concerns are taken into account, the costs of onsite devices are competitive, if not cheaper. Because of federal grants, the real cost of conventional systems is not readily visible. Tables IV-VII compare various onsite systems and their costs. The incinerating onsite toilet appears to have the greatest potential in the urban environment. The potential would be increased if it were manufactured in volume.

CONCLUSIONS

It is apparent that onsite treatment is competitive except in very large cities, and the economic incentive would be reduced if effluent acceptance and real costs were considered in the evaluation. Unfortunately, energy-dependent onsite treatment requires toilet flush reductions and alternative methods of greywater handling. In large cities in developing countries, or any site where water is short, this concern is reduced by reduced volumes, but in

Table V. Cost Estimates for Water-Saving Alternatives [3]

Alternative	Soil	Capital Cost ($U.S.)	Operation and Maintenance Cost ($U.S./yr)	Total ($U.S./yr)
Large Biological Toilet + Septic Tank (ST)–Soil Absorption System (SAS)	Good	2900	20	244
	Fair	3200	20	268
	Poor	3500	20	291
Small Biological Toilet + ST-SAS	Good	1900	90	237
	Fair	2200	90	260
	Poor	2500	90	283
Incinerator Toilet + ST-SAS	Good	1650	180	308
	Fair	1950	180	331
	Poor	2250	180	354
Low-Flush Toilet + ST-SAS	Good	1400	96	210
	Fair	1700	96	234
	Poor	2000	96	257
Septic Tank–Conventional Soil Absorption System (SAS)	Good	975	10	85
	Fair	1288	10	109
	Poor	1600	10	134
Septic Tank–Pressurized Distribution (dosing)–SAS	Good	1317	35	134
	Fair	1641	35	159
	Poor	1964	35	194
Septic Tank–Alternating Beds	Good	1700	10	141
	Fair	2326	10	189
	Poor	2950	10	238
Septic Tank–Mound System	--	3500	35	305
Septic Tank–Evapotranspiration (ET)	--	4000	10	319
Septic Tank–Sand Filter–Disinfection	--	3415	150	421
Aerobic Unit–Pressurized Distribution (dosing)	Good	2347	122	326
	Fair	2671	122	351
	Poor	2994	122	376
Aerobic Unit–Sand Filter–Disinfection	--	3395	207	492
Aerobic Unit–Disinfection	--	2645	147	374

present U.S. urban environments it is a primary concern. As mentioned earlier, effective onsite treatment in an urban environment could be achieved through the combined use of biological, thermal and conventional systems, each applied where most economically feasible. Table VIII provides an interesting comparison of the major factors involved in various systems of waste disposal and treatment.

One could envision (1) a central city with a sewered system and

Table VI. Estimated Price List of Sewerless Systems with Volume Projections ($U.S.)[a]

	List Price	Wholesale Price	Estimated Unit Price–High Production (1000–5000 units/order)
Incinerating			
Destroilet	599	449	360
Xpurgator	2000[b]	800	700
Composting			
Clivus			
Community Production	1685	605	200
Toa-Throne	1045	952	806
Ecolet	736[b]		
Mull-Toa	795[b]		
Bio Loo	795[b]		
Biological			
Mod A	980		
Mod 75	1400–1700[b]		
Bio-Flow #512	402		

[a]Depending on the marketing strategy selected, profits could vary widely, thereby altering these figures.
[b]It is felt that large-scale production should provide a figure of from 30–40% less for these systems. This level has not yet been attempted.

Table VII. Estimated Total Annual Cost per Capita for Representative Sewerless and Conventional Waste Treatment/Disposal Methods ($U.S.)

Treatment Method	Process Number	Population Size			
		500–2500	2500–15,000	15,000–50,000	50,000–100,000
Incinerating Toilet	PSS2	38	38	38	38
Biological Toilet	PSS3	23	23	23	23
Composting Toilet	PSS4	8	8	8	8
Conventional System		70–44	63–37	35–25	33–25

conventional plant for itself and its large manufacturing component; (2) a commercial area with thermal units; (3) the suburban area using single thermal units and soil disposal of greywater; and (4) the rural fringe areas using any of the biological toilets (Table IX).

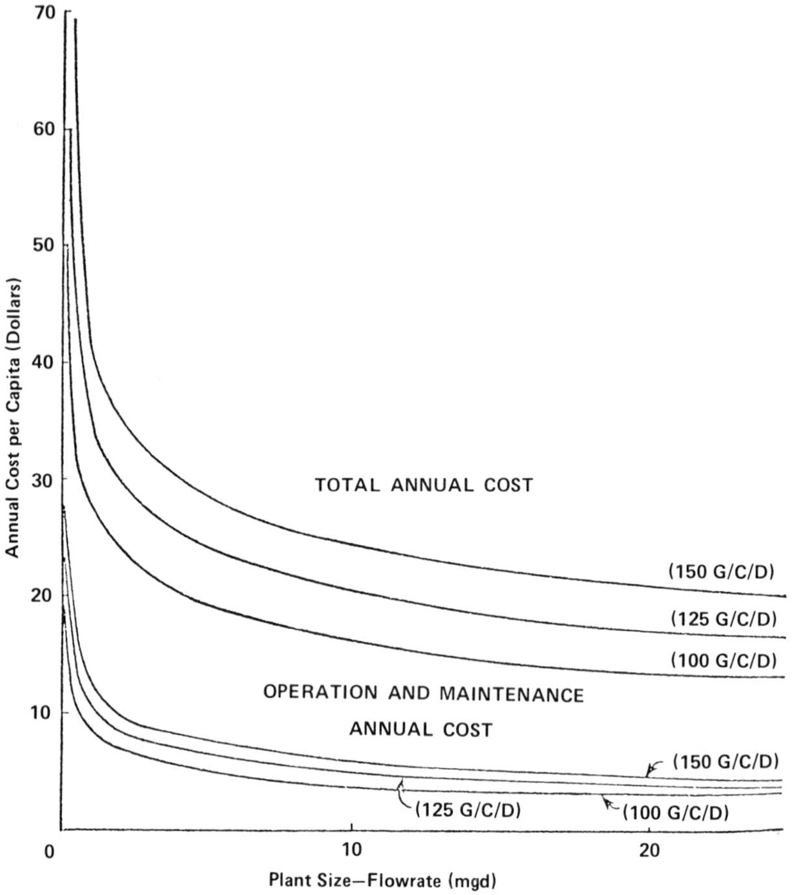

Figure 1. Annual per capita costs according to wastewater treatment plant size.

The primary ingredient needed at this point is to demonstrate the potential of onsite treatment under several real life situations, e.g., finding demonstration sites where such schemes can be tried.

REFERENCES

1. Brady, J., S. Goodman, K. Kerri and R. Reed. "Performance Indicators for Wastewater Collection Systems," paper presented at the Fiftieth Annual Water Pollution Control Federation Conference, Philadelphia, PA, October 2-7, 1977.

Table VIII. Assessment of Important Attributes Related to Systems of Waste Disposal/Treatment [4]

	System Type		
	Waterborne	Cartage	Onsite
Capital Cost	High	High/low	Low
Operating Cost	Low	High	Low
Offshore Cost Component[a]	High	High/low	Nil
Water Consumption	High	Low/nil	Low/nil
Optimal Density	High density (high rise)	High density (low rise)	High and low density (low rise)
Adaptability to Incremental Implementation	Nil	High	High
Adaptability to Self-Help	Nil	Low	High

[a]Offshore cost component refers to materials not available locally.

Table IX. The Combined Use of Various Waste Disposal/Treatment Methods in a Metropolitan and Surrounding Area

Site	Technology	
Central City	Sewered and treatment	
Second and Manufacturing Area	Plants	
Commercial Area	Single, thermal units	
Suburban Area	Single, thermal units	Soil disposal for greywater
Isolated Embedded Urban Cells	Larger, multiple-thermal units	Central laundries
Rural Fringe	Biological toilet	

2. U.S. Environmental Protection Agency. "O&M Considerations for Small Municipal Wastewater Treatment Facilities," Washington, D.C. (1977).
3. Krissel, J. "U.S. EPA Response to PL 92-500 Relating to Rural Wastewater Problems—Office of Research and Development (Sections 104 and 105)," in *Individual Onsite Wastewater Systems, Proceedings of the Third National Conference*, N. I. McClelland, Ed. (Ann Arbor, MI: Ann Arbor Science Publishers, Inc., 1977).
4. Rybczynski, W., P. Chrongrak and M. McGarry. "Stop the Faecal Peril: A Technology Review," International Development Research Centre, Ottawa (1977).

29

MICROBIAL ECOLOGY OF AN AEROBIC RECYCLING ONSITE TREATMENT PLANT

Paul G. Moe
Professor of Bacteriology
Division of Plant and Soil Sciences
West Virginia University
Morgantown, West Virginia 26506

William J. Shoupp
Research Assistant
Pittsburgh, Pennsylvania 15218

John M. Dingess
Graduate Research Assistant
School of Law
University of North Dakota
Grand Forks, North Dakota 58201

INTRODUCTION

As population densities increase, modern man is faced with two great problems. On the one hand, there is a finite supply of natural resources on this planet and we are rapidly approaching the point where shortages of resources may limit our further development. On the other hand, as the natural resources are being depleted, waste products are accumulating at an alarming rate and pollution of our environment is becoming a crucial concern.

One obvious answer to both problems is to recycle waste products into usable forms. Indeed, nature has been recycling elements from one form to another since the world began, but natural processes tend to be slow, and modern man is developing novel ways of speeding up the recycling processes. The rapid purification of wastewater to replace freshwater supplies again provides a good example of such a solution.

Recycling wastewater within an individual home so as to obviate the need for both freshwater supplies and wastewater disposal is a relatively novel idea that is currently being investigated. This report focuses on the results of our investigations into some of the biological problems associated with the operation of such a recycling unit.

BACKGROUND

The idea of recycling wastewater may, at first glance, be repulsive to many people; however, the issue can be placed in better perspective if one recognizes that even rain is recycled water from the best and worst sources. One must also consider that waste treatment plant effluents enter many streams and lakes, which serve as water sources for other municipalities downstream [1]. Indeed, one survey [2] showed that some American cities may have to use more than 18% raw sewage in their water supplies during dry seasons. Undeniably, the public attitude is changing in this regard. Kasperson [3], in a report on surveys taken in various locations in the U.S., states that from 45-75% of the respondents of an area would be willing to use recycled water for drinking. Others [4,5] have also observed ready acceptance of recycle systems in private homes. The potential for savings seems incredible. Gavis [6] states that an 80% reuse of wastewater would amount to a 400% increase in the available water supply.

In 1966, in a review of the microbiology of wastewater, Gaudy and Gaudy [7] stated that most studies of wastewater microbiology traditionally have centered on removing, killing or controlling microbes therein. They further stated that a more challenging and practical endeavor would be the description of the mechanisms and kinetics of the microbial population's growth in wastewater systems. In 1971 they went on to advocate that more attention should be paid to the biological principles involved [8]. They also stated that the potential for biological processing of waste had barely been tapped. Paynter and Bungay [9], in a contemporary report concerning studies of microbial interaction on the performance of waste treatment systems, also called for ecological studies of waste treatment processes.

Of all the operating parameters affecting the microbial ecology of a waste disposal system, the organic feedrate, aeration status, temperature and retention time were considered to be of most interest for this study. Unfortunately, there is relatively little information available in the literature on the effects of any of these variables on the microbial population in activated sludge or extended aeration systems.

It has been reported [10] that it is necessary to maintain a dissolved oxygen concentration of between 0.2 and 2.0 mg/l in the aeration tank of an activated sludge digestion system to maintain a predominance of aerobic microorganisms in the microflora. The level of dissolved oxygen present in the digestion tank represents a balance between the rate of dissolved oxygen utilization by microorganisms (usually between 10 and 100 mg/l/hr) and the oxygen transfer efficiency of the aeration system employed. Unfortunately, the oxygen transfer efficiency is quite low in domestic treatment systems, usually about 5%, so that only about 1% of the air pumped into the mixed liquor is absorbed [10, 11]. Thus, the aeration rate required to meet the needs of microbial metabolism can be calculated to be somewhere between 12 and 120 ml of air per liter of wastewater per minute. High aeration rates are known to create excessive turbulence, which prevents satisfactory floc formation [12]. Therefore, for efficiency as well as economic reasons, commercial units are designed to operate at the minimum aeration rate required to maintain aerobic conditions.

As in most living systems, an increase in temperature results in an increase in the reaction rate constants of some of the metabolic reactions occurring in activated sludge [13, 14]. Busch [15] suggested the use of the Arrhenius equation to predict this change, but quickly noted that in practice temperature effects are much less severe than predicted. He referred to microbial adaptability as a reason for this phenomenon.

The overall effect of temperature on growth of microorganisms is complicated by secondary effects of temperature on solubility of gases, especially oxygen, and other nutrients [16].

The retention time of the wastewater in the digestion tank, defined as the liquid volume contained in the tank divided by the flowrate through the tank, would also be expected to have an important influence on the makeup of the microflora population in the tank. Low retention times would select for the fast-growing organisms capable of maintaining a high population level in the tank, whereas longer retention times would allow a whole succession of microorganisms to develop.

Commercial household aeration units are usually sized for a 24- to 48-hour retention period [10]. Consequently, they likely would behave more like extended aeration systems than conventional activated sludge systems, which normally utilize aeration periods of 6–8 hours [10].

One concern with recycling units is the accumulation of salt in the system. While organic compounds are degraded mainly to CO_2 and H_2O, which are vented from the system as gases, mineral salts remain to recycle over and over in the system. Eventually salt concentrations will build up to toxic levels, which will inhibit biological activity. Whereas most bacteria are inhibited by salt concentrations of 2–3%, some can tolerate much higher concentrations. It has been reported [17] that activated sludge that has been developed in freshwater can recover quickly from slug doses of NaCl up to a mixed liquor concentration of 30,000 ppm. However, if the salt concentration goes as high as 45,000 ppm, the system efficiency is severely impaired.

In general, activated sludge systems are considered to be quite sensitive to shock loads of biochemical oxygen demand (BOD). Treatment efficiency is closely related to the food/microorganism ratio (F/M), which is upset by large fluctuations in BOD loading. Extended aeration systems are known to be more stable and can accept intermittent loads without upset [10].

Gaudy and Gaudy [8] stated that it is difficult to confidently predict the results of shock loads on an activated sludge system because the loads are generally imposed in combination and may change relative to the combination. Also, differences in the immediate past history of the sludge may dictate different reponses to the same shock. It has been reported [18-21] that a favorable system recovery to a qualitative shock often requires the addition of a nitrogen source, whereas a successful recovery to a quantitative shock does not. The time required for recovery is also shorter for quantitative shocks. The recovery time for qualitative shocks depends on the chemical nature of new compounds introduced.

As might be expected, many of the ecological studies that have been performed on activated sludge systems have concerned themselves with bacteria. Certainly it is an important consideration from a public health viewpoint, as several bacterial diseases are communicated by intestinal discharges [22]. One might expect the bacterial community of sewage and activated sludge to resemble the human intestinal flora. This is not the case. Several studies [23-30] have revealed the intestinal flora to be composed largely of obligate anaerobes. *Bacteriodies* and *Bifidobacterium* are usually the dominate genera, followed by smaller numbers of members of the family *Enterobacteriaceae* and gram-positive cocci. Because the activated sludge process is aerobic, obligate anaerobes persist only in the event of a malfunction in the aeration system [31]. Moreover, even in an anaerobic treatment process it has been reported that the dominant fecal flora are replaced by gram-positive rods and cocci [32, 33].

More in-depth studies of the bacteriology of activated sludge systems are presented by Prakasam and Dondero [34, 35], Banks and Walker [36, 37], Pike et al. [38], Lighthart and Oglesby [39] and Dias and Bhat [40,41]. It was generally found that *Zoogloea* was the dominant genus. High numbers of *Flavobacterium*, *Cytophaga* and *Achromobacter* were also found [39], with relatively few coliform species present [40]. *Bdellovibrio* and bacteriophages were not found to be active in activated sludge [41]. Pike [42] noted that most enteric organisms and pathogens grew more slowly and were overgrown by the dominant sludge species. They were not able to replenish their number after grazing by protozoa.

Bacterial predators are an important component of a properly functioning activated sludge system, and their necessity has been well established

[43-45]. Protozoa-free sludges produce effluents containing high levels of BOD, turbidity, organic carbon and suspended solids [44]. Such sludges are a clear demonstration of the importance of protozoa in removing the dispersed bacterial cells. Indeed, the dissolved oxygen demand level of a sludge is closely associated with the oxygen demand of the protozoa in it [46]. Grazing by protozoa prevents bacterial populations from reaching self-limiting numbers. This keeps the bacteria in a prolonged state of physiological youth, in which the rate of assimilation of organic material is at a maximum [47].

Fungi are certainly a part of any biological sewage treatment process and therefore are important to study. However, fungi are not normally found as dominant organisms in the activated sludge process [48]. A thorough review of the role of fungi in waste treatment processes is presented by Tomlinson and Williams [49], in which they identify *Penicillium*, *Cephalosporium*, *Cladosporium* and *Alternaria* as the four most common genera found in activated sludge plants.

MATERIALS AND METHODS

Equipment

The initial studies (runs I, II and III) were conducted using only one simple digestion tank constructed of plywood coated inside and out with fiberglass and epoxy resin. The total capacity of this tank was 1354 liters.

The top panel of the tank served as a mounting platform for a standard ceramic toilet bowl without an integral water closet. The toilet, flushed with recycled water, dropped its content of synthetic feces directly onto a stainless steel baffle, which hung 10 cm below the top panel inside the tank. The water supply to the toilet bowl was provided by recycling the water from the tank at the 91-cm depth level through a centrifugal pump up and into the toilet bowl through 1-inch-diameter piping.

The recycled water was flushed through the circuit 10 times daily at the rate of 19 liters per flush cycle. This simulated domestic toilet flushing and helped to aerate the contents of the digestion tank. A 24-hour timer in conjunction with a 15-minute reset timer were used to regulate the timing and duration of the flush-recycle periods.

In addition to the aeration provided via the flushing cycles, an aeration system utilizing the laboratory compressed air supply was fitted to the digestion tank. The air was first passed through a filter and a pressure regulator, then through a flowmeter and two lengths of tubing to two cylindrical diffusion air stones (25 × 22 m-diameter fused crystalline alumina). The air stones hung down perpendicularly into the water column of the tank at a depth of 40 cm.

In experimental runs I, II and III the digestion tank was filled with tap water to a depth of just over 185 cm. This amounted to 1020 liters of water. The tank was then loaded twice a day with an artificial waste material, which was accomplished with an automated tank loading device that was mounted on the top of the toilet bowl and supported by a wooden substructure that rested on the floor.

This loading system was activated twice a day by an automatic timing system, which allowed the motor to drive the rotating platform long enough to drop the contents of one beaker of waste material into the toilet bowl every 12 hours (at noon and at midnight each day). Then the next flushing-water cycle washed the waste material into the digestion tank. Weekly samples of the contents of the digestion tank were collected from six sampling ports arranged vertically along one face of the tank. Samples collected from the five upper sampling ports were uniform in their characteristics and were averaged together as being representative of the "mixed liquor" in the tank. Samples collected from the lowest port (7.5 cm above the bottom of the tank) were quite different and are reported below as being representative of the "sludge."

Because of difficulties experienced in reducing the content of suspended solids in these initial studies, the system was later modified to include a settling tank, filtration system, ultraviolet (UV) disinfection unit and storage tank. This modified system was used in runs IV through VIII (Figure 1).

The settling tank, when filled to a height of 2 meters, contained 100 liters of wastewater. The tank was fitted with a fiberglass baffle, which was mounted vertically through the center of the tank. Wastewater from the digestion tank entered the settling tank on one side of this baffle and was drawn out of the tank from the other side. Settled sludge was withdrawn from the bottom of the settling tank and pumped back to the digestion tank.

Supernatant wastewater from the quiescent side of the baffle plate was pumped through a filtering device (10-μ pore size) and an ultraviolet disinfection device (7.2 W of radiant energy at 2537 Å units) to a reservoir tank. This tank was of identical construction to the settling tank, except for the baffle plate. Water was pumped from the bottom of the reservoir tank back up to the commode on the flushing cycle to complete the circuit. A flexible immersion heating coil (240 V, 1000 W) was placed in the lower third of the digestion tank to allow operation of this unit at above ambient temperatures during run V. The entire assembly was located in an air-conditioned laboratory to facilitate temperature control.

To provide better aeration in the digester, the original air diffusion stones were replaced by larger aeration diffusers, which were 5 cm in diameter and

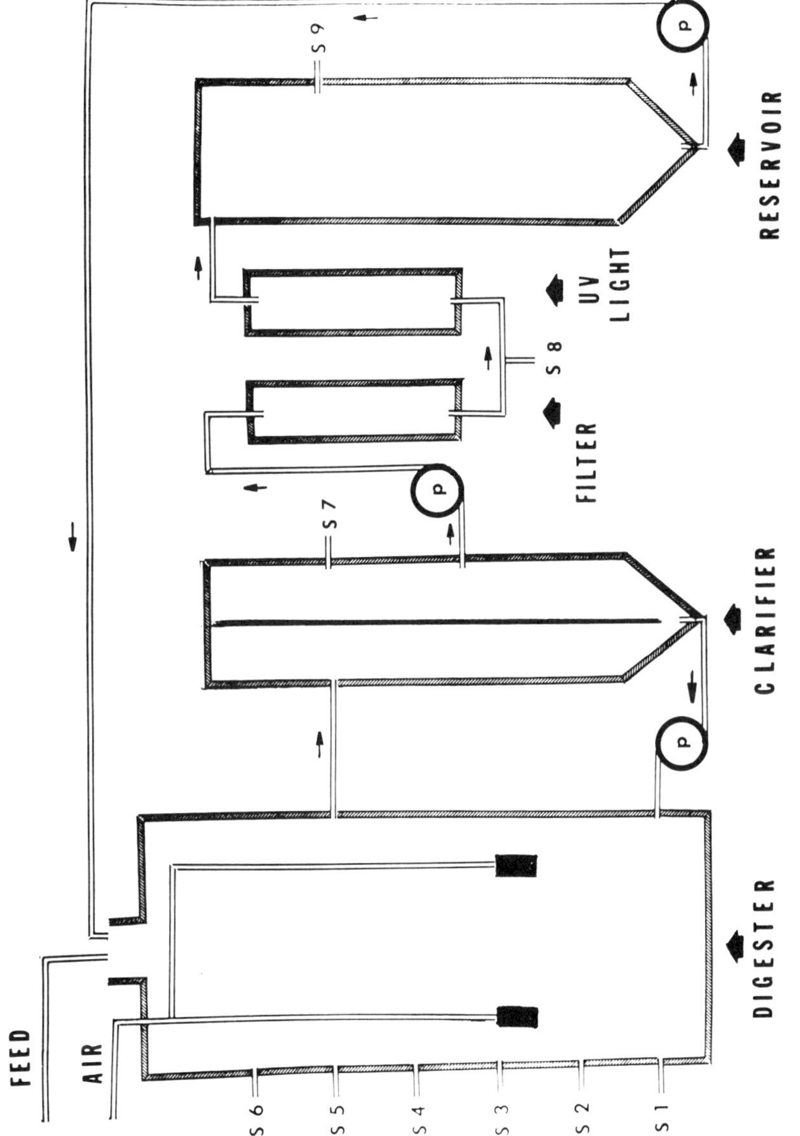

Figure 1. A schematic diagram of the revised experimental system.

15 cm long. These provided a diffusion surface of more than 300 cm^2, compared with the 9.5 cm^2 surface area of the original air diffusion stones.

For experimental runs IV, V, VII and VIII, 1098 liters of wastewater were retained in the digestion tank, giving a calculated retention time in the tank of 140 hours. During experimental run VI, where a shorter retention time was required, the volume of wastewater in the digester was reduced to 886 liters, resulting in a retention time of 112 hours.

Before each experimental run, an 18.9-liter seed of sludge obtained from the anaerobic digestion tanks of the Morgantown sewage treatment plant was added to the digestion tank. This seed was allowed to settle for five days before aeration and loading of waste material began.

During experimental runs IV–VIII, periodic samples were collected from the same six ports previously described in the digestion tank and from three additional ports: (1) in the settling tank, (2) between the filtering device and the UV disinfecting unit, and (3) in the reservoir tank. Tapwater was added to the system to replenish the water lost by sampling and evaporation whenever a noticeable decrease in the water level occurred.

Synthetic Sanitary Waste Material

An artificial waste material was used for the biodegradation studies. Its composition (Table I) was based on an artifical sewage concentrate employed by Hunter et al. [14] in their studies of the activated sludge process. The synthetic waste fell within the ranges for the major constituents of fecal and urinous wastes for an average human [50] (Table II). The dry weight

Table I. Composition of the Artificial Waste Material Used in this Study

Material	g/Person/day
Ferric Chloride	0.29
Magnesium Sulfate	0.84
Calcium Chloride	0.84
Sodium Chloride	1.35
Urea	5.10
Sodium Dihydrogen Phosphate	7.87
Sodium Bicarbonate	10.11
Toilet Tissue (shredded)	10.00
Dry Dog Food (ground)	33.70
	70.10 g total
Distilled water	60.06 ml

Table II. Partial Analysis of the Artificial Waste Material Used in this Study

Material	Artificial Feces
Nitrogen (wt%)[a]	2.4
Carbon (wt%)[b]	31.6
Hydrogen (wt%)	5.4
Phosphorus (%)[c]	0.35
Potassium (ppm)[d]	12.0
Sodium (ppm)	270.0
Magnesium (ppm)	18.0
Calcium (ppm)	150.0
Zinc (ppm)	1.5
Copper (ppm)	5.0
Iron (ppm)	5.0
Manganese (ppm)	0.2
BOD_5 (mg/l)[e]	6010.0

[a]By Kjeldahl method.
[b]By elemental analyzer (C and H).
[c]By colorimetric analysis.
[d]By atomic absorption (K, Na, Mg, Ca, Zn, Cu, Fe and Mn).
[e]By manometric method.

of the artificial waste material used to simulate the daily input of one person's sanitary wastes to the system was 70.05 g. This material was mixed with 66 ml of distilled water to form synthetic fecal pellets, which were introduced into the digestion tank via the automatic tank loading system.

Experimental Variables

The major objective of this project was to obtain some information on the effect of altering operating parameters of this recycling waste disposal system on the makeup of the microbial population in the system. The independent variables included organic feedrate, aeration rate, temperature and retention time. The survivability of pathogenic organisms in the system and the effect of shock loadings on the system were also studied. Several short (less than 30 days) experimental runs were made initially to test the operating efficiency of the system and to determine a suitable range of loading and aeration rates. It was found that a maximum of four persons per day loading rate could be used without anaerobiosis and a concomitant odor problem. The aeration system was found to be capable of supplying up to 15 liter/min of air reliably over a relatively long time span.

In light of the results from the preliminary runs, it was decided to conduct a long-term run (run I) to determine the long-term reliability of the entire system running at what were probably suboptimal loading and aeration rates. Data points were obtained over a period of 130 days for adenosine triphosphate content, pH and dissolved oxygen (DO) levels. This run proved that the system functioned reliably and provided some baseline data for the other experimental runs that were to follow.

The next two experimental runs employed loading rates of 2 (run II) and 3 (run III) persons per day and aeration rates of 6 and 12 liter/min. Each of these runs consisted of three distinct segments: (1) a 6-liter/min aeration rate with feed (72 days in run II and 56 days in run III); followed by (2) a 12-liter/min aeration rate with feed (39 days in run II and 31 days in run III); followed by (3) a 12-liter/min aeration rate without feed (35 days in run II and 42 days in run III).

Run IV was the first conducted after the system had been modified to include the water purification equipment and the improved aeration system. Operating conditions were maintained the same as in the second segment of run III, i.e., 3 persons per day loading rate and 12 liter/min of air aeration. When it was found that the additional equipment had only a minor effect on the operation of the original components, four more experimental runs to examine other variables were conducted.

In run V all factors were held constant with those of run IV, except the temperature of the digestion tank, which was increased from an average of 23°C to an average of 34°C.

To simulate what would occur in a smaller sized unit, it was decided to lower the level of water in the digestion and settling tanks during run VI. The change in the water level decreased the retention time in the digestion tank from about 140 hours to about 112 hours. All other parameters were held comparable with those of run IV.

For obvious health reasons an estimate of the survival of pathogenic bacteria in the system was desirable. Therefore, indicator organisms were added to the system and their survival monitored during run VII. Again, all other parameters were held constant with those of run IV.

During run VIII, the differences in experimental measurements that might be attributable to the time of sampling (i.e., sampling before feeding vs sampling after feeding) and the effect of shock loading, which might occur if a recycling system were used in a vacation home situation, were determined. This experimental run consisted of four segments: (1) a baseline period when experimental conditions were identical to those of run IV (35 days); (2) a period when conditions were equal to the baseline period, but experimental measurements were taken both before and after addition of waste material (21 days); (3) a chock loading sequence in which a 7-day portion of waste material was added once a week and experimental measurements were taken before and after loading (28 days); and (4) a period in which loading and sampling regimes returned to those of the baseline period (21 days).

Experimental Measurements

During runs II and III, 50-ml samples were taken weekly from the six sampling ports in the digestion tank. These samples were analyzed using standard methods for aerobic and anaerobic total plate counts (4), adenosine triphosphate (ATP) assay (83), total carbon and inorganic carbon (by combustion), organic carbon (by difference) and pH.

In all the other experimental runs, samples were taken from the nine ports described previously. In addition to the abovementioned measurements, these samples were also analyzed for the following: ciliated protozoa (using a Wipple ocular micrometer) and ammonia-nitrogen and nitrate-nitrogen (using a Technicon Autoanalyzer II system). During all of the runs, measurements of salinity, conductivity, temperature and dissolved oxygen were made in situ using portable meters. Whenever these sampling periods occurred, an additional one sample of liquid was removed from the digestion tank and used for BOD determinations (measured manometrically).

Cultural Procedures

The *Escherichia coli* used as an indicator organism during run VII were grown in batch cultures using nutrient broth (BBL) medium. Samples of 410 ml of 24-hour cultures of the organism (10^7–10^8 cells/ml) were loaded on a daily basis during a four-week period in the run. Fecal coliform populations of both the batch cultures used for loading and samples taken from the six locations in the system were measured using the presumptive and confirmed tests.

The original isolate used for the batch cultures was obtained from samples of the raw sewage influent of the Morgantown sewage treatment plant. The organism was isolated using the presumptive, confirmed and complete (plating on EMB Agar) tests [51]. The identification was further confirmed by gram-staining and various biochemical tests (indole production, methyl red reaction, Voges-Proskauer reaction, Simmon's citrate test, sulfide production, urease production, and glucose, lactose, mannitol, sucrose and arabinose fermentation tests [52].

During runs II and III, an attempt was made to isolate and then characterize the most prevalent bacterial forms present in the mixed liquor in the digestion tank. The initial isolations were made by aseptically picking out the most prevalent colonial forms developing on the standard plate count agar. This was done five times in each of the experimental runs. Four colonial biotypes predominated. These were subcultured on BBL nutrient agar and examined for microscopic morphology, gram-stain reaction and reactions to standard biochemical tests for bacteria. The source of inoculum for each of the biochemical tests was a 24-hour nutrient broth culture of a colony picked from a standard plate count agar pour plate and incubated at 30°C. The following tests were conducted [53, 54]:

- acetate utilization
- casein hydrolysis
- catalase production
- citrate utilization
- fat hydrolysis
- gelatin liquefaction
- sulfide production
- indole production
- litmus milk reaction
- methyl red reaction
- nitrate reduction
- oxidase production
- carbohydrate fermentation
- starch hydrolysis
- Voges-Proskauer test

During runs IV–VIII, attempts were made to characterize the microbial populations in the entire system. Twice during each experimental run samples were collected from each of the nine sampling ports and the following groups of microbes were enumerated: gram-negatives, gram-positives, lipolytic, proteolytic, cellulolytic, urea hydrolyzers, fecal coliforms and fungi, all using standard procedures [51, 52, 55].

RESULTS AND DISCUSSION

Replication of experimental runs, although desirable, was not practical in this study as only one system was available and the experimental runs themselves were quite lengthy. Therefore, only limited use could be made of statistical analyses of the data. Whenever possible, analysis of variance and simple correlation analyses were conducted, using higher order interactions as estimates of error terms.

Comparisons Between Runs I, II and III

The first three runs were run on the same equipment under similar conditions, and similar measurements were made. Typical analytical results are presented graphically in Figures 2-7. The data indicate that the system was seriously underpopulated in terms of total biomass at loading rates of one and two persons per day. Peak populations attained in runs I, II and III were approximately 10^5, 10^7 and 10^8 cells/ml, respectively (Figure 2). Only in run III, where the loading rate was equivalent to three persons per day, were normal size populations achieved even after three months of operation. These differences also show up nicely in the ATP assays (Figure 4).

A correlation coefficient of 0.65 was obtained between total aerobic plate counts and ATP assay. D'Eustachio et al. [56] extracted ATP from samples of pure bacterial cultures by a variety of methods and obtained excellent correlation (0.93) with the number of cells in samples determined by standard plate count techniques. While the correlation obtained in this study is not as strong, a heterogeneous bacterial system is involved rather than pure

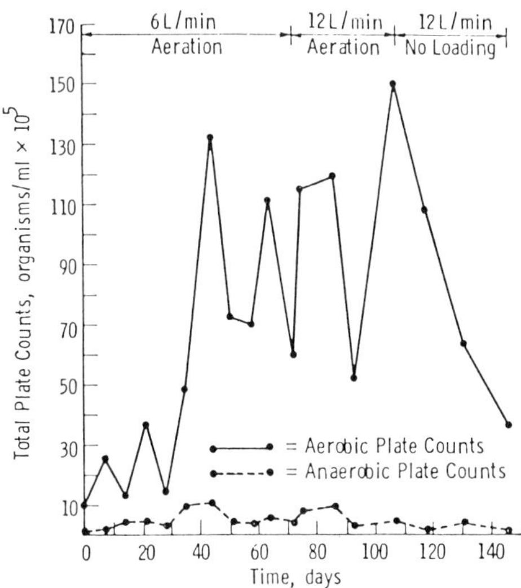

Figure 2. Variations observed over time in total plate count enumerations of aerobic bacteria in the mixed liquor in the digestion tank (data from run II).

cultures. This agrees with a study by Patterson et al. [57]. Their study confirmed previously published reports of a relatively constant pool of ATP under endogenous cellular conditions and indicated that the ATP pool in activated sludge is significantly lower than that reported for pure culture experiments.

Obviously the microbial population in the digestion tank was made up predominantly of aerobic organisms (Figure 2), as might be expected from the DO levels maintained. Anaerobic plate counts averaged one to two orders of magnitude lower than aerobic counts, and many of these organisms found to be capable of producing colonies under anaerobic conditions were undoubtedly facultative anaerobes.

The wide fluctuations noted in size of population with time are not at all unusual in studies such as this. Others [9,58] have observed such random variations, which simply reflect the complexity of activated sludge systems. Indeed, "mixed culture systems are very dynamic and the phenomena of selection and predomination strongly influence their behavior contrary to the assumptions [true for] steady-state [systems]" [58]. However, large fluctuations of the population can occur without affecting the overall process of activated sludge digestion [9]. Reid [59] stated that antibiotics produced by some activated sludge bacteria could affect predacious protozoa. If predator numbers dropped off, then the numbers of bacteria should logically increase until substantial predation occurs again. However, others [43,46] have stated that activated sludge population fluctuations cannot be predicted as simply a function of the wax and wane of predacious protozoa. The results of the present study show no obvious correlation between size of bacterial populations and numbers of protozoa.

It is of considerable interest to note the accumulation of organic carbon in each run (Figure 3). Unfortunately, organic carbon data are lacking for run I, but the rate of accumulation in run II is very similar to that observed in run III. Again there is considerable fluctuation, but after 100 days of operation, about 200 mg/l organic carbon had accumulated in both runs, in spite of 50% more carbon being fed into the system in run III. It was calculated that the organic carbon present in the digestion tank at the conclusion of the feeding cycle in run II amounted to 4.24% of the total carbon fed into the system, as compared with 2.54% in run III. This would indicate that the system was operating more efficiently at the higher loading rate utilized in run III.

Some workers have reported good correlations between organic carbon levels and bacterial counts [60]. In the present study, however, a correlation of less than 0.20 was obtained. This is most likely explained by the recycling of the organic carbon in this system.

The inorganic carbon levels roughly paralleled the organic carbon, with much greater fluctuations. Large temporary accumulations of inorganic

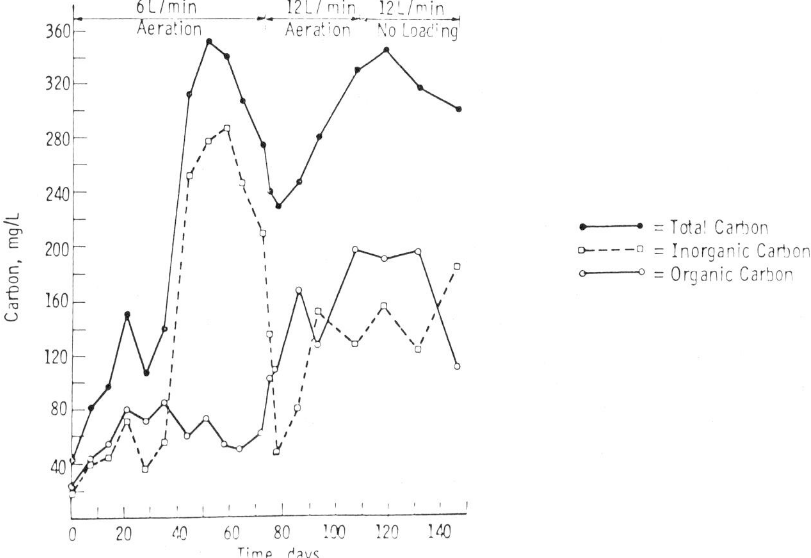

Figure 3. Variations observed over time in total, organic and inorganic carbon concentrations of the mixed liquor in the digestion tank (data from run II).

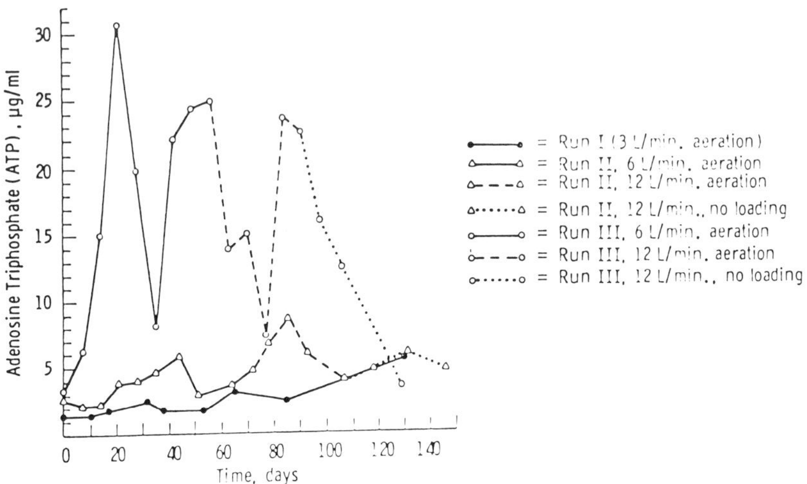

Figure 4. A comparison of variations observed over time in the adenosine triphosphate concentration (a measurement of total biomass) of the mixed liquor in the digestion tank during runs I, II and III.

carbon, such as occurred in run II from day 30 to day 50, probably resulted from drastic changes occurring in the makeup of the microbial population, perhaps the result of predation. Organisms with high metabolic efficiency could have been replaced by less efficient organisms, which assimilated less of the substrate carbon and produced more carbon dioxide; however, such perturbations had little apparent effect on the overall operation of the system. It was calculated that the total carbon remaining in the digestion tank at the conclusion of the feeding cycle in run II amounted to 6.99% of the total carbon added to the system. The comparable figure for run III was 5.85%. The other 93-95% of the carbon fed to the system was lost in volatile gases, presumably mainly in the form of carbon dioxide.

As expected, both organic and total carbon began dropping off rapidly after daily feeding was terminated in both runs. This was also correlated with a decrease in size of the microbial population. Apparently the microorganisms quickly consumed the remaining organic compounds circulating in the system and then starved to death. Predation may have been an important factor here also.

The pH of the mixed liquor in the digestion tank gradually increased with time in all three runs (Figure 5), probably because of the accumulation of mineral bases in the system. The higher pH values obtained with the higher feedrates, further supports this theory. It is of interest to note the rapid rise in pH that occurred on cessation of the feeding cycles in both runs II and III.

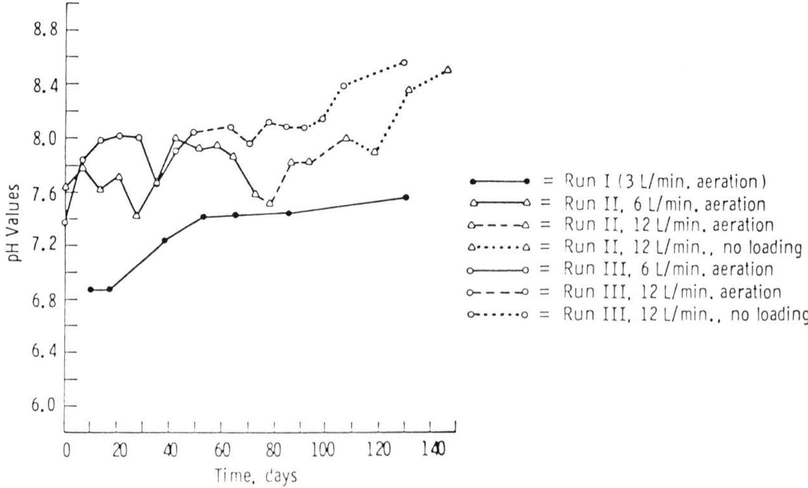

Figure 5. A comparison of variations observed over time in the pH of the mixed liquor in the digestion tank during runs I, II and III.

This suggests that some organic buffering system was operating along with the carbonate-bicarbonate system as long as the microbial population was active. No doubt some changes in the makeup of the microbial population resulted from the increasing pH, but the levels are within the satisfactory range for most microorganisms. According to Rheinheimer [61], the upper limit for optimal growth for most aquatic bacteria is around 8.5. This suggests that if these observed trends continued over a long period of time, high pH levels could limit the biological activity in the digester.

The DO curves (Figure 6) show what would be expected during both runs. There was an initial high oxygen saturation (8.0 ppm) of the water before loading was initiated. After loading with the artificial waste material was begun, the DO levels dropped within the 6 liter/min aeration regime until a low plateau level of DO was reached (approximately 2-3 ppm) because of the rapid consumption of oxygen by the bacterial population in the aerobic metabolism of available substrates. When the 12 liter/min aeration segment of each run was initiated, the DO levels predictably rose until another fairly constant level of DO was achieved (about 4 ppm). These relatively high DO concentrations indicated that DO was not a limiting factor to the bacterial population at the loading rates, which were imposed on the system. After loading was terminated, the DO curves showed a rapid climb back to levels seen at the initiation of the experimental runs.

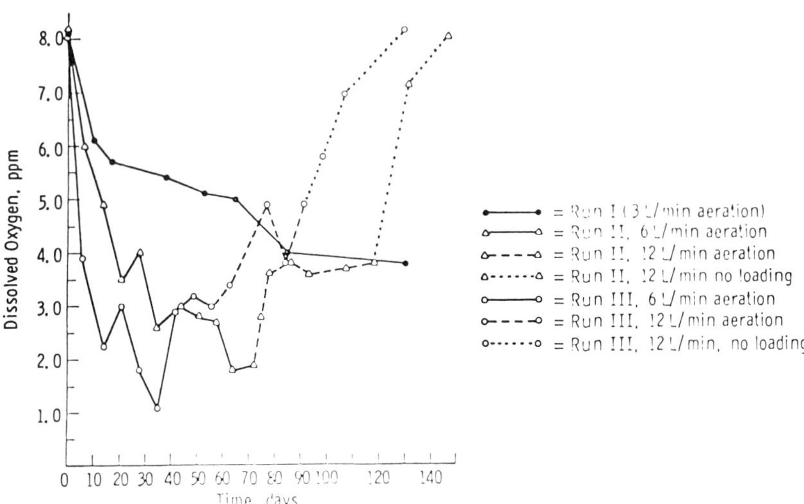

Figure 6. A comparison of variations observed over time in the dissolved oxygen content of the mixed liquor in the digestion tank during runs I, II and III.

It was calculated that an aeration rate of 12 liter/min to the digestion tank was actually supplying about 200 mg/hr of oxygen gas per liter of mixed liquor in the tank. Assuming a 5% oxygen transfer efficiency, this means that oxygen was being utilized at a rate of about 10 mg/hr/l at equilibrium conditions. This is well in line with other reported observations [10].

The conductivity of the mixed liquor predictably increased directly with time and loading rate (Figure 7), reflecting the accumulation of mineral salts in the system. This would most likely be one of the major factors limiting the length of time that such a system could operate successfully. Although many microorganisms are surprisingly tolerant of relatively high salt concentrations, eventually the salt accumulation would be expected to reach toxic levels.

The sludge samples obtained from the bottom of the digestion tank reflected trends similar to the mixed liquor samples. They contained about three times as much organic carbon as the mixed liquor samples, presumably because of the settling out of suspended particles of the synthetic feces and dead bacterial cells. This resulted in larger bacterial populations and lower

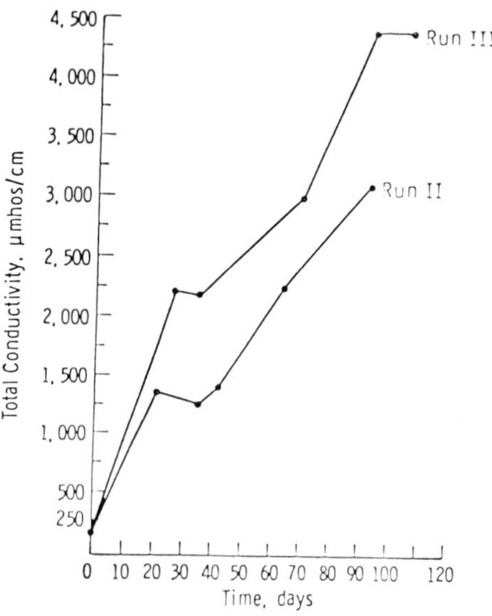

Figure 7. A comparison of variations observed over time in the electrical conductivity (a measurement of salinity) of the mixed liquor in the digestion tank during runs II and III.

dissolved oxygen levels in this region. Here again, the system remained aerobic throughout both runs. The rate of sludge accumulation was very slow. Unfortunately measurements were not made on the rate of accumulation of suspended solids, but it was apparent that this would not impose any limitation on the operation of the system. Four bacterial biotypes were found to predominate in the digestion tank. Isolations were not made from the sludge material.

From the results of the morphological, growth and biochemical studies conducted and comparisons made with generic characteristics reported by Skerman [62] and Buchanan and Gibbons [63], the four bacterial biotypes were identified as follows: Biotype #1 = an *Enterobacter* sp. (but with only slight lactose fermentation ability); Biotype #2 = *Pseudomonas* sp.; Biotype #3 = *Pseudomonas* sp.; Biotype #4 = *Flavobacterium* sp. These organisms have been commonly reported by other workers [64] and are not considered to be unusual. It was decided that the biological system was much too complex to attempt to characterize it in terms of individual species. In the following runs, therefore, the microflora was characterized only with regard to broad physiological groups.

Comparisons Between Runs IV, V, VI, VII and VIII

The results of these five runs are grouped together because they were conducted under similar operating conditions using the modified system. Because qualitative changes in the various parameters with time exhibited the same patterns as previously presented in Figures 2–7 for runs II and III, interest was mainly in quantitative differences observed between these runs.

Essentially two types of responses were observed in the dependent variables measured. For those variables that exhibited definite trends over a time interval, results are compared on the bases of linear regression coefficients indicating the weekly rates of change in the variable over the experimental period (Table III). For variables that remained essentially constant throughout the experimental period, arithmetic means were compared (Table IV).

Run IV

Experimental run IV, conducted to evaluate the influence of the added water purification equipment (settling tank, filter, disinfection unit and reservoir tank) on the performance of the system's original components, established that the additions had only a minor effect. For example, note the following comparisons of parameter values from run IV and those obtained

Table III. Effect of Experimental Conditions on the Weekly Rate of Increase–Linear Regression Coefficients–of Various Chemical and Physical Parameters Measured During Runs IV, V, VI, VII and VIII

Sample Site	Weekly Rates of Increase					Treatment Response[a]			
	Run IV	Run V	Run VI	Run VII	Run VIII	Run V	Run VI	Run VII	Run VIII
			(ppm/wk)		Salinity		(%)		
Sludge	144	143	281	154	180	−0.7	+95.1	+6.9	+25.0
Digester	150	143	281	154	137	−4.7	+87.3	+2.7	−8.7
Clarifier	144	132	207	148	132	−8.3	+43.8	+2.8	−8.3
Filter	–	–	–	–	–	–	–	–	–
Reservoir	144	114	207	143	132	−20.8	+43.8	−0.7	−8.3
			(μmhos/cm/wk)		Conductivity		(%)		
Sludge	353.3	205.5	424.3	301.2	187.1	−41.8	+20.1	−14.8	−47.0
Digester	307.1	205.5	424.3	301.2	98.9	−33.1	+38.2	−1.9	−67.8
Clarifier	310.0	222.7	402.7	291.7	226.2	−28.2	+29.9	−5.9	−27.0
Filter	–	–	–	–	–	–	–	–	–
Reservoir	315.0	238.5	381.8	208.5	229.6	−24.3	+21.2	−33.8	−27.1
			(ppm/wk)		Inorganic Carbon		(%)		
Sludge	19.2	31.4	20.4	6.5	11.1	+63.5	+6.2	−66.2	−42.2
Digester	13.6	27.7	19.3	4.1	6.8	+103.7	+41.9	−69.8	−50.0
Clarifier	16.8	29.0	20.1	4.6	6.4	+72.6	+19.6	−72.6	−61.9
Filter	18.5	39.5	19.5	3.0	5.8	+113.5	+5.4	−83.8	−68.6
Reservoir	19.0	33.3	17.9	3.3	5.7	+75.3	−5.8	−82.6	−70.0

			(ppm/wk)		Organic Carbon		(%)		
Sludge	11.1	4.3	9.4	15.7	7.4	−61.3	−15.3	−41.4	−33.3
Digester	5.3	5.1	6.9	14.2	6.8	−3.8	+30.2	+167.9	+28.3
Clarifier	1.9	4.6	9.0	15.7	4.9	+142.1	+373.7	+726.3	+157.9
Filter	2.5	4.9	10.0	15.0	5.3	+96.0	+300.0	+500.0	+112.0
Reservoir	4.1	3.2	9.4	17.5	3.9	−22.0	+129.3	+326.8	−4.9
			(ppm/wek)		Ammonia–Nitrogen		(%)		
Sludge	16.1	−0.5	19.4	18.1	10.5	−103.2	+20.5	+12.4	−34.8
Digester	11.6	−0.6	17.4	12.3	10.5	−105.5	+50.0	+6.0	−9.5
Clarifier	11.9	0.1	17.3	12.5	10.3	−98.8	+45.4	+5.0	−13.4
Filter	12.4	0.6	17.4	12.6	9.9	−95.5	+40.3	+1.6	−20.2
Reservoir	12.7	0.9	16.8	11.7	10.1	−93.0	+32.3	−7.9	−20.5
			(ppm/wk)		Nitrate–Nitrogen		(%)		
Sludge	0.80	0.74	1.35	1.38	1.44	−7.5	+68.8	+72.5	+80.0
Digester	0.84	0.61	1.01	0.93	1.07	−27.4	+20.2	+10.7	+27.4
Clarifier	0.56	2.02	1.94	1.87	1.08	+260.7	+246.4	+233.9	+92.9
Filter	0.69	2.17	1.79	1.72	1.06	+214.5	+159.4	+149.3	+53.6
Reservoir	0.40	2.18	2.09	2.01	1.21	+445.0	+422.5	+402.5	+202.5

[a]Treatment response is defined here as the difference between a run IV parameter value and a parameter value from a succeeding run, expressed as a percentage of the run IV value.

Table IV. Effect of Experimental Conditions on the Mean Values of Various Biological, Chemical and Physical Parameters Measured During Runs IV, V, VI, VII and VIII (weekly measurements averaged together over entire run)

Sample Site	Means of Weekly Measurements					Treatment Response[a]			
	Run IV	Run V	Run VI	Run VII	Run VIII	Run V	Run VI	Run VII	Run VIII
			(ppm)		Dissolved Oxygen		(%)		
Sludge	1.05	1.51	1.45	1.59	0.99	+43.8	+38.1	+51.4	-5.7
Digester	5.93	4.56	5.28	6.40	4.85	-23.1	-11.0	+7.9	-18.2
Clarifier	3.10	0.88	1.71	3.12	2.09	-71.6	-44.8	+0.6	-32.6
Filter	–	–	–	–	–	–	–	–	–
Reservoir	1.72	1.62	1.53	1.94	1.47	-5.8	-11.0	+12.8	-14.5
			(units)		pH		(%)		
Sludge	7.45	7.01	7.50	7.05	7.31	-5.9	+0.7	-5.4	-1.9
Digester	7.60	7.20	7.60	7.40	7.60	-5.3	0	-2.6	0
Clarifier	7.58	7.34	7.65	7.38	7.63	-3.2	+0.9	-2.6	+0.7
Filter	7.58	7.48	7.58	7.41	7.64	-1.3	0	-2.2	+0.8
Reservoir	7.55	7.34	7.61	7.32	7.71	-2.8	+0.8	-3.0	+2.1

	(CFU/ml × 10^6)				Aerobic Plate Counts		(%)		
Sludge	240.0	46.0	57.0	14.0	118.0	−80.8	−76.2	−94.2	−50.8
Digester	70.0	48.0	22.0	24.0	21.0	−31.4	−68.6	−65.7	−70.0
Clarifier	49.0	160.0	24.0	17.0	82.0	+226.5	−51.0	−65.3	+67.4
Filter	49.0	36.0	3.7	1.1	19.0	−26.5	−92.4	−97.8	−61.2
Reservoir	2.5	2.0	3.0	0.1	1.7	−20.0	+20.0	−96.0	−32.0
	(organisms/ml × 10^4)				Ciliated Protozoa		(%)		
Sludge	2.60	2.40	0.85	2.50	2.40	−7.7	−67.3	−3.8	−7.7
Digester	2.80	2.70	1.20	2.70	2.50	−3.6	−57.1	−3.6	−10.7
Clarifier	1.40	0.71	0.27	1.10	0.90	−49.3	−80.7	−21.4	−35.7
Filter	–	–	–	–	–	–	–	–	–
Reservoir	0.12	0.09	0.06	0.05	0.12	−25.0	−50.0	−58.3	0

[a]Treatment response is defined here as the difference between a run IV parameter value and a parameter value from a succeeding run, expressed as a percentage of the run IV value.

in run III during an experimental period with conditions equivalent to those of run IV:

Parameter	Run IV Value	Run III Value
Total Carbon (weekly increase in ppm)	30	27
Aerobic Plate Counts (mean CFU/ml × 10^6)	70	81
Dissolved Oxygen (mean ppm)	5.9	3.5
pH (mean)	7.6	8.1

Good agreement existed between all parameters with the exception of dissolved oxygen, which averaged about 40% higher in run IV. The higher run IV value was undoubtedly attributable to the more efficient air diffusion system employed in this run.

Values obtained for various parameters from run IV are used hereafter in this report as a basis for comparison of the effects of different experimental conditions. Responses are defined as the differences between a run IV parameter value and a parameter value of a succeeding run, as expressed as a percentage of the run IV value (e.g., Table III, Salinity, run VI, Digester: 0.281 − 0.144/0.144) × (100) = +95.1% response).

Run V

The most outstanding effect produced by increasing the temperature of the digester from 23°C to 34°C was a dramatic reduction in ammonia-nitrogen levels. The concentration of ammonia-nitrogen remained at approximately 2 ppm throughout run V, whereas ammonia-nitrogen increased steadily with time in all other runs. This difference between runs IV and V becomes more apparent when they are compared graphically, as in Figure 8. The decreased solubility of ammonia in water at the higher temperature alone would not account for the difference noted. Other more complex factors are involved. It is quite likely that the higher temperature resulted in an increased rate of nitrification. Such a hypothesis is strengthened by the more rapid rate of nitrate-nitrogen accumulation observed in run V when compared with run IV. Lijklema [65] has stated that high temperatures are favorable for nitrification. However, similarly high rates of nitrate-nitrogen accumulation occurred during runs VII and VIII, which were conducted under similar conditions at lower temperatures. Also, the decrease observed in the rate of ammonia-nitrogen accumulation in run V is not balanced by the increased rate of nitrate-nitrogen accumulation. Apparently a large portion of the ammonia-nitrogen in run V was either transformed into other unidentified forms or lost from the system through volatilization.

The increased operating temperature of the digestion tank also decreased the solubility of oxygen in some parts of the system (Table IV). The DO

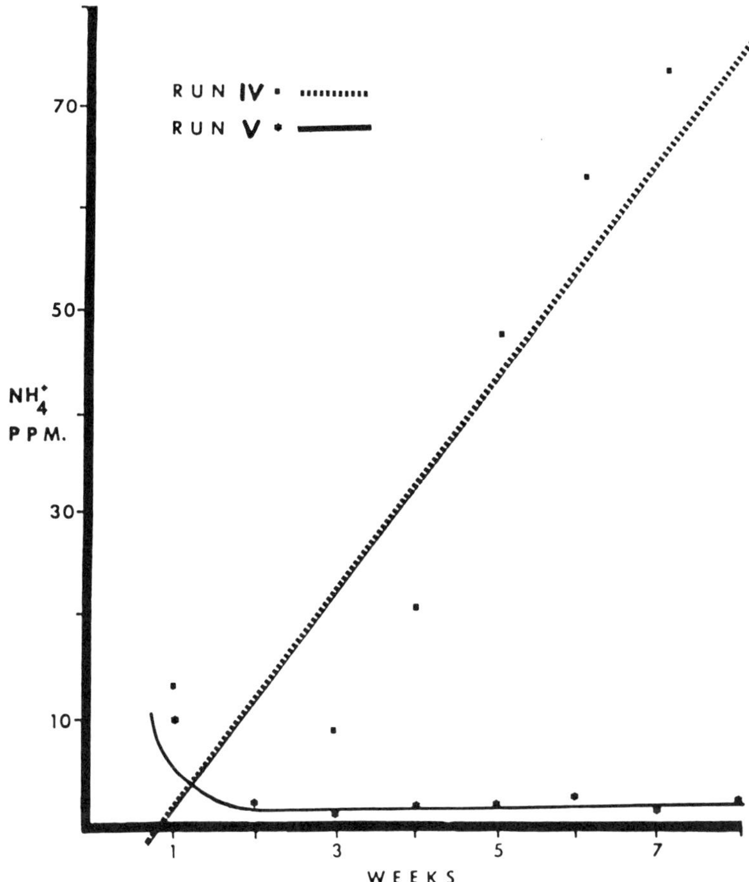

Figure 8. A comparison of the rates of ammonia–nitrogen accumulation observed in the mixed liquor in the digestion tank during runs IV and V.

content of the mixed liquor was an average of 1.3 ppm lower during run V than in run IV, and the DO in the settling tank fell an average of 2.1 ppm. The sludge layer and reservoir tank dissolved oxygen levels were similar to those of run IV.

The original reasoning behind run V justified the added expense of heating the digestion tank on the premise that the higher temperature would increase the metabolic rate of the activated sludge organisms, thereby accelerating substrate removal. This did occur to some extent as evidenced by the 60% decrease in the rate of organic carbon accumulation in the sludge layer at the

Table V. Comparison of the Efficiency of the System over Time as Measured by the Percent Reduction in Biological Oxygen Demand of Wastewater Passing Through the Digestion Tank in Runs IV, V, VI, VII and VIII (percent BOD reduction calculated as influent BOD − effluent BOD × 100/influent BOD)

	Run				
Week	IV	V	VI	VII	VIII
0	–	–	–	98.5	99.5
1	98.5	98.2	97.5	97.7	98.6
2	–	97.8	96.0	96.5	97.9
3	95.9	96.2	94.3	96.2	97.0
4	94.9	95.4	93.5	95.6	93.1
5	93.5	94.4	90.9	93.1	85.1
6	94.2	93.5	90.3	90.7	90.0
7	93.5	92.5	89.0	92.8	88.8
8	–	90.9	–	91.3	87.0
9	–	–	–	–	86.1
10	–	–	–	–	86.1
11	–	–	–	–	86.1
12	–	–	–	–	84.9
14	–	–	–	–	84.4
16	–	–	–	–	83.3
Average Weekly Decrease in BOD Reduction	0.8%	1.0%	1.4%	0.9%	1.1%

bottom of the digestion tank. However, no effect was noted in the efficiency of BOD reduction of the system (Table V). Others [15, 66] have also reported that fluctuations of temperature within the mesophyllic range have very little effect on metabolic rates in activated sludge systems.

Run VI

The smaller volume of water in the digestion tank during run VI (18% less than run IV) led to a faster rate of accumulation of many of the concentration parameters (Table III).

The figures indicate there is an inverse relationship between system volume and the rate of increase of these parameters. However, even at the rate of salt accumulation experienced during run VI, it would take more than three years for salinity to reach toxic levels [17]. This has practical implications in that a smaller system, presumably built for a smaller price, could be installed in a

Table VI. Effect of Experimental Conditions on the Mean Size of Various Segments of the Microbial Population Observed During Runs IV, V, VI, VII and VIII

Sample Sites	Experimental Run IV	V	VI	VII	VIII	Means of All Runs
	Gram-Negative Bacteria (CFU/ml × 10^5)					
Sludge	180.00	6.00	3.70	0.26	1.22	38.25
Digester	18.54	2.30	1.52	0.33	0.15	4.57
Clarifier	4.25	3.10	0.75	1.00	0.08	1.84
Filter	1.90	2.80	0.08	1.21	0.04	1.21
Reservoir	0.20	0.12	0.24	0.02	0.01	0.12
	Gram-Positive Bacteria (CFU/ml × 10^5)					
Sludge	47.00	0.33	5.10	0.36	33.00	17.16
Digester	1.28	0.03	0.43	0.06	0.75	0.51
Clarifier	3.50	0.01	0.09	0.01	0.39	0.80
Filter	0.25	0.02	0.01	0.01	0.02	0.06
Reservoir	0.10	0.01	0.01	0.01	0.01	0.02
	Lipolytic Bacteria (CFU/ml × 10^4)					
Sludge	100.00	0.02	0.26	0.19	22.50	20.14
Digester	100.00	0.02	0.38	0.33	0.27	20.20
Clarifier	0.01	0.01	0.40	0.01	0.40	0.16
Filter	0.01	0.01	0.42	0.01	0.72	0.23
Reservoir	0.01	0.01	9.60	0.01	0.01	0.19
	Proteolytic Bacteria (CFU/ml × 10^5)					
Sludge	93.50	40.00	18.50	40.00	65.50	51.50
Digester	21.14	36.10	73.14	34.70	13.58	35.73
Clarifier	33.00	105.00	82.00	56.50	33.50	62.00
Filter	23.50	12.00	4.05	64.00	16.00	23.91
Reservoir	4.00	0.01	4.10	6.05	9.85	4.80
	Cellulolytic Bacteria (CFU/ml × 10^2)					
Sludge	25.00	25.00	0.10	1.10	1.10	10.45
Digester	2.17	2.22	0.12	0.14	0.12	0.93
Clarifier	13.00	13.00	0.10	0.04	0.03	5.23
Filter	77.50	80.00	0.22	0.02	0.02	31.55
Reservoir	0.01	0.01	0.11	0.01	0.01	0.03
	Urea-Hydrolyzing Bacteria (MPN/ml)					
Sludge	50.00	0.01	0.01	2.30	19.15	14.29
Digester	120.00	0.01	0.01	0.57	0.12	24.14
Clarifier	0.01	0.01	2.15	1.40	0.01	0.71
Filter	0.01	0.01	0.01	0.01	0.01	0.01
Reservoir	0.01	0.01	1.45	0.01	0.01	0.29

Table VI, continued

Sample Sites	Experimental Run IV	V	VI	VII	VIII	Means of All Runs
	Coliform Bacteria (MPN/ml × 10^2)					
Sludge	8.70	2.30	0.01	3.45	19.50	6.79
Digester	5.42	1.68	0.04	2.47	0.74	1.59
Clarifier	6.10	0.02	0.10	3.45	0.56	2.05
Filter	5.70	0.01	0.02	1.21	0.02	1.39
Reservoir	0.10	0.36	0.01	0.01	0.01	0.09
	Fungi (CFU/ml)					
Sludge	11.50	7.00	45.00	75.00	8.00	29.30
Digester	6.30	5.20	21.25	27.33	51.00	22.22
Clarifier	4.50	5.00	1.50	6.50	15.00	6.50
Filter	4.00	1.00	1.40	2.00	2.05	2.09
Reservoir	1.00	1.00	1.10	0.50	3.25	1.37

household and still operate for a reasonable length of time before cleaning would be required.

Ammonium-nitrogen accumulated at a faster rate during run VI, but the actual difference in the rate of increase was only at most about five ppm/wk. The rate of increase for nitrate-nitrogen was also higher in run VI, but here again the actual difference between run IV and run VI values is small, a few tenths of a ppm per week and probably not significant (see run V).

Run VII

During runs IV, V, VI and VII, coliform populations in the digestion tank averaged a few hundred cells per ml (Table VI). In run VII, from day 29 to day 54 an average of 18.0 × 10^4 coliform cells/ml of digester tank volume were added daily. Samples taken throughout the system during that same time period recovered only an average of 64.0 × 10^2 cells/ml and, importantly, only two samples from the reservoir tank contained any coliform cells. After the addition of indicator organisms was discontinued, their recovery from the system was rapidly diminished (Figure 9), indicating that the coliforms were not able to establish themselves in the microbial population inhabiting the system.

The lack of change in the system attributable to the addition of indicator organisms is not surprising. In general, cultures of organisms added to sewage disposal systems disappear quickly [67, 68] and specifically fecal

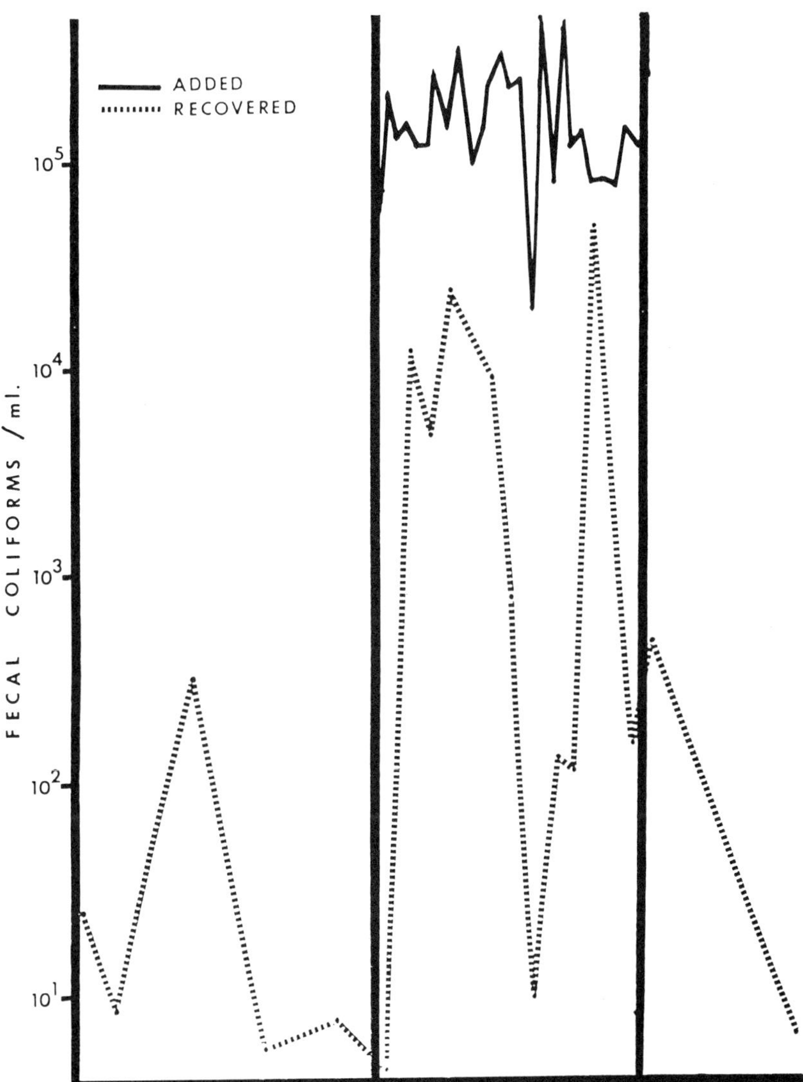

Figure 9. A comparison of the numbers of coliform bacteria added to and recovered from the mixed liquor in the digestion tank during run VII.

coliforms and enteric pathogens have not been found to persist in other activated sludge systems [40, 42]. Because other bacteria and protozoa persisted in the reservoir tank, the ultraviolet light disinfection unit was probably not very effective in killing the coliforms. The decline in their population must therefore be caused by unfavorable ecological conditions within the system.

The addition of the indicator organisms only slightly altered most of the chemical and physical parameters of the system (Tables III and IV). Inorganic carbon did not increase as fast as in the previous runs, but organic carbon accumulated at a more rapid rate. The addition of the coliforms in nutrient broth is undoubtedly responsible for this. Presuming that 50% of the dry weight of nutrient broth is carbon, the daily introduction of 410 ml of culture media into the system would amount to an increase of approximately 9 ppm/wk of organic carbon. Table III shows that the organic carbon concentration increased by approximately 5-14 ppm/wk. This additional carbon might have also altered the ecological balance and produced the lower inorganic carbon levels.

Run VIII

It was thought that some of the unexplained differences in experimental measurements obtained in the earlier runs might be attributable in part to variations in the time of sampling, but the results of the sample variation period in run VIII (Table VII) do not indicate this. The data reveal that the differences in parameter measurements taken before and after feeding were very small for most sampling sites. There was a slight increase in carbon in the sludge layer immediately after feeding, but that was expected to occur as feed material would first fall to the bottom of the digestion tank.

During the actual shock loading sequence (weeks 9 through 12), the various parameters displayed a great deal of variation, but this occurred as a response to feeding. After regular daily feeding was resumed, stability was quickly reestablished. Table VIII shows that shock loading had its greatest effect on the sludge layer of the digestion tank during weeks 9 through 12. Salinity, conductivity, organic carbon, ammonia-nitrogen, nitrate-nitrogen and aerobic plate counts all increased substantially after a shock load; however, after six days time these parameters all returned to the preshock levels.

Efficiency ratings for the system, as measured by the decrease in BOD of the effluent from the digestion tank compared with the BOD of the waste material, are presented in Table V for runs IV-VIII. In the initial stages of operation, the decrease in the BOD of the effluent from the digestion tank compared with the BOD of the waste material is very great, but this is an artifact of the system attributable to the dilution of the influent entering the digestion tank (189 liters diluted to 1098 liters) and the fact that many of the suspended solids settled to the bottom of the digestion tank and did not pass through the system. As the system continued to operate, the BOD of the recirculating water increased as the more recalcitrant organic compounds circulated throughout the system. The effects

Table VII. Observed Mean Differences in Various Biological, Chemical and Physical Measurements Taken Before and After Regular Daily Feeding During Run VIII

Parameter Measured	Sampling Site				
	Sludge	Mixed Liquor	Settling Tank	Filter	Reservoir Tank
Salinity (ppm $\times 10^3$)	+0.07	+0.05	+0.06	–	–0.03
Conductivity (mohms/cm)	+58.00	+43.00	–16.00	–	+200.00
Dissolved Oxygen (ppm)	–0.30	–0.90	+1.30	–	+0.10
pH	+0.20	+0.30	–0.10	–0.10	0
Inorganic Carbon (ppm)	+27.30	–3.70	–5.30	–12.60	–13.00
Organic Carbon (ppm)	+59.30	+7.80	–5.00	+1.30	+5.70
Ammonia (ppm)	–0.10	–0.10	+0.20	+0.20	+0.20
Nitrate (ppm)	–1.00	+0.80	+1.30	–0.70	+1.00
Aerobic Plate Counts (CFU/ml $\times 10^6$)	+20.00	–21.00	–7.30	+11.00	–1.30
Ciliate Protozoa (organisms/ml $\times 10^4$)	0	–0.03	0	–	–0.03

of experimental conditions on the mean values of various microbial populations were calculated and are presented in Table VI.

The data indicate that while large fluctuations took place in the makeup of the population, most of the components remained active under all conditions. In the digestion tank itself, the gram-negative organisms consistently numbered in the hundreds of thousands per ml, while the gram-positives ranged in the tens of thousands per ml. These estimates are obviously much too low because total plate counts (Table IV) were up in the tens of millions. This is no doubt attributable to the toxicity of the selective media used for these differential counts (deoxycholate Agar for gram-negatives and Phenylethyl Alcohol Agar for gram-positives). Lipolytic organisms generally number only a few thousand per ml except in run IV, when for some unknown reason they reached a million cells per ml. The proteolytic organisms were consistently the most abundant, numbering in the millions per ml. This was not surprising considering the high protein content of the feed. The other groups of organisms were quite scarce, rarely exceeding a few hundred per ml.

In general, except for the protozoa which were consistently more numerous in the mixed liquor, microbial populations attained their largest numbers in the sludge layer. In most cases microbial populations were smaller in the filtered water and reached their lowest numbers in the reservoir tank. An interesting exception occurred with the cellulolytics, which in runs IV, V and VI reached their highest numbers in the filtered water. This was no doubt attributable to the colonization of the cellulose filter by these organisms. In later runs the filter was cleaned and disinfected with chlorine at frequent intervals.

The only evident difference between runs appears to be a higher number of all organisms present in run IV than in the later runs. This may have been attributable to a buildup of predators in the system with time. Although the system was cleaned out before the start of each run, it was impossible to completely sterilize it and undoubtedly there was some carryover of organisms from one run to the next.

Obviously the microbial population is very dynamic, and many unknown factors affecting the makeup of the population could not be adequately controlled or monitored in this study.

CONCLUSIONS

As is often the case with exploratory research such as this, many new questions are generated. It is obvious, for instance, that normal criteria used to evaluate the performance of activated sludge systems are not directly applicable to recycling systems. The question remains, however, as to what

Table VIII. Observed Mean Differences in Various Biological, Chemical and Physical Measurements Taken Before and After Shock Loading During Run VIII

	Sampling Site				
Parameter Measured	Sludge	Mixed Liquor	Settling Tank	Filter	Reservoir Tank
Salinity (ppm × 10^3)	+4.2	+0.3	+0.1	–	+0.1
Conductivity (mohms/cm)	+7662.0	+287.0	+138.0	–	+200.0
Dissolved Oxygen (ppm)	−0.1	−3.0	−1.8	–	−0.5
pH	−0.6	−0.3	−0.2	−0.1	−0.1
Inorganic Carbon (ppm)	−4.3	+8.9	+10.0	+13.3	+2.7
Organic Carbon (ppm)	+18.0	+11.1	+5.5	+8.3	−2.0
Ammonia–Nitrogen (ppm)	+5.5	+4.9	+5.5	+6.7	+12.5
Nitrate–Nitrogen (ppm)	+4.9	+1.8	+1.8	+2.0	+2.0
Aerobic Plate Counts (CFU/ml × 10^6)	+130.0	+7.6	+12.0	–	+2.2
Ciliate Protozoa (organisms/ml × 10^4)	+0.06	+0.18	0	–	0

criteria would be suitable. If one accepts the proposal that the main criteria should be: (1) to stabilize organic wastes, (2) to provide an aesthetically acceptable water product, and (3) to present no unusual health hazards to the users of the system, then the system described here would be considered satisfactory. Approximately 95% of substrate carbon was converted to carbon dioxide. As long as aeration was sufficient to maintain an aerobic condition in the digestion tank, no objectionable odors were detected. The product water exhibited only a slight color and turbidity, which were not deemed objectionable. Seeding of the system with pathogenic-like organisms indicated that health hazards with such a system would most likely be minimal because of the inability of such organisms to establish themselves in the microbial population. This problem of establishing suitable standards for the performance of recycling waste disposal systems has recently been addressed by the National Sanitation Foundation, and standards have now been published [69].

The specific findings of this project were as follows:

1. Organic loading rates equivalent to the waste disposal needs of up to three adult persons per day were processed by the system satisfactorily. Presumably much higher loading rates could have been accommodated if a more efficient aeration system had been employed. The system operated more efficiently at a loading of three persons per day than at one or two persons per day.

2. Aeration requirements increased in proportion to the organic loading rates within the range of operating conditions employed in this study.

3. Small changes of temperature within the mesophyllic range had minimal effect on the operation of the system. One important effect noted was a lower rate of ammonia accumulation associated with the higher operating temperature, but the cause of this phenomenon was not determined. This could have practical implications if accumulations of ammonia inhibited biological activity in the digestion tank. The rate of sludge accumulation was also significantly reduced at the higher operating temperature.

4. Reducing the retention time in the digestion tank by reducing the volume of mixed liquor in the tank resulted in the predictable effect of increasing the accumulation rate of residuals. Actually this system was operated at retention times far in excess of normal commercially available units, which are usually designed for retention times of no more than 48 hours. The data indicate that retention time could easily be reduced considerably without jeopardizing the operation of the system and thereby reduce the size and cost of the system.

5. Coliforms introduced into the digestion tank as indicators of pathogenic survivability were unable to establish themselves within the microbial population of the tank and their recovery from the system dropped rapidly

after each inoculation—a strong indication that the system could not support the growth of any enteric pathogens that might be introduced.

6. In experiments designed to simulate sporadic use, it was found that shock loading produced brief perturbations in the system. However, the overall stability of the system was quickly reestablished. This recovery ability is certainly a necessary requirement for any system in actual use.

7. The microbial population inhabiting the digestion tank was extremely complex, exhibiting violent fluctuations in total numbers as well as in makeup. These changes often appeared to be in response to competition for substrate and predation rather than to operational variables. Overall, the microbial population exhibited an amazing resiliency and was able to survive over a wide range of conditions. In light of this it is felt that the detailed study that would be required to fully characterize the microbial ecology of the system could not be justified at this time.

8. There are a number of engineering improvements that could be made to improve the operation of the system. For instance, it was felt that the filtering device was inadequate; daily monitoring and frequent replacement of filter cartridges were necessary. A larger filtration system with provisions for automatic backwashing would be necessary before the system could go into actual residential use. Another feature that might alleviate part of the filtration problem would be to establish a timed aeration-quiescent sequence in the digestion tank. The absence of turbulence would allow some settling of suspended particles, and by withdrawing water from the digestion tank only after a period of quiescence, the operation of the settling and filtering devices should be improved.

The installation of a simple baffling system in the digestion tank to prevent short-circuiting of added fecal material directly to the settling tank would be an improvement. Better placement of more efficient aerators, perhaps using oxygen-enriched air, would also be beneficial.

Another part of the system in need of improvement is the disinfection unit. The ultraviolet light device was not very effective in disinfecting the processed effluent. A chemical sterilizer such as an iodater or chlorinator might improve effluent quality. However, chemical-type disinfecting units would require the addition of another filter, such as activated charcoal, to remove the sterilizing agent before the processed wastewater could be introduced into the digestion tank, because of the danger of killing the beneficial organisms in the system.

ACKNOWLEDGMENTS

This research was supported in part by grants from the Westinghouse Electric Corporation and the Water Research Institute, West Virginia University, with funds allotted under the Water Resources Act of 1964 (PL 88-379) administered by the Office of Water Research and Technology, U.S. Department of the Interior.

REFERENCES

1. Graeser, H. J. "Water Re-Use," *J. Am. Water Works Assoc.* 66:575-578 (1974).
2. Sebastian, F. P. "Purified Wastewater, the Untapped Resource," *J. Water Poll. Control Fed.* 46:239-246 (1974).
3. Kasperson, R. E. "Public Acceptance of Water Re-Use. A State-of-the-Art Analysis," in *Water Re-use and the Cities*, R. E. Kasperson and J. X. Kasperson, Eds. (Hanover, NH: University Press of New England, 1977), pp. 121-141.
4. Bailey, J. R., R. J. Benoit, J. L. Dodson, J. M. Robb and H. Wellman. "A Study of Flow Reduction and Treatment of Wastewater from Households," Federal Water Control Administration Report No. 11050 FKE, U.S. Government Printing Office, Washington, D.C. (1969).
5. Cover, A., and F. Lucicain. "An Operator's View of Performance. Sanitation District No. 3, Boyd County, Kentucky," in *Individual Onsite Wastewater Systems. Proceedings of the Fourth National Conference, 1977*, N. I. McClelland, Ed. (Ann Arbor, MI:Ann Arbor Science Publishers, Inc., 1978), pp. 135-143.
6. Gavis, J. "Wastewater Re-use," National Water Commission Report No. NWC-ESS-71-003, National Water Commission, Arlington, VA (1971).
7. Gaudy, A. F., and E. T. Gaudy. "Microbiology of Waste Waters," *Ann. Rev. Microbiol.* 20:319-336 (1966).
8. Gaudy, A. F., and E. T. Gaudy. "Biological Concepts for Design and Operation of the Activated Sludge Process," EPA Office of Research and Monitoring Project No. 17090FQJ, U.S. Government Printing Office Washington, D.C. (1971).
9. Paynter, M. B. J., and H. R. Bungay. "The Effect of Microbial Interactions on Performance of Waste Treatment Processes," in *Biological Waste Treatment*, R. P. Canale, Ed. (New York. John Wiley & Sons, Inc., 1971), pp. 51-61.
10. Hammer, M. J. *Water and Waste-Water Technology* (New York: John Wiley & Sons, Inc., 1975).
11. Stafford, R. T. "Keynote Address to the Fourth National Conference on Individual Onsite Wastewater Systems," in *Individual Onsite Wastewater Systems. Proceedings of the Fourth National Conference, 1977*, N. I. McClelland, Ed. (Ann Arbor, MI: Ann Arbor Science Publishers, Inc., 1978), pp. 5-14.
12. McKinney, R. E. *Microbiology for Sanitary Engineers* (New York: McGraw-Hill Book Co., 1962).
13. Eckenfelder, W. W., and D. J. O'Connor. *Biological Waste Treatment* (Elmsford, NY: Pergamon Press, Inc., 1961).
14. Hunter, J. V., E. J. Genetelli and M. E. Gilwood. "Temperature-Retention Time Relationships in the Activated Sludge Process," *Proc. 21st Ind. Waste Conf.* 50:953-963 (1966).

15. Busch, A. W. *Aerobic Biological Treatment of Waste Waters, Principles and Practice* (Houston: Oligodynamic Press, 1971).
16. Ludzack, F. J., R. B. Schaffer and M. B. Ettinger. "Temperature and Feed as Variables in Activated Sludge Performance," *J. Water Poll. Control Fed.* 33:141-156 (1961).
17. Kincannon, D. F., and A. F. Gaudy. "Some Effects of High Salt Concentration on Activated Sludge," *J. Water Poll. Control Fed.* 38:1148-1159 (1966).
18. Gaudy, A. F., and R. S. Engelbrecht. "Quantitative and Qualitative Shock Loading of Activated Sludge Systems," *J. Water Poll. Control Fed.* 33:800-816 (1961).
19. Gaudy, A. F., and B. J. Turner. "Effects of Air Flow Rate on Response of Activated Sludge to Quantitative Shock Loading," *J. Water Poll. Control Fed.* 36:767-781 (1964).
20. Thabaraj, G. J., and A. F. Gaudy. "Effect of Dissolved Oxygen Concentration on the Metabolic Response of Completely Mixed Activated Sludge," *J. Water Poll. Control Fed.* 41:R323-R335 (1969).
21. Thabaraj, G. J., and A. F. Gaudy. "Effect of Initial Biological Solids Concentration and Nitrogen Supply on Metabolic Patterns During Substrate Removal and Endogenous Metabolism," *J. Water Poll. Control Fed.* 43:318-334 (1971).
22. Ehlers, C. E., and E. W. Steel. *Municipal and Rural Sanitation* (New York: McGraw-Hill Book Co., 1958).
23. Drasar, B. S., M. Shiner and G. M. McLeod. "Studies on the Intestinal Flora," *Gastroenterology* 56:71-79 (1969).
24. Finegold, S. M., and L. G. Miller. "Normal Fecal Flora of Adult Humans," *Bacteriol. Proc.* 68:93 (1968).
25. Floch, M. H., W. Gershengoren and L. R. Greedman. "Methods for the Quantitative Study of the Aerobic and Anaerobic Intestinal Bacterial Flora of Man," *Yale J. Biol. Med.* 41:50-61 (1968).
26. Gorback, S. L. "Studies of Intestinal Microflora," *Gastroenterology* 53:845-855 (1967).
27. Haenel, H. "Some Rules in the Ecology of the Intestinal Microflora of Man," *J. Appl. Bacteriol.* 24:242-251 (1961).
28. Mata, L. J., C. Carrillo and E. Villatoro. "Fecal Microflora in Healthy Persons in a Pre-industrial Region," *Appl. Microbiol.* 17:596-602 (1969).
29. Moore, W. E. C., and L. V. Holdeman. "Human Fecal Flora: The Normal Flora of 20 Japanese-Hawaiians," *Appl. Microbiol.* 27:961-972 (1974).
30. VanHoute, J., and J. Gibbons. "Studies of the Cultivatable Flora of Human Feces," *Antoni van Leewenhoek; J. Microbiol. Serol.* 32:212-222 (1966).
31. Crowther, R. F., and N. Harkness. "Anaerobic Bacteria," in *Ecological Aspects of Used-Water Treatment*, C. R. Curds and H. A. Hawkes, Eds. (London: Academic Press, Inc., 1975), pp. 65-91.
32. Mah, R., and C. Sussman. "Microbiology of Anaerobic Sludge Fermentation," *Appl. Microbiol.* 16.358-361 (1967).
33. Toreien, D. F. "Direct-Isolation Studies on the Aerobic and Facultative Anaerobic Bacterial Flora of Anaerobic Digesters Receiving Raw Sewage," *Water Res.* 1:55-59 (1967).
34. Prakasam, T. S. B., and N. C. Dondero. "Aerobic Heterotropic Bacterial Populations of Sewage and Activated Sludge. I. Enumeration," *Appl. Microbiol.* 15:461-467 (1967).

35. Prakasam, T. S. B., and N. C. Dondero. "Aerobic Heterotropic Bacterial Populations of Sewage and Activated Sludge. II. Method of Characterization of Activated Sludge Bacteria," *Appl. Microbiol.* 15:1122-1127 (1967).
36. Banks, C. J., M. Davies, I. Walker and R. D. Ward. "Biological and Physical Characterization of Activated Sludge: A Comparative Experimental Study of Ten Different Treatment Plants," *J. Water Poll. Control Fed.* 48:492-509 (1976).
37. Banks, C. J., and I. Walker. "Sonication of Activated Sludge Flocks and the Recovery of Their Bacteria on Solid Media," *J. Gen. Microbiol.* 98: 363-368 (1977).
38. Pike, E. B., E. C. Carrington and P. A. Ashburner. "An Evaluation of Procedures for Enumerating Bacteria in Activated Sludge," *J. Appl. Bacteriol.* 35:309-321 (1972).
39. Lighthart, B., and R. T. Oglesby. "Bacteriology of an Activated Sludge Waste Treatment Plant–A Guide to Methodology," *J. Water Poll. Control Fed.* 41:R267-R281 (1969).
40. Dias, F. F., and J. V. Bhat. "Microbial Ecology of Activated Sludge. I. Dominant Bacteria," *Appl. Microbiol.* 12:412-417 (1964).
41. Dias, F. F., and J. V. Bhat. "Microbial Ecology of Activated Sludge. II. Bacteriophages, Bdellovibrio, Coliforms and Other Organisms," *Appl. Microbiol.* 13:412-417 (1965).
42. Pike, E. B. "Aerobic Bacteria," in *Ecology Aspects of Used-Water Treatment*, C. R. Curds and H. A. Hawkes, Eds. (London: Academic Press, Inc., 1965), pp. 1-63.
43. Curds, E. R., and A. Cockburn. "Studies on the Growth and Feeding of *Tetrahymena pyriformis* in Axenic and Monoxenic Culture," *J. Gen. Microbiol.* 54:343-358 (1958).
44. Curds, C. R., A. Cockburn and J. M. VanDyke. "An Experimental Study of the Role of Ciliated Protozoa in the Activated Sludge Process," *Water Poll. Control* 67:312-329 (1968).
45. Curds, C. R., and G. C. Fey. "The Effect of Ciliated Protozoa on the Fate of *Escherichia coli* in the Activated Sludge Process," *Water Res.* 3:853-867 (1969).
46. Canale, R. P., T. D. Lusting, P. M. Kehrbegre and J. E. Salo. "Experimental and Mathematical Modeling Studies of Protozoan Populations on Bacteria," *Biotechnol. Bioeng.* 15:707-728 (1973).
47. Johannes, R. E. "Influence of Marine Protozoa on Nutrient Regeneration," *Limnol. Oceanog.* 10:434-442 (1965).
48. Cooke, W. G. "A Laboratory Guide to Fungi in Polluted Waters, Sewage and Sewage Treatment Systems. Their Identification and Culture," Public Health Service Publication No. 999-WP-1, U.S. Dept. of Health, Education and Welfare, Cincinnati, OH (1963).
49. Tomlinson, T. C., and I. L. Williams. "Fungi," in *Ecological Aspects of Used-Water Treatment*, C. R. Curds and H. A. Hawkes, Eds. (London: Academic Press, Inc., 1975), pp. 93-152.
50. Vysotsky, V., T. Vlasova, A. Kochetkova, A. Ushakova and S. Shishkina. "Normal Composition of Urine and Feces in Healthy Subjects," *Vopr. Pitan.* 6:35-38 (1974).
51. *Standard Methods for the Examination of Water and Wastewater, 14th ed.* (New York: American Public Health Association, 1976).

52. Pelczar, M. J., and E. C. S. Chan. *Laboratory Exercises in Microbiology* (New York: McGraw-Hill Book Co., 1972).
53. Collins, C. H., and P. M. Lyne. *Microbiological Methods, 3rd ed.* (Baltimore: University Park Press, 1970).
54. MacFaddin, J. F. *Biochemical Tests for Identification of Medical Bacteria* (Baltimore: Williams and Wilkins Co., 1976).
55. Rodina, A. G. *Methods in Aquatic Microbiology* (Baltimore: University Park Press, 1972).
56. D'Eustachio, A. J., D. R. Johnson and G. V. Levin. "Rapid Assay of Bacterial Populations," *Bacteriological Proceedings* (Washington, D.C. American Society for Microbiology, 1968), p. 13.
57. Patterson, J. W., P. L. Brezonik and H. D. Putman. "Measurement and Significance of Adenosine Triphosphate in Activated Sludge," *Environ. Sci. Technol.* 4:569-575 (1970).
58. Cassell, E. A., F. T. Sulzer and J. C. Lamb. "Population Dynamics and Selection in Continuous and Mixed Cultures," *J. Water Poll. Control Fed.* 38:1398-1406 (1966).
59. Reid, L. R. "Design of Wastewater Disposal Systems for Individual Dwellings," *J. Water Poll. Control Fed.* 43:2004-2010 (1971).
60. Yoshikura, T. "Rapid Determination of Total Organic Carbon and Its Application to Water Research," *Bull. of Jap. Soc. Sci. Fish.* 42(12: 1423-1429 (1976).
61. Rheinheimer, G. *Aquatic Microbiology* (New York: John Wiley & Sons, Inc., 1974).
62. Skerman, V. B. D. *A Guide to the Identification of the Genera of Bacteria* (Baltimore: Williams and Wilkins Co., 1967).
63. Buchanan, R. E., and N. E. Gibbons. *Bergy's Manual of Determinative Bacteriology, 8th ed.* (Baltimore. Williams and Wilkins Co., 1974).
64. Shoupp, W. J. "A Recycled-Water Sanitary Waste Disposal System," Ph.D. Thesis, West Virginia University, Morgantown, WV (1978).
65. Lijklema, L. "Model for Nitrification in Activated Sludge Processes," *Environ. Sci. Technol.* 7:429-433 (1973).
66. Ludzack, F. J., H. L. Kreiger and M. B. Ettinger. "Interactions of Waste Feed, Activated Sludge and Oxygen as Traced by Radioactive Carbon," *J. Water Poll. Control Fed.* 36:782-788 (1964).
67. Grumman Aerospace Company. "Development of Immobilized Enzyme Systems for Enhancement of Biological Waste Treatment Processes," EPA Water Quality Office, Program No. 16050DXN, Contract No. 14-121562, U.S. Government Printing Office, Washington, D.C. (1970).
68. Heulelekion, H., and M. Berger. "Value of Culture and Enzyme Additions in Promoting Digestion," *Sewage Ind. Wastes* 25:1259-1267 (1953).
69. "National Sanitation Foundation Standard No. 41 for Wastewater Recycle/Reuse and Waste Conservation Devices" (Ann Arbor, MI: National Sanitation Foundation, 1978).

30

USE OF SHALLOW, LOW-PRESSURE INJECTION SYSTEMS IN LARGE AND SMALL INSTALLATIONS

B. L. Carlile
Extension Soil Specialist
Soil Science Department
North Carolina State University
Raleigh, North Carolina 27607

INTRODUCTION

A low-pressure pipe system (LPP) is a network of small-diameter perforated pipes placed 10–18 inches deep in narrow trenches 5–12 inches wide in natural soil. Septic tank effluent is pumped through the LPP system in controlled doses to ensure uniform distribution throughout the entire soil absorption field. Figure 1 illustrates the following basic components of the LPP system:

- septic tank
- pumping chamber
- submersible effluent pump, level controls
- high water alarm, level switch
- supply manifold
- perforated distribution laterals

The perforated laterals are placed shallowly in soil material suitable to receive and treat septic tank effluent, as shown in Figure 2. The soil material may be natural soil or a combination of natural soil and suitable fill material of sufficient depth to effect treatment before the effluent reaches a water table or other restrictive horizon. The LPP system is designed to produce even distribution of the effluent, maintain maximum separation of

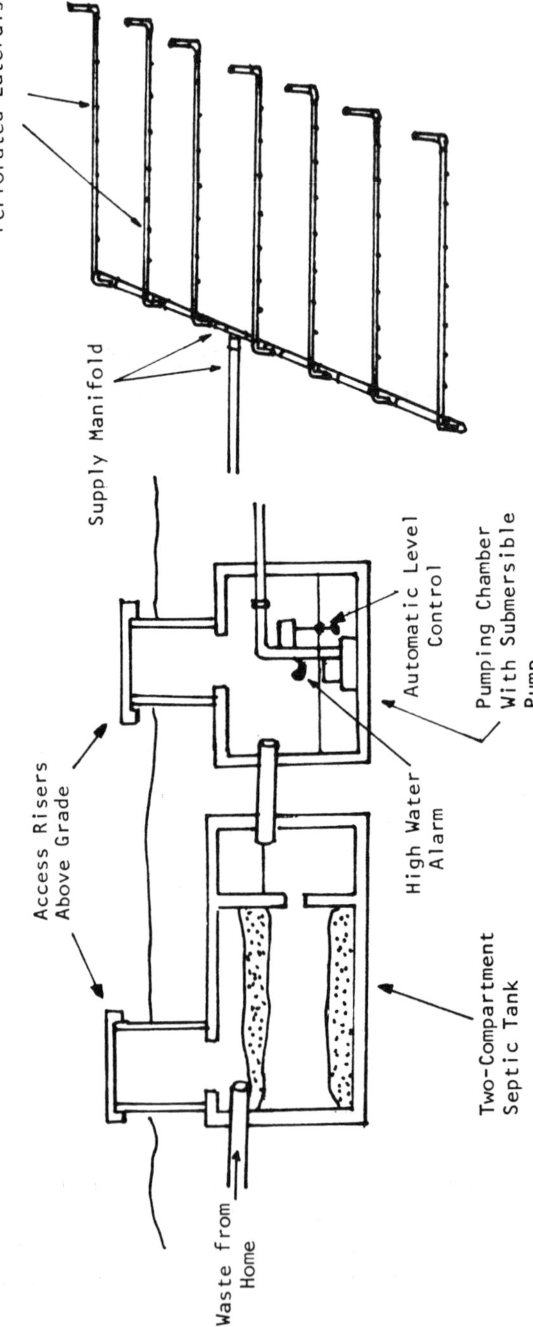

Figure 1. Basic components of a low-pressure pipe (LPP) system.

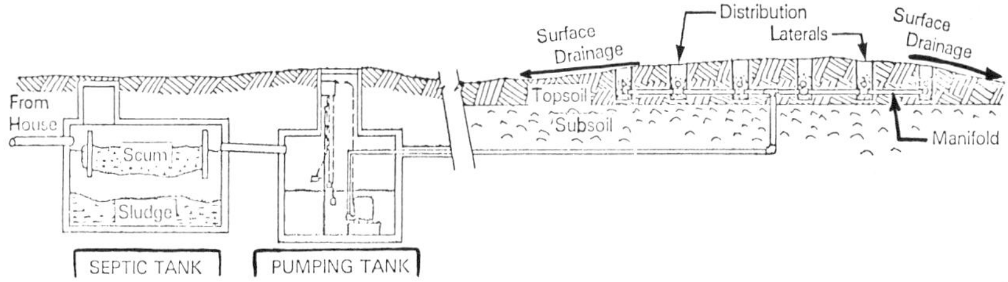

Figure 2. Cross section of a pressure distribution system in natural soil.

the distribution lines above water tables and control dosing of effluent throughout the soil absorption area for optimum dosing and resting cycles.

SOIL AND SITE CONDITIONS FOR LPP SYSTEMS

The LPP system was designed and tested in North Carolina to overcome several soil, site and space limitations that prohibit the successful operation of a conventional gravity-fed septic tank–soil absorption system. These conditions include:

1. rapidly permeable coastal sands;
2. inland coastal soils with shallow water tables;
3. sites with restrictive horizons at shallow depths;
4. steeply sloped sites; and
5. large wastewater flows.

North Carolina State University soil scientists have developed design requirements for the LPP system by evaluating the performance of more than 200 LPP systems installed under various conditions across the state. These include more than 150 systems installed and evaluated in coastal sites through a four-year cooperative project funded by the North Carolina Sea Grant Program. Some 25 systems have been installed in Piedmont sites of the state during the past two years as part of the Triangle J Council of Government Individual Wastewater Project funded by the U.S. Environmental Protection Agency (EPA). These systems, as well as several others in the mountain regions of the state, include small systems designed to serve private homes with 300 gpd waste discharge and large systems designed to serve schools, small communities and industries with wastewater flows of more than 20,000 gpd.

Rapidly Permeable Coastal Sands

The use of conventional, gravity-fed septic tank–soil absorption systems in coastal areas of the eastern seaboard presents some severe problems. Such sites are usually characterized by soils with rapid permeability and water tables within 2–5 feet of the surface. With a conventional septic tank system, portions of the soil absorption trench become overloaded, creating saturated flow through the trench bottom until some clogging of the soil occurs. In sands, the clogging may not be enough to prevent continued saturated flow through portions of the trench bottom, with the resulting effect of wastewater contaminants reaching the water table below, and possibly migrating to, nearby wells or surface waters. This condition is believed to be partly responsible for the high coliform counts measured in some areas of shellfish waters in North Carolina, which has resulted in the closure of several hundred thousand acres of such waters for shellfish harvesting.

The LPP system minimizes these kinds of problems because with pressure distribution no portion of the system is overloaded, optimum dosing and resting minimize saturated flow through the soil, and shallow placement increases the travel path from the point of injection to the water table. Extensive monitoring studies are currently underway in North Carolina to determine the effectiveness of LPP systems to reduce levels of contaminants in coastal waters in comparison with conventional systems.*

Inland Soils with High Water Tables

High water tables create problems with conventional septic tank–soil absorption systems when the water table submerges the distribution lines and prevents sewage absorption, creates total anaerobic conditions in the soil surrounding the trench, and prevents adequate treatment of the effluent prior to reaching nearby surface water or wells. In many areas of the lower coastal plain of North Carolina, where high water tables are prevelant, there is evidence of improperly treated sewage in roadside ditches during wet periods of the year. Some of these sites can be used safely for onsite waste disposal by raising the soil absorption trenches so that there is a minimum of a foot separation between the trench bottom and the seasonal high water table. This often requires a pump to lift the sewage above the septic tank, a situation where the LPP distribution system is best used to improve system performance.

---

*This is a cooperative study of the North Carolina Department of Human Resources, North Carolina State University and University of North Carolina-Chapel Hill through a grant from the Coastal Plains Regional Commission.

Restrictive Horizons

Many Piedmont and mountain sites in the state have restrictive horizons at shallow depths in the soil that prevent the proper discharge of septic tank effluent through conventional soil absorption trenches. These horizons may be impervious clays, cemented hardpans or fractured rock. As conventional absorption lines are normally placed 2- to 3-feet deep, restrictive horizons should not occur within 3 feet of the surface for proper functioning of the system. Problems caused by restrictive horizons include the contamination of wells by improperly treated sewage moving through rock fractures, the movement of sewage along the top of hardpans and subsequent breakout, and the perching of sewage by clay horizons with subsequent flooding of the absorption trenches. Because the LPP system can be installed at depths as shallow as 10 inches, many sites with restrictive horizons at depths of 20–36 inches can be used safely for subsurface sewage disposal. On level or gently sloping lots, cross trenching (or "herring-bone" trenching) has been used successfully to increase the trench area and, thus, the absorptive capacity of the site for sewage (Figure 3).

Steeply Sloped Sites

Conventional absorption lines can, and have been, successfully used on sloping sites if certain criteria are met. These include sufficient soil depth (32–40 inches); equal loading of soil trenches; slopes suitable for equipment; and sites downslope from the waste source. If these criteria cannot be

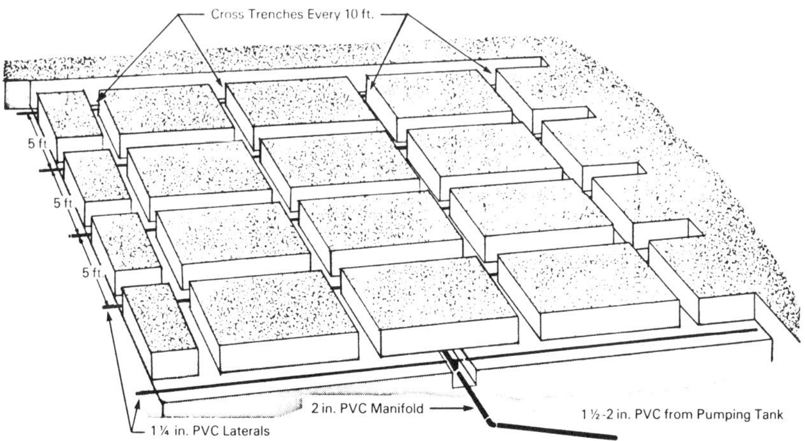

Figure 3. LPP system with cross trenching to increase sewage absorption.

met, a pressure distribution system may be needed to enhance the safe disposal of sewage on the site. Such systems have been used successfully on slopes up to 20% in North Carolina, particularly to repair failing systems where all of the suitable area downslope is occupied by the failing conventional system and the only suitable repair area or replacement area is upslope of the house. The only suitable area for waste disposal for many new building sites in the mountains of the state may be upslope from the house and require a lift pump. Current recommendations are that if a lift pump is required, the use of pressure distribution will enhance the effectiveness of the system.

Sloping lots do present particular design problems for the successful use of the LPP system. Pressure heads within the field laterals should be between 2 and 6 feet (0.87–2.60 psi), requiring an elevation differential of less than 4 feet from the top to the bottom lateral. However, on slopes exceeding this limit, special methods can be used to reduce these pressure differentials and distribute effluent equally among the laterals. The most common method used is to split the manifolds into two or more fields and install pressure-reducing values in the lower manifolds to bring pressure heads within acceptable limits. On larger systems, dual alternating pumps may be used to feed upper and lower fields to further split slopes and reduce pressure differentials.

Large Wastewater Flows

A problem inherent in the use of conventional gravity-fed absorption lines for large flows is the unequal distribution of sewage between and within the field absorption trenches. This results in overloading and subsequent clogging of portions of the soil absorption trenches and possibly eventual failure of the system. Pumps are often used to deliver sewage to distribution boxes where gravity flow is then responsible for distribution in each trench. This still results in overloading of sections of each trench, a problem that is easily overcome with total pressure distribution. There are some economics of scale for the design of larger LPP systems, although experience has shown that for wastewater flows above 2000-4000 gpd, multiple pumps serving separate fields are most economical and more easily managed. This unit size normally requires a 3/4- to 1-hp submersible effluent pump for optimum dosing pressures throughout the system.

DESIGNING A LOW-PRESSURE PIPE SYSTEM

After determining that a specific site is acceptable for an LPP system, the system must be designed for that site. Such a design involves a sequence of three steps, which must be followed for any LPP system design. These are:

1. determining the area needed for the absorption lines;
2. laying out and locating the system; and
3. designing the dosing system.

The design sequence is illustrated in the following step-by-step example.

A. Determine the Area Needed

The total amount of absorption area depends on two factors: (1) the daily wastewater flow to be disposed of; and (2) the absorptive capacity of the soil. Waste flow estimates are derived by the local health department according to state regulations. Soil loading rates are determined according to estimated soil permeability of the most restrictive zone in the upper 30 inches of soil (Table I).

Step 1: Determine the daily wastewater flow for the system. For residential systems, North Carolina regulations estimate flow at 150 gpd for each bedroom in the house. These regulations also contain flow estimates at facilities other than homes.

Step 2: Estimate soil permeability according to a soil evaluation and/or properly conducted percolation tests. Determine the wastewater loading rate from Table I.

Step 3: Compute total area needed for the absorption system: Divide daily wastewater (from Step 1) by the loading rate (Step 2).

Table I. Maximum Loading Rates for Low-Pressure Pipe Systems in Soils of Certain Textures and Estimated Permeabilities

Estimated Permeability (min/in.)	USDA Soil Texture[a]	Maximum Loading Rate (gpd/ft^2)[b]
20	Sand, loamy sand	0.50–0.40
20–40	Sandy loam, silt loam	0.40–0.30
40–60	Sandy clay loam, clay loam	0.30–0.20
60–90	Silty clay loam, sandy clay	0.20–0.10
90–120	Silty clay, clay	0.10–0.05

[a]This table does not consider the effects of clay mineralogy on soil permeability. A sandy clay composed of 1:1 clays may in fact be more permeable than a clay loam composed of 2:1 clays. It is very important that soil permeability, total daily wasteflow and loading rate be determined by the local health department before the LPP system is designed.

[b]These loading rates should be used only for calculating the size of LPP systems as presented in this document. These rates must *not* be used for sizing mounds or other soil absorption systems.

Example: a) Wastewater flow for 3 bedroom home = 450 gpd.

b) Estimated soil permeability = 50 min/in.
Loading rate = 0.25 gpd/ft².

c) Total area needed = 450 gpd ÷ 0.25 gpd/ft² = 1800 ft².

B. Laying Out and Locating the Distribution System

Once the required absorption area has been computed, it is necessary to fit the required area to the actual site. The major considerations are that the lateral lines should not extend more than 70 feet in either direction from the manifold, and lateral lines are placed on the contour and spaced a minimum of 5 feet apart. The final shape and configuration of the absorption field will depend on several factors, including slope, drainage, trees and horizontal setback requirements on the lot. Wooded lots will require more than the computed absorption area because of the extra room needed to "fit" the distribution laterals around trees, while still maintaining a separation of at least 5 feet between laterals.

Step 4: Determine the linear feet of laterals required ("laterals" are 1.25-inch polyvinylchloride (PVC) distribution pipes with drilled holes). If the lines can be spaced 5 feet apart, simply divide the total absorption area (Step 3) by 5 feet.

Example: Absorption area of 1800 ft² ÷ 5 ft = 360 linear feet of laterals.

Step 5: Determine the best configuration and orientation of the 1800-ft² distribution on the given site. Lateral lines should be placed *parallel* to the elevation contours.

Examples: Each of the following are possible layouts for an 1800-ft² dosing system. The total linear footage of lateral lines will be the same regardless of shape (Figure 4).

a) 30 ft × 60 ft
b) 40 ft × 45 ft
c) 90 ft × 20 ft

NOTE: For examples a and b, the manifold (supply line) can be located at either end of the laterals, whereas for c, for example, the manifold must be located in the center of the laterals to feed both directions.

Step 6: Designate the exact location of the septic tank, pumping tank and distribution field. Specify exactly what provisions are necessary for landscaping, drainage and diversions. On the site, stake out the area to be used for the distribution field. This area *must* be protected from disruption during construction activities.

C. Designing the Distribution System

The purpose of the low-pressure dosing is to provide uniform distribution of septic tank effluent over the entire soil absorption system. The proper dosing involves balancing the size of the distribution system with the dosing

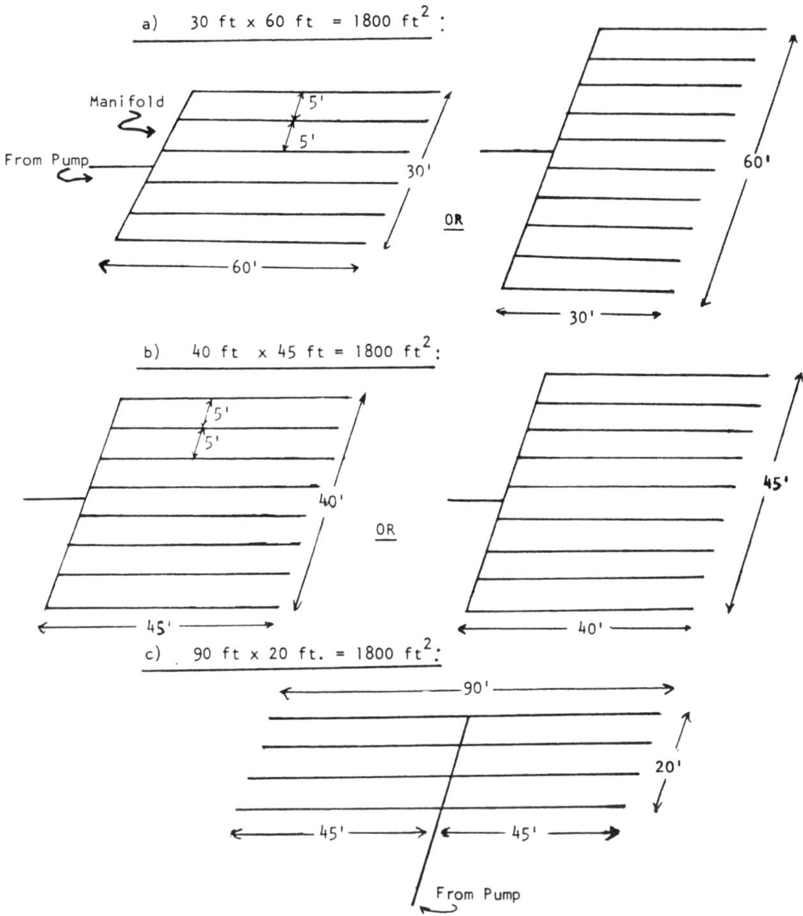

Figure 4. Various configurations for an 1800-ft^2 distribution field containing 360 linear feet of lateral lines.

volume, pumping capacity, desired pressures and flowrate. The best dosing is achieved at a pressure head between 2 and 6 feet (0.87 and 2.60 psi). Lower pressures do not provide uniform delivery of effluent, while higher pressures may cause excess velocities from the holes resulting in surfacing of the effluent.

Step 7: Determine the size of the septic tank and pumping chamber. Septic tank volume is the same as for a conventional system and is determined according to appropriate state and local regulations. The pumping chamber should provide for at least one day of emergency storage capacity; therefore, it must contain at least twice the daily waste flow.

Example: 2 × 450 gal = 900-gal pumping chamber

Step 8: Determine the hole size and spacing for the distribution laterals. Holes are generally spaced 2.5- to 5-feet apart and are of 1/8- to 1/4-inch in diameter. Certain exceptions to these dimensions may be made within a given system, such as 3/32-inch holes at wider spacing in one or two lower laterals, but *not* in the entire distribution system.

Example: a) For 360 linear feet of laterals (Step 4) at 5-foot hole spacing, the distribution system will have 360 ÷ 5 = 72 holes.

At 2.5-foot hole spacing, the distribution system will have 360 ÷ 2.5 = 144 holes.

b) Table II indicates that a 1/8-inch hole will discharge 0.26 gpm at a 2-foot head and 0.37 gpm at a 4-foot head, while a 3/16-inch hole will discharge 0.59 gpm at a 2-foot head and 0.83 gpm at a 4-foot head. Any of these combinations may be selected.

c) Summarizing steps a and b will result in total flow through the system for each condition as follows:

1. 72 holes × 0.26 gpm/hole = 19 gpm
2. 144 holes × 0.26 gpm/hole = 37 gpm
3. 72 holes × 0.37 gpm/hole = 27 gpm
4. 144 holes × 0.37 gpm/hole = 53 gpm
5. 72 holes × 0.59 gpm/hole = 42 gpm
6. 144 holes × 0.59 gpm/hole = 85 gpm
7. 72 holes × 0.83 gpm/hole = 60 gpm
8. 144 holes × 0.83 gpm/hole = 120 gpm

d) For level lots, the system will require a pump with a capacity equal to whichever condition is selected from above when operating against a certain total head (to be determined in the following steps).

NOTE: Special considerations must be made for distribution systems on sloping ground. It is very important that hole sizes and spacings provide for equal flow per unit length of each lateral. It is necessary to compensate for the difference in elevation head between the uppermost and lowermost laterals through proper choice of hole sizes and spacings in each lateral line.

A distribution system with more than 4 feet of elevation between the upper and lower laterals should not be designed with a single manifold, but will require separate (split) manifolds for upper and lower laterals with separate valves for pressure adjustment.

Step 9: Determine the total pumping head of the system. "Total head" is the amount of work (expressed in feet) that the pump must do to overcome:

a) the difference in elevation from the pump to the end of the supply manifold,

Table II. Flowrate as a Function of Pressure Head and Hole Diameter in Drilled PVC Pipe

Pressure Head		Drilled Hole Diameter (in.)					
		3/32	1/8	5/32	3/16	7/32	1/4
(ft)	(psi)	Flowrate (gpm)					
1	0.43	0.10	0.18	0.29	0.42	0.56	0.74
2	0.87	0.15	0.26	0.41	0.59	0.80	1.04
3	1.30	0.18	0.32	0.50	0.72	0.98	1.28
4	1.73	0.21	0.37	0.58	0.83	1.13	1.48
5	2.16	0.23	0.41	0.64	0.93	1.26	1.65
6	2.60	0.25	0.45	0.70	1.02	1.38	1.81

$Q = 449\ CA\ (2gh)^{1/2}$

where Q = flow per orifice (gpm),
C = 0.6 for sharp-edged orifices,
A = cross-sectional area of orifice (ft^2),
g = gravitational constant = 32.2 ft/sec^2, and
h = pressure head (ft).

b) the frictional resistance of the pipe, and

c) the pressure head required in the lateral lines.

Total Head = Elevation Head + Friction Head + Pressure Head

a) Elevation Head: difference in elevation from the pump to the end of the manifold. (Remember that the pump will be 4 or 5 feet *below* ground level in the pumping chamber.)

b) Friction Head: loss of pressure due to friction in the total length of pipe from the pump to the end of the supply manifold (use only the length of the supply and manifold lines, not the length of lateral lines). Table III gives friction losses for different sizes of schedule 40-PVC pipe at various pumping rates.

c) Pressure Head: pressure required for even distribution through the perforated lateral lines, usually between 2 and 6 feet.

Step 10: Select proper supply manifold diameter. This will depend on allowable friction loss in the pipe when matched with the pump capacity to be used.

Example: If an elevation head of 10 feet for the sample system discussed and a pressure head requirement of 4 feet are assumed, as well as a horizontal distance from the pump to the end of the manifold of 100 feet, total head requirement can now be estimated:

Elevation head = 10 feet

Pressure head = 4 feet

Friction head = ?

Table III. Friction Loss per 100 feet of Schedule 40-PVC Pipe

Friction Loss (feet of head)

Flow (gpm)	Pipe Diameter (in.) 1	1.25	1.5	2	3	4	6	8	10
1	0.07								
2	0.28	0.07							
3	0.60	0.16	0.07						
4	1.01	0.25	0.12						
5	1.52	0.39	0.18						
6	2.14	0.55	0.25	0.07					
7	2.89	0.76	0.36	0.10					
8	3.63	0.97	0.46	0.14					
9	4.57	1.21	0.58	0.17					
10	5.50	1.46	0.70	0.21					
11		1.77	0.84	0.25					
12		2.09	1.01	0.30					
13		2.42	1.17	0.35					
14		2.74	1.33	0.39					
15		3.06	1.45	0.44	0.07				
16		3.49	1.65	0.50	0.08				
17		3.93	1.86	0.56	0.09				
18		4.37	2.07	0.62	0.10				
19		4.81	2.28	0.68	0.11				
20		5.23	2.46	0.74	0.12				
25			3.75	1.10	0.16				
30			5.22	1.54	0.23				
35				2.05	0.30	0.07			
40				2.62	0.39	0.09			
45				3.27	0.48	0.12			
50				3.98	0.58	0.16			
60					0.81	0.21			
70					1.08	0.28			
80					1.38	0.37			
90					1.73	0.46			
100					2.09	0.55	0.07		
125						0.85	0.12		
150						1.17	0.16		
175						1.56	0.21		
200							0.28	0.07	
250							0.41	0.11	
300							0.58	0.16	
350							0.78	0.20	0.70
400							0.99	0.26	0.90
450							1.22	0.32	0.11
500								0.38	0.14
600								0.54	0.18
700								0.72	0.24
800									0.32
900									0.38
1000									0.46

A pumping capacity must now be selected before the friction head can be calculated. Because most small, economical submersible effluent pumps (0.3-0.4 hp) will supply 20–30 gpm against nominal heads, condition C-3 from Step 8 is selected for total pumping requirement of the system. Therefore, the sample system will require a pump with a capacity of 27 gpm. If 1.5-inch pipe is used for the supply line, the friction head for 100 feet at 27 gpm will be about 4.5 feet. So, the total head requirement is:

10 feet + 4 feet + 4.5 feet = 18.5 feet

This means that the sample system will require a pump with a capacity of 27 gpm at a total head of 18.5 feet. It is always necessary to specify the *total head* when selecting a pump of a certain capacity. This can be checked against the performance curve provided by the pump manufacturer.

Step 11: Select a pump of proper capacity. Consult the pump performance curve. The system requirements of flow and total head (27 gpm) and 18.5 feet) intersect at a point that must fall *on* or *below* the performance curve. If the point falls *above* the curve, then this pump is too small for the dosing system selected. There are several options for correcting this problem:

a) Select a larger pump.

b) Reduce total head through use of larger supply line and thus reduce friction head.

c) Reduce total head by selecting a lower pressure head (e.g., decrease pressure in the laterals from 4 feet to 2 feet).

d) Reduce the total flow requirements by designating smaller hole sizes or by increasing hole spacing to effect fewer total holes in the system.

A combination of choices can be made. The goal is to design a system that works properly for the lowest possible price. Reduction in pressure heads and hole sizes and increases in hole spacings should still be within the limits as listed in previous steps.

Step 12: Calculate the total storage volume of the pipes in the distribution system (see Table IV for storage capacities of different pipe sizes).

Example: The sample LPP dosing system includes 100 feet of 1.5-inch supply manifold and 360 feet of 1.25-inch laterals. Table IV indicates that 100 feet of 1.5-inch pipe contains a volume of 9.2 gallons and 100 feet of 1.25-inch pipe contains 6.4 gallons or 23 gallons per 360 feet.

Total storage = 9.2 gal + 23 gal = 32.2 gal

Step 13: Select the proper dosing volume or the volume to be pumped to the distribution field during each pumping cycle.

Optimal performance of an LPP system is achieved with two to four dosing cycles per day (112–225 gallons per dose for a 450-gpd

Table IV. Storage Capacity per 100 feet of Different Pipe Sizes

Inside Diameter (in.)	Storage Volume (gal)
1	4.1
1.25	6.4
1.5	9.2
2	16.2
3	36.7

system). However, each dose should supply enough effluent to provide uniform delivery through all holes or at least five times the volume of the lateral network.

Dosing volume = supply line volume + 5 × lateral volume

For the sample system, this would be

$$9.2 + 5 \times 23 = 124.2 \text{ gal/dose}$$

An actual volume of 150 gallons per dose would be appropriate for this system and would result in 450 ÷ 150 = 3 pumping cycles per day. (Note that a pump delivering 25 gpm would only operate for 6 minutes per cycle, or a total of 18 minutes per day.)

Step 14: Determine whether a check valve (one-way valve) is needed in the supply manifold. Any effluent that remains in the supply and lateral lines of a properly sited system will drain back to the pumping chamber when the pump shuts off. If this volume is too large, it can cause excessive use of the pump and of power. Check valves may be needed on large systems with long pumping distances. However, check valves should be avoided if possible since they tend to malfunction when used for septic tank effluent. In general, a check valve should only be used if the *total storage volume* (Step 12) is greater than *25% of the total daily waste flow.*

Step 15: Determine the *depth* of water in the pumping chamber to be pumped per dose.

Example: For a 900-gallon rectangular pumping tank, a 150-gallon dose is equal to 1/6 of the total volume or 1/6 of the total liquid depth of the tank. If that depth were 5 feet, the depth of water per 150-gallon dose would be:

$$5 \text{ feet} \times 1/6 = 5/6 \text{ feet} = 10 \text{ inches}$$

Therefore, the float control switch for the pump should be set for a 10-inch drawdown to provide automatic doses of 150 gallons.

Step 16: Accurately list all the design specifications for the LPP system and list all necessary materials for construction.

CONCLUSIONS

The low-pressure pipe distribution system appears to offer an alternative to some problems of wastewater disposal in North Carolina. By following simple design procedures, a system that has sound hydraulic operating principles can easily be built onsite at a cost at least competitive with conventional systems in similar problem areas. This system is *not* suited to all soils, all problems or all sites. It is an alternative, not a panacea, for those who wish to live in problem areas unserved by public treatment facilities.

31

THE GRAVITY-FLOW SEPTIC TANK–AN INNOVATIVE, NO-CLEANING, NO-PROBLEM SYSTEM

Oliver Marcotte, M.D.
25000 W. Ten Mile
Southfield, Michigan 48034

INTRODUCTION

This investigation was made in response to a request that this author evaluate residential sewage problems in Southfield, Michigan.

THE SEPTIC TANK–CODE DEVELOPMENT BAFFLE ADDED

In 1881 a patented baffle was added to the regular septic tank to help protect the trench. Since then there has been no change except that from time to time the Health Department has authorized that the trench(es) and tank be enlarged. This enlargement developed into a standard code. However, standard codes can often delay the acceptance of new workable ideas.

SCUM IS THE CULPRIT

Today, because approximately one-third of American housing units use the septic tank, it is accepted as the alternative of choice. However, problems arise because this septic tank system has unpredictable failures (Figure 1). Why? The cause of failure is the development of scum in the tank (Figure 2). Without a heavy scum, decomposition of organic material

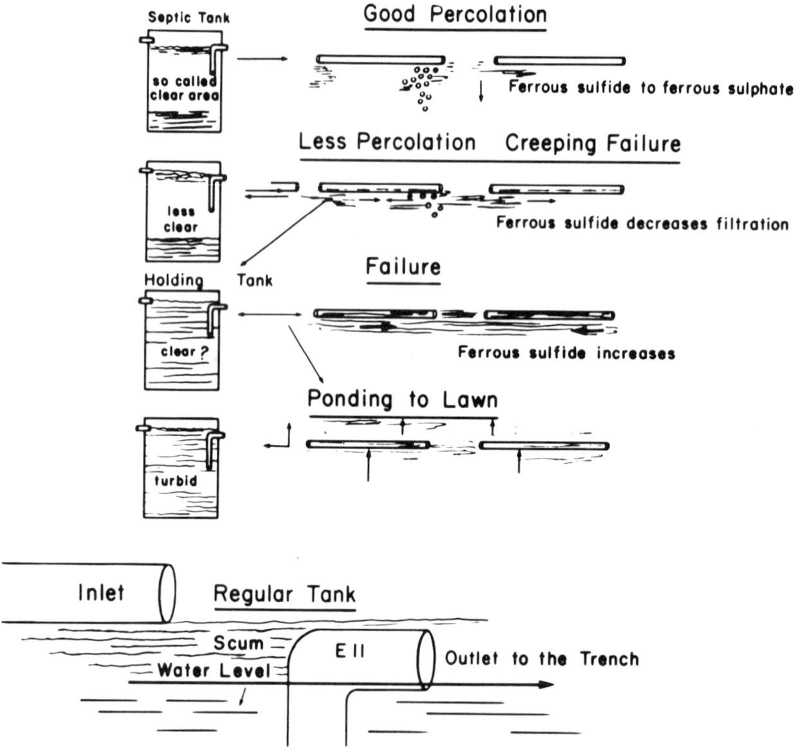

Figure 1. Septic tank failure.

can take place and problems are no longer a threat—action is dynamic. With a heavy scum, toxic gases cannot exit so the amount of decomposition decreases, increasing organic matter. Finally, the septic tank merely becomes a "holding" tank, causing many problems. These problems are passed on to the trench; then, on to the resident for special attention.

HOW TO IMPROVE THE SEPTIC TANK SYSTEM

Sewage is organic matter, a temporary product that continuously decomposes to gas, water and chemicals. Nature does this on a permanent basis and has no unpredictable failures. This indicates that there must be a better way of solving today's sewage problems.

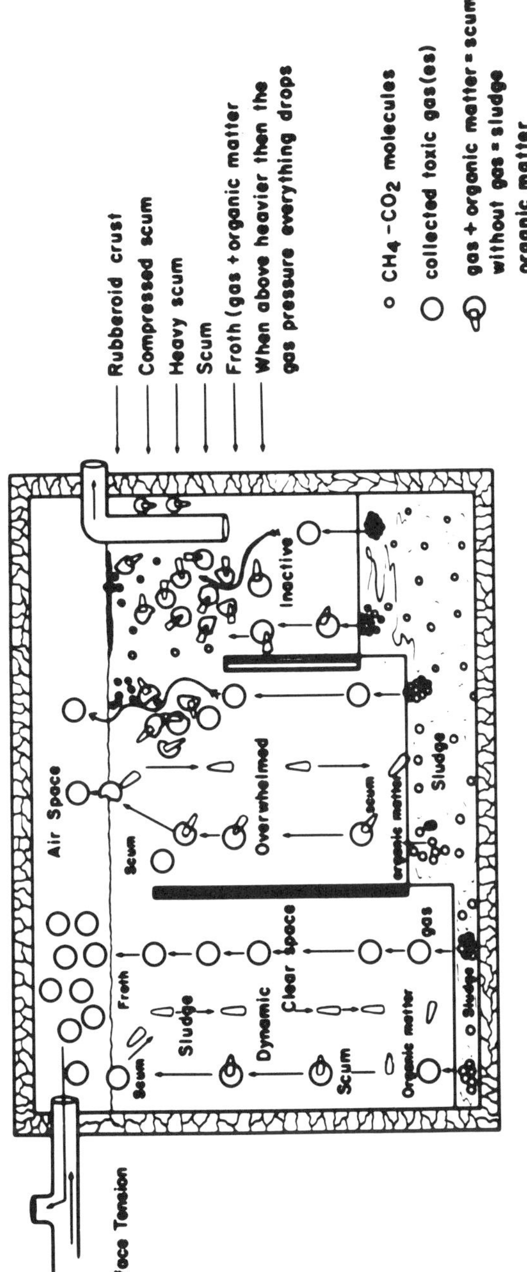

Figure 2. The effect of scum in a regular septic tank.

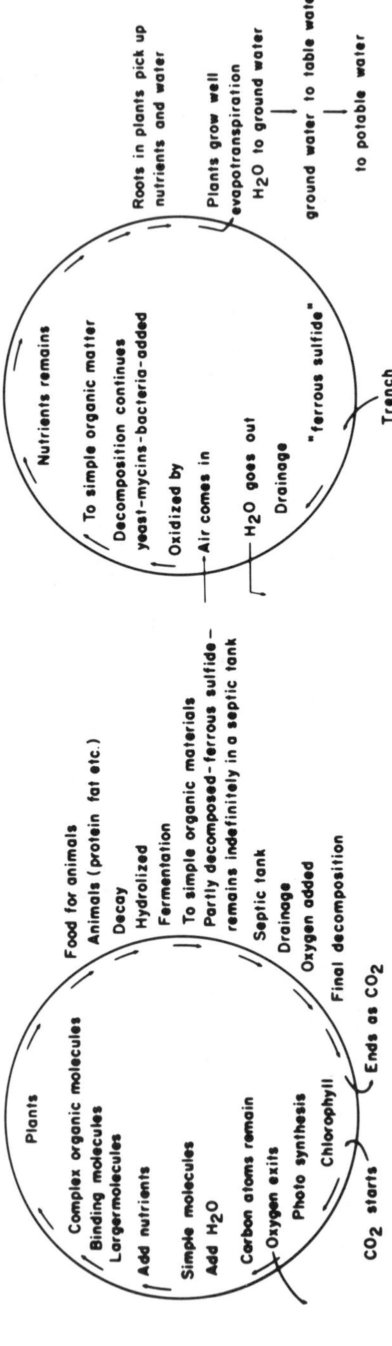

Figure 3. The carbohydrate cycle.

Use of the Baffle in a Septic Tank

In the regular septic tank the carbohydrate cycle (Figure 3) completely stops at the halfway station. Here it remains indefinitely as scum above and sludge below. The baffle is good and bad (Figure 4). It is good because raw scum is held back giving retention time to further decompose the sewage. In the clear space, suspended solids go by means of hydraulic power to the trench. It is bad when scum and sludge are overwhelmed and the tank becomes a holding tank with no clear space. The hydraulic power then sends the heavy black particulate matter to the trench.

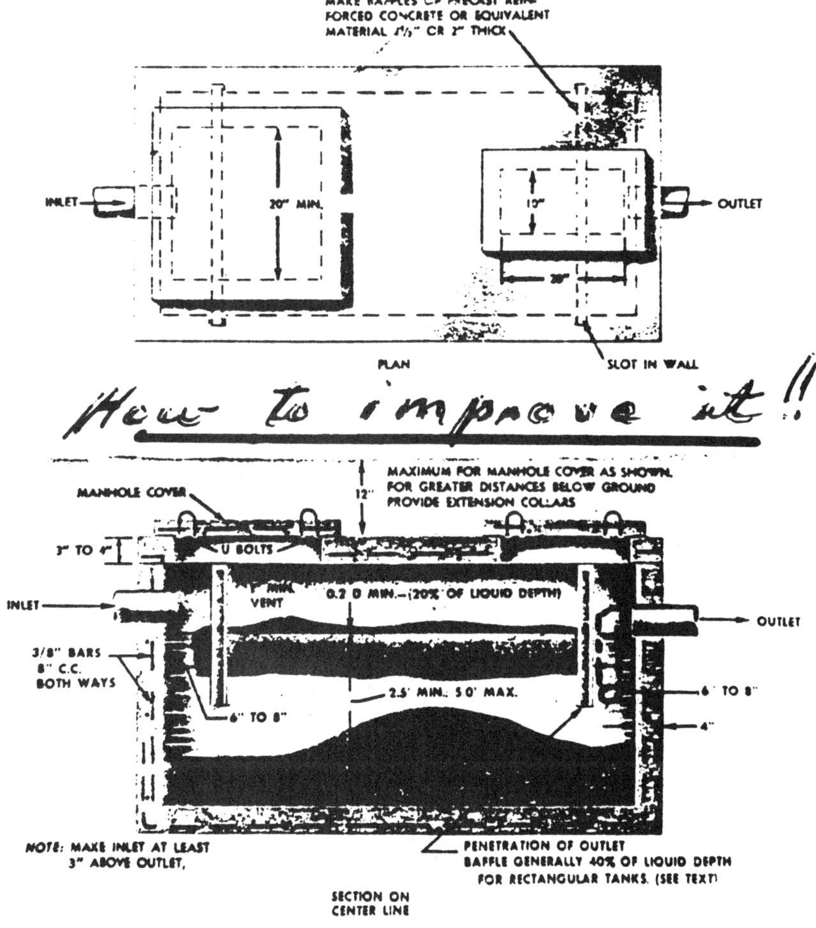

Figure 4. Improvements on the septic tank.

Drainage and Oxidation

If the drainage and oxidation in the trench are adequate, the black particulate matter goes on to gas, water and nutrients. If inadequate, the black particulate plugs up and ponds on the lawn, causing trouble for the unhappy resident.

DEVELOPMENT OF THE GRAVITY-FLOW SEPTIC TANK SYSTEM

The Gravity-Flow Septic Tank System (patent #415-4685) is a system that effectively mimics nature's way of disposing of sewage (Figure 5).

No Scum Problem Because of Slotted Pipe Inserts

This system is ideal because there is no scum problem. What scum does develop exits through the multiple slits in the pipe inserts. By action

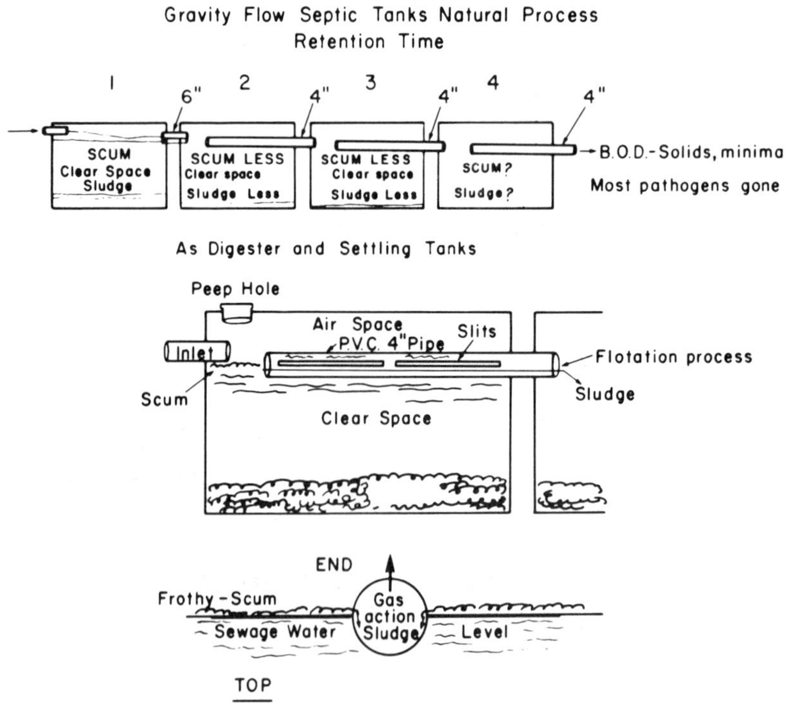

Figure 5. The gravity-flow septic tank system.

in the pipe the scum loses its gas, becoming sludge, then goes on to the next tank. Four tanks are used (Figure 6). The anaerobic bacteria and natural dynamic processes, without holding back for stabilization of sewage, go on to 85–90%. The minimal "ash" is not a problem. The sewage stabilization problem of the regular septic tank is well known.

Pathogens

With this system, if pathogens are present they are subjected to treatment by many other bacteria. Most, if not all, die; however, to be sure there is no health hazard remaining, a small trench is added (Figure 7).

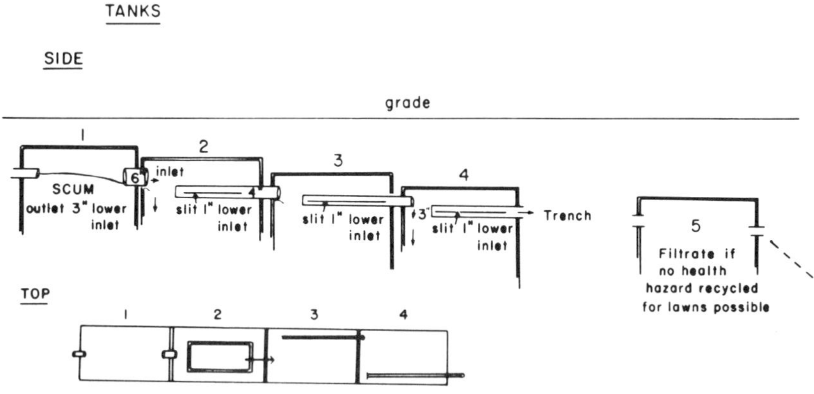

Figure 6. Example of four-tank system.

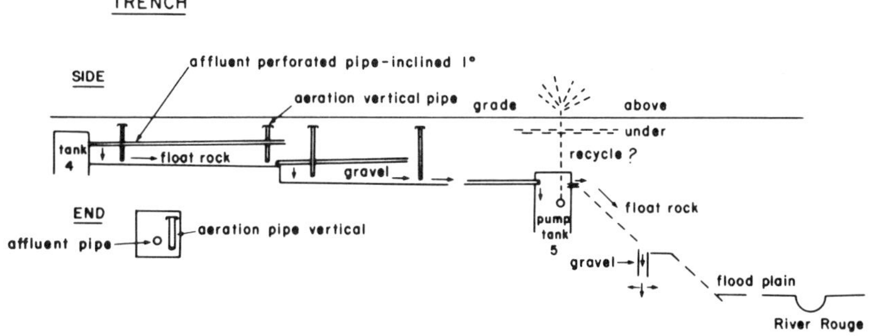

Figure 7. Septic tank trench.

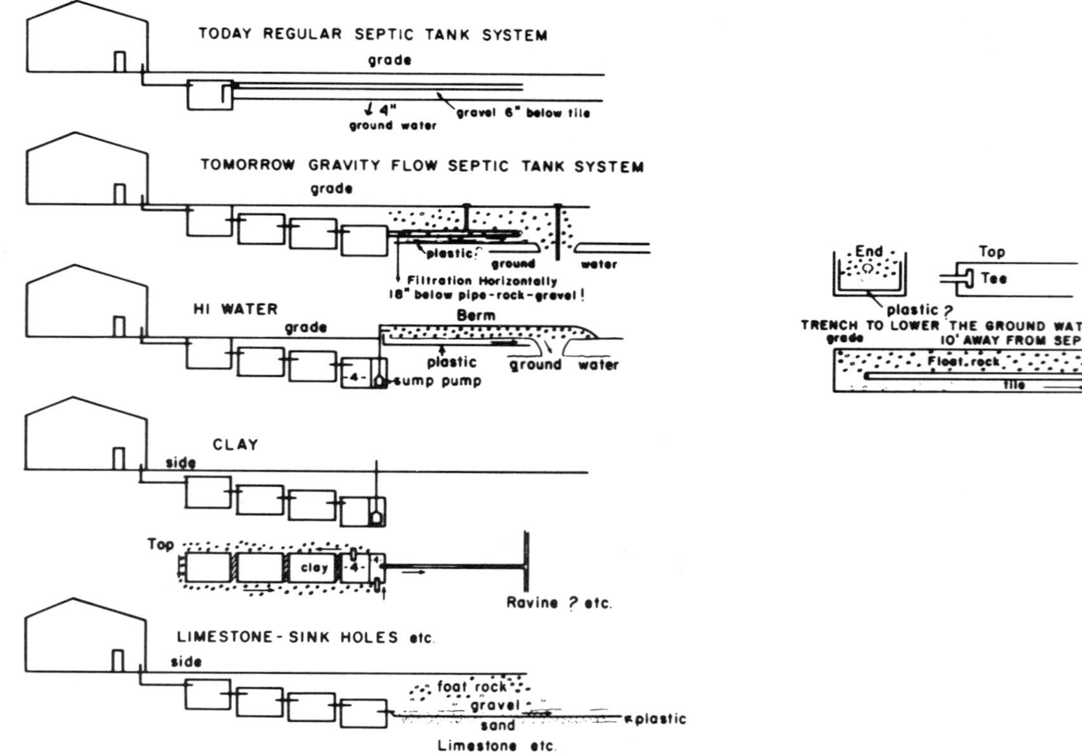

Figure 8. Septic tank variations for various soil conditions.

Variant is Used for Clay and High-Water Areas

In areas of clay, high water, limestone, etc., a simple variant is added (Figure 8). This is not a problem; it only demands a little thought.

Thirteen Repair Jobs Installed With Permits

To date, 13 systems have been installed in residential areas as repair jobs with permits–some in clay, some in high-water areas. All of the customers have been happy with the system because their sewage problem has been eliminated.

Tank Added at End of Trench Recycling Water

For a possible fourteenth installation, a fifth tank may be added at the end of the small trench. This added tank will permit the use of the filtrate for the lawn sprinkler. However, this idea is presently still in the experimental stage.

Testing

In developing this system, laboratory technicians at the Southeastern Oakland County Sewage Disposal System in Madison Heights tested more than 100 effluent samples for coliform bacteria, suspended solids and biochemical oxygen demand (BOD). All these test samples were taken from the exit of the system, and suspended solids were found to be minimal. Moreover, these 100 samples were all taken from units installed for residents with large families.

CONCLUSIONS

What the Health Department and society at large have been looking for these past 98 years is now a reality in the Gravity-Flow Septic Tank System–an onsite, no-problem, no-cleaning sewage disposal system for all residents. What the system does *not* handle are disposable diapers, sanitary napkins, facial tissues, paper towels, etc.

This system is already available to residents in Oakland County as a repair job. It is hoped that its installation for new housing areas will soon be permitted all over the U.S. The system can be built on most types of land, thereby opening areas never before opened to new construction.

32

ROLE OF PUBLIC AGENCIES AND PRIVATE INTERESTS IN IMPLEMENTING ONSITE AND SMALL COMMUNITY WASTEWATER MANAGEMENT PROGRAMS

Peter A. Ciotoli, AICP, Senior Planner
Glenn M. Johnson, P.E., Group Manager
Roy F. Weston, Inc.
West Chester, Pennsylvania 19380
Don C. Niehus
Environmental Planner
Municipal Environmental Research Laboratory
U.S. Environmental Protection Agency
Cincinnati, Ohio 45268

INTRODUCTION

As evidenced by the information presented in the preceding National Sanitation Foundation (NSF) conferences [1,2], federal and state policies and regulations regarding onsite and small community (i.e., noncentral) wastewater systems have changed dramatically. At the national level, these changes are reflected in the 1977 Clean Water Act Amendments, in the most recent U.S. Environmental Protection Agency (EPA) memorandum (PRM 79-8), and in the newly formed "White House Rural Water and Sewer Initiatives" [3]. At the state level, state agency organizational changes, numerous state-sponsored workshops and conferences on noncentral wastewater management issues, and changes in state sewerage construction grant allocation policies have helped alter and refocus state responsibilities toward the management of onsite and small community systems. At the local level, the responsibility for managing, operating and regulating onsite and small community systems has undergone equally dramatic changes over the past several years, with management responsibilities shifting from state to local levels, and new specialized wastewater management agencies and service districts being created.

This presentation provides an overview of typical wastewater management program activities and participants at national, state, regional and local levels [4-7]. Both public and private sector entities are identified as participants in the overall management of onsite and small community systems. The purpose of this management agency overview is threefold:

1. It identifies and examines the involvement of various agencies in the management process.
2. It highlights those problems and constraints associated with the organization of the current management program structure that affect the performance and implementation of onsite and small community wastewater management program objectives.
3. It offers general observations, recommendations and guidance on how various management responsibilities can be provided by entities at the national, state, regional and local levels.

MANAGEMENT FUNCTIONS

To properly manage noncentral wastewater systems, an administration, operation and implementation program with sufficient technical, financial and legal capabilities must be developed to perform selected functions. These functions, which ensure the adequate performance of a noncentral wastewater system, fall into these major categories:

- Planning
- Regulation and enforcement
- Financing
- Technical assistance/public education
- Operation and maintenance (O&M)

DESCRIPTION OF ROLES AND RESPONSIBILITIES

National Role

At the national level, activities by agencies to improve onsite and small community system management fall into four categories: grant assistance, planning, research and technical assistance/information transfer.

Since the passage of the Clean Water Act Amendments of 1977 (PL 95-217), federal interest in the wastewater management problems of small communities has increased dramatically. Prior to that, federal water pollution control efforts were focused on conventional centralized collection and treatment facilities for large- and medium-sized communities. As these needs are being met, attention can be turned to the problems of smaller communities. The new amendments also recognize the need to give greater consideration to using lower cost or more environmentally sensitive wastewater systems.

Grant Assistance

The Clean Water Act of 1977 and subsequent regulations (PRMs 78-9 and 79-8) require greater consideration of onsite and alternative systems through the 201 Construction Grants Program. The major changes are summarized in Table I. To encourage implementation of nonconventional systems, part of

Table I. Clean Water Act Amendments–Impacting Small Flows Seminar

Amendment	Section
A set-aside of 2% for innovative and alternative sytems; 85% funding (as opposed to the usual 75% for capital costs of alternative technologies).	17; 202_A
A cost-effectiveness bonus of 15% for such technologies; that is, they can be 15% more costly and still be selected.	16; 201_J
A set-aside of up to 4% of the total grant amount for grants to rural areas (fewer than 3500) implementing alternative technologies. The set-aside will be 4% in the states with 25% or higher rural population, and may be negotiated at up to 4% for states with lower rural populations.	27; 205_H
Creation of a clearinghouse for information on alternative technologies to aid in technology transfer.	7; 104_Q
A requirement that such technologies be more systematically considered in the grants process, specifically in the facilities plans.	12 and 41; 201_G and 217
Revised procedures for the evaluation of collection systems.	36; 211
Provisions making individual systems grant eligible for rehabilitation under certain conditions.	14; 201_H
Provisions to reduce water consumption and sewage flow.	21; 204_A
Provisions to study requirements for coordinating water supply and wastewater treatment.	72; 516
Eligibility of alternative systems to serve existing private homes and businesses if public agency applies for grant, gives assurances of adequate maintenance, develops a monitoring program and initiates a user charge and cost recovery system. Publicly owned alternative systems are also grant eligible.	14; 201_H

the construction grant fund has been "set-aside" for alternative and innovative systems. In addition, some states are modifying 201 project priority lists to increase the number of fundable small community systems.

Step 1 Facilities Plans for small communities must now do a more adequate analysis of existing system conditions; possible repair or replacement of existing systems; various configuration of alternative and conventional systems; and the relative cost-effectiveness of different schemes. Where alternative technologies are partially or wholly the selected alternative, the grant application must develop an O&M management plan, a user charge and cost recovery system, and a water quality monitoring program.

Although the EPA 201 Construction Grants Program is of primary importance, other federal agencies may also provide funding for small community wastewater systems. Other programs for facilities construction include the following:

1. Farmers Home Administration (FmHA), Department of Agriculture, "Water and Waste Disposal Systems for Rural Communities," (PL 92-419).
2. Department of Housing and Urban Development (HUD). "Community Development Block Grants–Discretionary," (PL 93-383).
3. Economic Development Administration, Department of Commerce. "Grants and Loans for Public Works and Development Facilities," (PL 89-136).

Some communities have met some personnel costs through participation in the Department of Labor's Comprehensive Employment and Training Act program (CETA, PL 93-203). According to the "White House Rural Development Initiatives," the federal government was to spend about $2.5 billion in the 1979 fiscal year to help small communities construct or upgrade their water and sewer systems.

Planning

Wastewater facilities planning is an integral part of the 201 Construction Grants program just discussed. Another important EPA planning program is the 208 areawide and state water quality management planning program. Increasing awareness of the needs of small communities, the appropriateness of alternative technologies, and alternative institutional and management arrangements is evident among 208 agencies. The 208 agency should be consulted early in the 201 Facilities Planning process for assistance in developing facilities and management strategies for small communities.

Research

EPA's research on small community wastewater systems is centered within the Municipal Environmental Research Laboratory (MERL) in Cincinnati. Its current work involves:

1. summarizing the performance and cost characteristics of alternative onsite, cluster and community systems;
2. updating and expanding the Public Health Service *Septic Tank Manual*;
3. developing the methodology for conducting facilities planning for small communities;
4. evaluating septage management practices; and
5. analyzing institutional arrangements for management of onsite and alternative wastewater systems.

Other federal research on small community wastewater technology is undertaken by the FmHA, Forest Service, National Park Service, HUD, Office of Water Resources Technology (Department of Interior) and the National Science Foundation.

Technical Assistance/Information Transfer

Technical assistance (e.g., application assistance, plan review, referral, design, guidance model codes) is available from EPA's 10 regional offices, Facility Requirements Division (Office of Water Program Operations) in Washington and MERL in Cincinnati. Available publications include those from MERL (i.e., Office of Research and Development), Water Planning Division (208 staff), Water Program Operations (201 program) and Technology Transfer. Seminars are held regularly to transfer research findings and program requirements. EPA has also provided funds to the University of West Virginia to operate a Small Flows Clearinghouse. Publications and technical assistance are also available from other federal agencies. These sources include the FmHA, Forest Service, Soil Conservation Service (SCS) and HUD.

Various national organizations have been active in publishing reports and holding conferences on small community wastewater systems. These groups include the National Sanitation Foundation, National Environmental Health Association, National Association of Homebuilders and American Society of Agricultural Engineers.

State Role

State involvement in implementing onsite and small community wastewater management programs to a large extent parallels that of the federal government by promulgating and enforcing regulations, and providing technical and financial assistance to individual communities. The concern for proper wastewater management has long been vested with state government, particularly with public health authorities, and more recently with water pollution control agencies, planning organizations and other environmental management and regulatory agencies.

Regulation/Enforcement

State public health authorities have traditionally been responsible for setting and enforcing standards. Some states have retained all regulatory authority over noncentral wastewater systems, while others have delegated all or part of the responsibility to local governments. Table II summarizes the regulatory approach toward onsite and small community systems regulation assumed by several states investigated in the EPA study entitled "Management of On-site and Small Community Systems" [6].

Public health laws and codes in states that share regulatory responsibilities with local governments are usually viewed as minimum standards to be adopted by local jurisdictions (which additionally have the right to establish regulations more restrictive than the state minimum). This regulatory arrangement can be structured in several ways. The most popular arrangement (as depicted in Table II) is for local governments to review plans and permit individual onsite systems, while the state retains the right to review and approve larger systems (and sometimes innovative and experimental systems as well). Under this shared arrangement, some states, e.g., Wisconsin, reserve the right to review and approve subsurface wastewater disposal systems in

Table II. State Case Studies

	Onsite Programs		Small Community Programs	
	State/Local Institutional Arrangement	Program Approach[a]	State/Local Institutional Arrangement	Program Approach[b]
New Hampshire	State	TR & EN	State	SR
Illinois	State/local	TR	State	FP
Maine	State/local	TR & EN	State/local	FP
Pennsylvania	State/local	TR & EN	State/local	FP
Washington	State/local	TR	State/local	COM
California	Local	ADM	State	EL
Vermont	Local	TR & EN	State/local	FP
Maryland	Local	TR	State	EL
Minnesota	Local	TR & EN	State	COM

[a]ADM = administrative; TR = technical review; and TR & EN = technical review and enforcement.

[b]SR = subdivision review only; EL = enabling legislation only; FP = facilities planning provisions; and COM = combination of programs.

subdivisions. The state of Washington exercises regulatory authority over multilot developments by requiring formation of a management agency to oversee maintenance and operation of subsurface wastewater disposal systems in subdivisions.

The state of New Hampshire is one that has retained all regulatory authority over onsite and small community systems; furthermore, it has consolidated most functions dealing with subsurface wastewater disposal into a single agency—the New Hampshire Water Supply and Pollution Control Commission.

Financing

The states (along with EPA regional offices) are responsible for administering the EPA construction grants program. These funds are typically allocated via a priority list developed and maintained by a state water pollution control agency, which is not necessarily the same state entity that regulates onsite systems. The priority lists and state construction grants programs must now recognize the needs of rural communities and investigate alternative technologies where appropriate.

The states of California and Wisconsin illustrate interesting state financing programs applicable to rural areas. The State of California Water Resources Control Board (SCWRCB) is funding a portion of the O&M costs in three communities applying alternative systems. One of these communities is Stinson Beach, whose program was described in Chapter 22. Wisconsin has recently created a state fund to finance the rehabilitation of failing industrial onsite systems. Under this financing program, individual homeowners may apply for loans through county health departments to correct failing systems.

Technical Assistance/Public Education

As part of wastewater management programs in many states, certification and licensing of wastewater system designers and installers has provided needed technical guidance and education to both public and private sector entities. States like Illinois, Minnesota and Pennsylvania have conducted training programs for system designers and installers for many years.

Complementary state educational program activities include preparation and dissemination of technical manuals for wastewater system evaluation and design, and pamphlets outlining recommended homeowner maintenance practices for onsite systems. The technical manuals and pamphlets prepared by the Pennsylvania DER are noteworthy for their quality and comprehensiveness.

Financing community alternative wastewater management projects in California should also result in needed information on the actual costs of building, operating and maintaining these types of programs.

Regional Role

Agencies operating at the regional level, i.e., at a multistate, multicounty or multimunicipal basis, also have a major role to play in the management of onsite and small community systems. Types of agencies that operate at the regional level include:

- Regional planning commissions
- Regional sewer authorities, districts or utilities
- Interstate cooperatives
- Watershed associations

These different types of agencies have been involved in planning, technical assistance/public education and operation of noncentral systems.

Planning

Regional planning commissions and watershed associations are examples of multimunicipal and multicounty entities involved in the preparation of water quality management plans that, in many cases, address the need for noncentral system management programs. For the past several years, regional planning commissions in Vermont, New Hampshire and Maine have been involved in preparing 201-type wastewater facilities plans for participating local governments through the statewide 208 areawide water quality management planning program. While these plans do not establish regulations or capital improvement projects to be adhered to by the member local governments, they do serve as a guide on common problems, such as developing model or prototype onsite management programs, regional septage management strategies and model ordinances for regulating onsite wastewater systems siting and design.

Watershed associations, in the form of lake management districts, are popular in the states of Wisconsin, Minnesota, Michigan and Maine. In Maine, for example, the Cobbossee Lake Watershed District Association was created to investigate areawide nonpoint water pollution problems and to develop and implement plans to abate them. This multitownship organization has been conducting sanitary surveys of the lakeshore residences and been active in developing uniform procedures for siting and design of subsurface systems within its jurisdiction.

Technical Assistance

Interstate cooperatives, such as the Northwest States Task Force for On-Site Disposal (made up of Oregon, Idaho, Washington, Alaska and the province of British Columbia), and the Ten-State Standards Committee on Individual Sewage Systems of the Great Lakes–Upper Mississippi River Board of State Sanitary Engineers (represented by Illinois, Indiana, Iowa, Michigan, Minnesota, Missouri, New York, Ohio, Pennsylvania, Wisconsin and the province of Ontario) are examples of regional entities involved in technical assistance. These cooperatives are involved in evaluating research and developing criteria and standards for onsite systems.

Operation and Maintenance

Regional sewer authorities have traditionally been involved in providing conventional sewerage services in urban and suburban areas. These entities have recently recognized their role in onsite and small community wastewater management by providing O&M services and septage treatment facilities to small communities. Examples of regional sewer agencies that are investigating opportunities for the management of noncentral systems include the Washington Suburban Sanitary Commission in the Washington, DC area, the St. Paul–Minneapolis (Minnesota) Metropolitan Council, and the Seattle (Washington) METRO. Generally, an entity with a broader jurisdictional base than a single town and available technical resources and expertise, such as regional sewer utilities, may be better suited than independently operated utilities to provide operation and maintenance services because of economies of scale and efficiency.

Local Role

Municipalities, towns, counties and special districts have traditionally been the primary focus (in conjunction with state and regional agencies) of onsite wastewater management programs. Management activities of local agencies include planning, regulation, operation and technical assistance. In addition to these public agencies, onsite system designers, installers, septage haulers and site evaluators are also involved in local wastewater management activities.

Planning

The wastewater facility plan (e.g., the 201 Facility Plan), local comprehensive plan and zoning map are principal tools of local government to guide the direction and character of future growth and wastewater management services within a community. As mentioned before, the 201 Facility Planning Program requires communities to perform analyses of the condition of existing systems to determine the need for new facilities, as well as an investigation of alternative technologies, including noncentral wastewater systems.

Regulation and Enforcement

Local governments are increasingly assuming the enforcement role in implementing onsite wastewater management programs. Typical local enforcement agencies include town health departments, county health departments, or special wastewater management districts (e.g., sanitary districts, soil and water conservation districts, and onsite management districts). Regulations are implemented by county and local health officers, district sanitarians or certified "agents" of the state.

Illinois, California, Minnesota, Virginia, Maryland and Washington are examples of states that have delegated much of their regulatory authority over individual systems to county health departments. In these states, the counties are free to develop more restrictive standards than the prescribed state minimum (except in California where there are no approved statewide minimum standards), and can develop staff and resource capabilities to implement onsite regulations. As mentioned earlier, in most state–local arrangements, the states usually delegate authority to regulate only small systems to local governments.

The state–local arrangements formulated in Pennsylvania and Maine illustrate programs that place the enforcement role with the township and the private sector through state-certified sewerage agents, who are authorized to perform site evaluations, system designs and installations. In Pennsylvania, the Sewage Enforcement Officer (SEO) is hired by the municipality (or the county) to evaluate site conditions, review and approve onsite system designs, and inspect the system installation. The SEO is certified by the state after taking qualification exams and attending training seminars.

Special management districts organized in California have also assumed authority for regulating system location and design, as well as supervising or providing maintenance. The Stinson Beach and Georgetown Divide (California) onsite management programs are examples of special approaches to approvals for system regulation.

Technical Assistance/Public Education

As mentioned in the discussion of state technical assistance programs, manuals, brochures and educational materials prepared by state agencies are important complements to local public education efforts to educate the public concerning design and maintenance of onsite systems. This can be done on a one-to-one basis at the local level, particularly through onsite management districts. The public education procedures of the Stinson Beach onsite management program offer a good approach to follow.

Operation and Maintenance

In areas where physical conditions warrant a closer evaluation of wastewater system design, installation and operation, a wastewater management district has been created to direct and assume the supervision and enforcement roles. There is a growing number of special district programs organized on a communitywide or subdivision basis that provide continuous maintenance and monitoring of onsite and small community systems. Such management programs are administered by newly formed or preexisting sanitary districts, special management districts, public authorities, county and municipal public works agencies and private entities such as homeowners associations, publicly regulated utilities, rural cooperatives and private installers/septage haulers. These locally organized management programs can own, operate and maintain noncentral wastewater systems, or can contract with individual homeowners to provide maintenance services.

ISSUES, PROBLEMS, CONSTRAINTS AND SOLUTIONS

Based on the research work to date and a review of the literature regarding onsite systems management, the following are major issues inhibiting the implementation of successful management programs and should be of concern to individuals interested in this concept (applicable management functions are highlighted):

1. inadequacies in wastewater facilities *planning*;
2. deficiencies in legislative authority and intergovernmental conflict regarding the *regulation* of onsite and small community systems;
3. lack of a uniform *financing* policy toward noncentral systems construction and maintenance;
4. reluctance of the general *public* to accept noncentral systems technology; and
5. lack of a uniform strategy for *operation and maintenance* of noncentral wastewater systems.

Changing Attitudes Toward Wastewater Facilities Planning

The Clean Water Act and subsequent regulations and PRM outline a number of specific requirements for an approvable noncentral management program. A major requirement is the need for a comprehensive wastewater facility plan that addresses existing wastewater system problems, investigates alternative solutions, and incorporates areawide and local policies regarding land use growth and development. In a small community facility plan, the planner or engineer must first identify existing institutional relationships, determine problems, evaluate and select regulatory and operational approaches, examine enabling legislation, and outline an implementation program to secure necessary legislative and organizational changes.

These various activities should be undertaken to ensure that the completed wastewater facilities plan becomes usable, accurate and locally acceptable, and gives guidance to developing wastewater management policies and programs for the community. Several statewide and areawide 208 planning agencies (as mentioned earlier) have recognized the critical role of the wastewater facilities plan as a basis for developing community wastewater management programs.

In conjunction with the increased emphasis on the wastewater facility plan, adjustments to statewide plan review procedures are being considered in several states. For example, Illinois has recently created an Innovation and Alternative Design Review Panel on which are represented numerous departments of the State Water Pollution Control and Health Agencies. California has created an Alternative Systems Unit to specifically review small community facility plans. Within the past few months, New Hampshire has designated one individual within the state's water pollution control agency as a small community assistance representative. The California and New Hampshire experiences illustrate the recognition on the part of these states that an individual or group of "experts" in facility plan preparation and federal funding policies would be necessary to implement noncentral wastewater management programs.

State–Local Conflicts Regarding Noncentral System Regulation

The successful experience of management programs rests largely on their ability to enforce uniform design standards and site evaluation requirements. The enforcement responsibility is often shared between state and local governments, which occasionally results in jurisdictional conflicts and time delays in issuing permit approvals. A frequent problem that arises under this shared arrangement is that an individual or a community may attempt to satisfy two or more regulatory agencies desiring different outcomes to obtain permit approval [8].

A growing concern in states in which regulatory responsibilities are shared between state and local government is the realm of explicit interagency or intergovernmental agreements, which outline the responsibilities of the state and local regulatory bodies. In the state of Washington, for example, the resulting confusion and conflict in enforcing regulations has prompted several sessions of the State House Committee on Ecology to review current regulatory responsibilities and administrative practices.

Other states in similar situations have consolidated multiple agency responsibilities in water pollution control. After the EPA was created, many states reorganized to centralize state water resource management responsibilities. Effective water resources management (and, in this case, the management of onsite and small community systems) can be provided through an integrated coordinated process, which recognizes available expertise at various levels of government.

Lack of a Uniform Federal Financing Policy

The EPA, through federal legislation and PRM, has developed cost-effectiveness guidelines to be applied in reviewing and selecting alternative wastewater management technologies for small communities. The standard procedure for the EPA is to provide grant assistance to only the most cost-effective alternative (based on a thorough analysis of community need and alternative choices). As mentioned in the previous section, however, there are several grant assistance programs available through the federal government (e.g., EPA and FmHA). In addition, states may also have parallel grant assistance programs in the form of grants, loans, tax supports or other transfer payments, which can be applied to implement wastewater management projects.

In this situation, an individual with favorable "grantsmanship" skills could develop a financial package (of federal and state revenues) to implement projects that are not the most cost-effective in the EPA analysis. Thus, the cost-effectiveness of different alternatives can be ignored through various means of financing, which may result in low cost to the homeowner even with a project that is more costly than some of the alternatives investigated. Community preferences for traditional technologies (e.g., gravity sewers and a standard treatment plant) obviously contribute to this situation and are common occurrences in small communities.

From this illustration, it appears that a uniform, consistent policy toward determining cost-effectiveness and financing small community projects is needed. The "White House Rural Development Initiatives" represents an attempt by the federal government to coordinate the numerous agencies involved in financing small community wastewater management projects through a series of interagency agreements. For example, through this cooperative effort by federal agencies, development of common criteria for conducting cost-effectiveness analysis and coordination procedures for interagency facility plan review has been proposed. Should such a program be implemented at the federal and state level, low-cost technologies may be given greater preference in small towns and rural areas.

Public Attitudes Toward Noncentral System Technology

The key to success of a wastewater management program is public acceptance of the applied sewerage technology. In dealing with nonconventional approaches to wastewater management, it is very important to educate the public and explain the service being provided. In most cases, it is necessary to convince service area residents that the proposed system is feasible, applicable and necessary.

The job of disseminating information about available technologies is shared by agencies such as NSF, EPA, FmHA and the Alternative Wastewater Management Association (AWMA) at the national level, as well as state and local entities. From experience, the most effective means of disseminating information and raising public awareness concerning the applicability of low-cost technologies is through implementation of projects in small community and rural situations.

Projects such as these that have been implemented are a result of federal, state and local cooperation and interaction. Despite the participation of many agencies in organizing these demonstration programs, it is the local agency (e.g., the county or town health department, special management district or utility) that provides the necessary one-to-one interaction with the service area resident. The visibility and performance of the local representative is a key ingredient to developing, initiating and operating a successful management program. In most instances, the local representative is a necessary component of the management program.

Establishing Operation and Maintenance Programs—A Frequently Overlooked Management Function

The poor performance of onsite systems in the past is partly a result of inadequate maintenance, design and/or installation. Typical management programs concentrate on enforcing regulations dealing with site evaluation, system design and installation supervision, leaving system operation and maintenance to the homeowners. Proper maintenance of onsite and small community systems can be provided through a variety of methods, depending on the willingness of the local government and general public to accept this responsibility. Shifting the responsibility of providing periodic system maintenance from the homeowner to the public sector has been suggested as a solution; however, there are several problems associated with this approach:

1. Voluntary approaches to periodic maintenance of systems by homeowners may not ensure that work is actually being accomplished.
2. Public maintenance of systems through organized maintenance districts may be unpopular because it involves another function to be performed by local governments.
3. Contracting with private septage haulers is a possibility; however, some controls are necessary to ensure that an adequate and fair service is being provided.
4. Inspection of system operation requires routine surveillance of the system with limited spot-checking and testing of system performance. Relying totally on complaints or references of system malfunction by neighbors or community residents generally is not an effective approach. Some form of scheduled inspection or maintenance is usually required.

Many of the existing wastewater management programs, particularly those using onsite systems, continue to place maintenance responsibilities on the homeowner. In fact, even such onsite management programs as that in Georgetown Divide Public Utility District, California, the homeowner owns the onsite system and consequently is responsible for repairing or replacing the system should a malfunction occur. The service charge levied by the district provides necessary funds to perform periodic maintenance and inspection of system operation.

This issue of system ownership and liability for repair or replacement is a key concern to be addressed when organizing a management program. Typically, the long-term satisfactory performance of an onsite system is difficult to guarantee, and onsite management programs have elected to leave the burden of system repair/replacement with the homeowner. Some private septic tank installers and cleaners are evaluating the feasibility of offering maintenance services to individual homeowners on a contract basis; however, it remains to be seen how interested the private sector and homeowner are in entering into service contracts of this type.

CONCLUSIONS

Onsite and small community management programs have proved to be cost-effective and viable solutions to wastewater needs in a number of communities across the U.S. Implementing this type of wastewater management program is a difficult task in most communities, largely because of (1) the unwillingness of the public to accept noncentral system technology; (2) difficulties in properly enforcing regulations concerning noncentral system siting, design and operation; and (3) legislative deficiencies inhibiting the initiation of management programs. These issues are not independent, but rather are interrelated because of the participation of numerous agencies at national, state, regional and local levels in carrying out various management functions. These constraints can be overcome through:

1. better cooperation among participating agencies;
2. documentation of existing management program performance costs and effectiveness;
3. education of project reviewers, site evaluators, system designers and consumers;
4. clarification of state/local responsibilities;
5. adoption of state enabling legislation for creation of noncentral wastewater management districts; and
6. development of mechanisms to improve the delivery of federal and state rural wastewater management programs through model codes, cost-effectiveness guidelines, job and training programs, and demonstration and pilot projects.

It is hoped that a large number of communities across the U.S. will be able to meet their wastewater needs through improved management of existing and upgraded onsite and small community wastewater systems. It remains to be seen how many communities will participate directly in the federal grants program to meet their needs. States and EPA regional offices are attempting to streamline grant and facility review procedures to provide assistance in a more timely fashion.

Local governments are becoming interested in applying noncentral wastewater system technologies to existing systems and developing areas. Even so, in view of the great needs, it is unlikely that all communities will be able to be assisted in the near future. In the meantime, the states and the communities themselves can do much to alleviate their wastewater problems at low cost by adopting some of the management approaches discussed here.

REFERENCES

1. Plews, G. D. "The Adequacy and Uniformity of Regulations for On-Site Wastewater Disposal-A State Viewpoint," in *Individual Onsite Wastewater Systems, Proceedings of the Second National Conference*, N. I. McClelland, Ed. (Ann Arbor, MI: Ann Arbor Science Publishers, Inc., 1975).
2. Stewart, D. E. "Alternative Methods of Regulating On-Site Domestic Sewerage Systems," in *Individual Onsite Wastewater Systems, Proceedings of the Third National Conference*, N. I. McClelland, Ed. (Ann Arbor, MI: Ann Arbor Science Publishers, Inc., 1976).
3. The White House Rural Development Initiatives. "Making Water and Sewer Programs Work" (1978).

4. "Management of Small Waste Flows," EPA 600/2-78-173, Municipal Environmental Research Laboratory, Cincinnati, OH (1978).
5. "Legal and Institutional Approaches to Water Quality Management Planning and Implementation," EPA 68-01-3564, Washington, DC (1977).
6. Roy F. Weston, Inc. "Management of On-Site and Alternative Wastewater Systems," Technology Transfer Seminar, Wastewater Treatment Facilities for Small Communities, U.S. Environmental Protection Agency (July 1979).
7. Niehus, D. C. "Institutional Arrangements for the Management of On-Site and Alternative Systems," paper presented at Alternative Wastewater Treatment System Workshop, University of Illinois, June 1979.
8. Urban Systems Research and Engineering, Inc. "Planning Wastewater Facilities for Small Communities," Technology Transfer Seminar, Wastewater Treatment Facilities for Small Communities, U.S. Environmental Protection Agency (July 1979).

33

INNOVATIVE AND ALTERNATIVE TECHNOLOGY FOR EPA'S CONSTRUCTION GRANTS PROGRAM

Robert M. Southworth, P.E., Sanitary Engineer, Municipal Technology Branch
Alan B. Hais, Chief, Municipal Technology Branch
Office of Water and Waste Management
Environmental Protection Agency
Washington, D.C. 20460

INTRODUCTION

The U.S. Congress placed new emphasis on restoring and maintaining the chemical, physical and biological integrity of the nation's waters when it passed the Federal Water Pollution Control Act Amendments of 1972 (PL 92-500). As part of that Act, Congress established the Construction Grants Program to fund the planning, design and construction of publicly owned treatment works (POTW) and authorized the U.S. Environmental Protection Agency (EPA) to administer it. Of the eligible capital costs of a POTW, 75% may be funded by EPA if all program requirements are met.

Public Law 92-500 requires the EPA Administrator to encourage the use of wastewater treatment processes that reclaim, recycle and reuse both wastewater and the pollutants removed from it. Congress restated its desire in the Clean Water Act of 1977 (PL 95-217) that such processes be used to treat municipal wastewater. This time, however, Congress emphasized its desire by providing "extra" funds for projects that have processes that reclaim, recycle and reuse wastewater. Those "extra" funds were authorized in the innovative/alternative (I/A) provisions of the Clean Water Act of 1977. Projects classified as innovative or alternative receive an 85% grant, rather than a 75% grant.

This chapter discusses the I/A provisions of EPA's Construction Grants Program, with particular attention given to alternatives to conventional treatment for small communities, onsite and individual systems.

CONSTRUCTION GRANTS PROGRAM

EPA's comprehensive Construction Grants Program requires grantees to follow a three-step procedure before municipal wastewater treatment facilities can be funded. In the first step, a planning study is conducted for a designated study area and concludes with the selection of a wastewater management system for implementation. Facilities in the selected system are designed in the second step of the program and constructed in the third step. Each step must be completed before the next step is initiated.

Many requirements must be met before a project is funded. Those requirements vary depending on what step the project is in; however, there are minimum requirements that all projects must meet before they are funded. They include the following:

1. Projects must be directed to pollution abatement or must eliminate a health hazard.
2. Projects must be on the fundable portion of a state's priority list.
3. Projects must be cost-effective.
4. Projects must meet all federal, state and local requirements.

A detailed discussion of these minimum requirements is beyond the scope of this chapter; however, all projects, including I/A projects, must meet the minimum requirements before they are eligible for funding through the Construction Grants Program.

INNOVATIVE/ALTERNATIVE TECHNOLOGY PROGRAM

The innovative/alternative technology provisions of the Clean Water Act of 1977 contain certain common goals for innovative and alternative technology. Even though those technologies have common goals, they also have some differences. Those similarities and differences were recognized by EPA when the Innovative and Alternative Technology Guidelines were developed. These guidelines contain criteria for identification of innovative and alternative technology and are incorporated as Appendix E to the overall Construction Grants Regulation (40 CFR Part 35, Subpart E).

"Alternative processes and techniques" are defined as proven methods that provide for reclaiming and reuse of water, particularly recycling of wastewater constituents or energy recovery. Because alternative processes and techniques are proven methods, EPA was able to specifically identify alternative technologies and list them in the Guidelines. Land treatment of effluent, beneficial utilization of sludges, energy recovery from sludge processing, onsite systems and individual systems are examples of identified alternative technologies.

"Innovative processes and techniques" are defined as developed methods that offer an advancement in the state-of-the-art, but *have not been fully* proven in the circumstances of their intended use. The "advancement in the state-of-the-art" is primarily directed toward reclamation, recycling and recovery of wastewater. However, it is also directed toward beneficial use of wastewater constituents, energy recovery, cost reduction, reduced uses of resources and other environmental benefits. Thus, in its simplest form, innovative technology is essentially an extension of alternative technology because it encourages new or improved methods for achieving reclamation or recycling.

Because innovative technology "has not been fully proven," EPA could not identify those technologies. Instead, criteria were developed to use as a basis for comparing a project to see if that project was innovative. Those criteria (also listed in Appendix E to the Construction Grant Regulations) require a grantee to demonstrate that certain benefits are achieved with respect to the goals of the Clean Water Act of 1977 before a project can be classified as innovative.

To implement the I/A provisions of the Clean Water Act of 1977, Congress authorized EPA to increase the federal share of a construction grant for an I/A project from 75% to 85%. States are required to "set aside" 2% of their Fiscal Year (FY) 1979 and 1980 allocations and 3% of their FY 1981 allocation for the Construction Grants Program to fund the 10% increase in the grant for an I/A project. At least 0.5% of the I/A set-aside for each of the three years must be used to fund innovative projects.

EPA's Construction Grant Regulations require that facilities plans; i.e., Step 1 of Construction Grants Program, begun after September 30, 1978, contain an analysis of innovative and alternative processes. These regulations also contain incentives for the use of I/A technology. A major incentive is that I/A projects receive a 15% cost preference in the cost-effectiveness analysis required in the facilities plan. The I/A project may cost up to 15% more than the most cost-effective non-I/A project, yet still be funded at the 85% level.

Another incentive for I/A projects is that they may be given a higher priority when the state prepares its priority list. This is significant because only projects on the fundable portion of a priority list can be funded. The higher the priority of the project, the better the chances are that it will be in the fundable portion of the list.

Congress realized that I/A projects may not be constructed because of concern that those projects may fail. As an incentive to overcome those concerns, Congress authorized EPA to fund 100% of the eligible costs to replace or to modify an I/A project that fails to meet design performance standards. Requirements that must be met before a replacement project can be funded by EPA are as follows:

1. Failure to meet design standards is *not* due to any person's negligence.
2. Correction of the failure requires significantly increased capital or operating and maintenance expenditures.
3. The failure occurred within the two-year period after final inspection by EPA.
4. The replacement project is on the fundable portion of the state's priority list.

The I/A provisions of the Clean Water Act of 1977 and EPA's I/A regulations are intended to overcome the impediments to implementation of innovative and alternative technology. Both "tools" afford grantees and their engineers the opportunity to take the lead role in implementing I/A technology as opposed to being identified as part of the reason that technology is not implemented.

ALTERNATIVES TO CONVENTIONAL TREATMENT FOR SMALL COMMUNITIES

The Clean Water Act of 1977 requires states with a rural population of 25% or more to set aside 4% of the state allotment of construction grant funds to fund alternatives to conventional treatment works for small communities. Congress added this requirement because of a concern that larger municipalities would receive the majority of a state allotment to fund large projects. As a result, no funds would be left for small communities.

Funds from the 4% set-aside can be used only to fund alternatives to conventional treatment works for small communities. Congress defined a small community as any municipality with a population of 3500 or less, or highly dispersed sections of larger municipalities. The EPA Regional Administrator is responsible for determining whether an area is a highly dispersed section of a larger municipality.

Funds from the 4% set-aside are used to fund 75% of the initial or capital costs of a project. However, because alternatives to conventional treatment are considered alternative technology, projects funded from the 4% set-aside are eligible for an increase in the grant from 75% to 85%. Funds for the additional 10% grant come from the I/A set-aside previously discussed.

Therefore, if a project contains alternatives to conventional treatment works for small communities, it is eligible for a 75% grant from the 4% set-aside and a 10% grant from the 2/3% I/A set-aside, for a total grant of 85%.

Technologies that are alternatives to conventional treatment works for small communities include onsite systems, individual systems, alternative collection systems and alternative technologies identified in Appendix E to the Construction Grant Regulations. Onsite and individual systems are discussed later in this chapter.

Alternative collection systems include collection systems that have pressure sewers, vacuum sewers or small-diameter gravity sewers. When those types of sewers are used in a small community, they are eligible for an 85% grant. Of course they must be cost-effective and meet the other basic construction grant requirements before they can be funded. Alternative sewers are exempt from the federal requirement that two-thirds of the expected flow in the collection system be wastewater generated by the community inhabitants in existence on October 18, 1972.

Pressure sewers, vacuum sewers and small-diameter gravity sewers are not eligible for an 85% grant if used in large communities; i.e., more than 3500 population or *not* a highly dispersed section of a larger municipality. However, those types of sewers may be eligible for a *75%* grant if they are cost-effective and meet all requirements.

Some of the techniques identified in Appendix E; e.g., self-sustaining incineration, are not generally appropriate for small communities. Although those techniques are identified as alternative to conventional treatment works for small communities, they would rarely be cost-effective for a small community. In most cases, such techniques would be too expensive and would require highly skilled operation and maintenance (O&M) personnel not normally available in small communities.

Small communities are areas that perhaps can most benefit from the I/A program. Not only do alternatives to conventional treatment works meet the reclamation, recycle and reuse objectives of the Clean Water Act of 1977, but they are also eligible for 85% funding; are low cost and reliable; and are not O&M-intensive processes.

ONSITE SYSTEMS

Onsite systems may be publicly or privately owned. When privately owned, they are classified separately as individual systems according to the Construction Grants Program.

Onsite systems are alternative to conventional treatment works for small communities; however, their use is not limited to small communities. If they are cost-effective and meet the other basic requirements, they can be used in any size community.

Numerous processes are available for onsite treatment of wastewater. They include septic tanks with soil absorption systems, aerobic units, mounds, sand filters and composting toilets, to name a few. Also included are processes needed to treat the septage from septic tanks. EPA does not prohibit the use of any onsite treatment process. However, as with other processes, an onsite treatment process must be cost-effective before it is eligible for construction grant funding.

In the past several years, onsite systems have not received adequate consideration when wastewater treatment facilities were planned. Now they must be evaluated as I/A technology during the facilities planning process, and adequate justification must be provided if those systems are considered unsuitable for the area being studied.

INDIVIDUAL SYSTEMS

Individual systems are defined as privately owned alternative wastewater treatment works that serve one or more principal residence (occupied 51% of the time by the voting resident) or small commercial establishments. As alternative technologies, these systems are eligible for 85% funding.

The following are the limitations on a grant for an individual system:

1. A public body must apply for the grant on behalf of the residence(s) or small commercial establishment.
2. The principal residence or small commercial establishment must have been in use on December 27, 1977.
3. Individual systems must be cost-effective.
4. The grantee must certify that public ownership of the treatment works is not feasible.
5. The grantee must certify the treatment works will be properly installed, operated and maintained.
6. The grantee must establish a comprehensive program for regulation and inspection of the individual systems.

The Construction Grant Regulations indicate that alternative technology receives a 15% preference in the cost-effectiveness analysis conducted during the facilities planning study, with one exception–individual systems. The Clean Water Act of 1977 states that the cost of privately owned treatment works "will be less than the cost of providing a system of collection and central treatment of such wastes." Therefore, individual systems have to be cost-effective without the 15% cost preference before they can be funded through the Construction Grants Program.

Technologies for individual systems are mainly technologies for onsite treatment. Processes such as septic tanks with soil absorption systems, aerobic units, composting toilets, dual waterless/greywater systems, mounds and evapotranspiration beds are eligible for use as individual systems. As with publicly owned onsite treatment systems, EPA does not prohibit the use of any technology for an individual system if it is cost-effective and meets the other applicable federal, state and local requirements. Cost-effective septage treatment processes may also receive 85% funding when used in conjunction with individual systems.

The definition of alternative technology that applies to individual systems indicates that alternative collection sewers (pressure sewers, vacuum sewers and small-diameter sewers) may receive 85% funding for an individual system. As with all alternative collection systems, they must be in a small community to receive 85% funding.

Wastewater-generating fixtures such as commodes, sinks, tubs and drains and associated plumbing are *not* grant eligible as part of an individual system. Conveyance pipes from those fixtures to the flange of a treatment unit are also not grant eligible. EPA will fund only the treatment unit; e.g., composting toilet, and sewers that convey treated or partially treated wastewater as part of an individual system.

Individual systems are viable wastewater management systems and should be adequately considered during the facilities planning process. The Clean Water Act of 1977 emphasized the viability of those systems by making them eligible for the incentives applied to innovative and alternative technology.

RESULTS OF THE FIRST-YEAR I/A PROGRAM

EPA's innovative/alternative program became effective on October 1, 1978. Since that time, several projects have been reviewed to determine whether they were innovative or alternative and several have been classified I/A. Table I presents the results of the first-year I/A program.

EPA's Technical Support Group (TSG) for the I/A program, located at EPA's Municipal Environmental Research Laboratory (MERL) in Cincinnati, Ohio, has classified 38 projects, or portions of projects, innovative and 218 projects, or portions of projects, alternative. Of the total, approximately one-third have actually received a Step 2 or Step 3 grant award for innovative or alternative technology.

Table I. Results of the First-Year I/A Program

	Projects Approved by TSG[a]	
	No.	Amount ($ thousands)
Innovative	38	11.1
Alternative	218	33.2

[a]TSG = Technical Support Group at EPA's Municipal Environmental Research Laboratory in Cincinnati, Ohio.

Several of the approved projects are alternatives to conventional treatment works for small communities. Some examples are given below:

Location	Type of Project
Patten, Maine	Septic tank, SAS and subsurface sand filter
Sherborn, Maine	Septic tank, SAS and sand filter
Fountain Run, Kentucky	Septic tank with SAS and small-diameter gravity sewer
Iberia, Missouri	Pressure sewer
Avery, Idaho	Small-diameter gravity sewer, pressure sewer, community SAS

EPA's innovative/alternative technology program, which is slated to last for three years, will expire with the utilization of FY'81 construction grant funds unless Congress renews the program. Congress may not renew the program unless it sees some convincing results that the program is working. Those convincing results will have to be in terms of the quality and quantity of projects funded through the program. Therefore, EPA, grantees and consulting engineers must enter I/A projects into the "review system" as quickly as possible. Otherwise, Congress may let the program "die" in 1981 before its true potential can be realized.

34

THE NATIONAL EPA SMALL WASTEWATER FLOWS CLEARINGHOUSE

Paul G. Moe, Senior Scientist (Agricultural Science)
Raul Zaltzman, Senior Scientist (Civil Engineering)
EPA-SWF Clearinghouse
West Virginia University
Morgantown, West Virginia 26506

INTRODUCTION

The National EPA Small Wastewater Flows Clearinghouse is administered by, and housed at, West Virginia University in Morgantown, West Virginia. It now operates under a grant funded by the U.S. Environmental Protection Agency (EPA) under the authority of, and as provided for by, the 1977 Clean Water Act Amendments. As stated in the Act, the main function of the Clearinghouse is "to develop and make available an information and data base system on practices, procedures, systems, materials, standards and applicability of alternatives to water pollution control in rural and other areas where collection and disposal of sewage in conventional community-wide sewage collection and disposal systems is impractical, uneconomical or otherwise unfeasible" [1].

SOURCES OF INFORMATION

The Clearinghouse is attempting to collect all pertinent information resulting from research, demonstration and wastewater management projects. The relevant periodical literature in this field is reviewed as soon as it becomes available (Table I). Other sources of information being monitored

Table I. Periodicals Monitored by the EPA Small Wastewater Flows Clearinghouse

1. *Effluent and Water Treatment Journal*
2. *Journal of the American Society of Civil Engineers* (ASCE)
3. *Environmental Pollution*
4. *International Journal of Environmental Studies*
5. *Journal of Environmental Health*
6. *Journal of Environmental Sciences*
7. *Pollution Engineering*
8. *Solid Wastes Management*
9. *Environmental Research*
10. *Journal of Soil and Water Conservation*
11. *Water Services*
12. *Water, Air and Soil Pollution*
13. *Water and Wastes Engineering*
14. *Groundwater*
15. *Journal of Chemical Ecology*
16. *Journal of Environmental Economics and Management*
17. *Water Research*
18. *Water Resources Bulletin*
19. *Journal of Bacteriology*
20. *Journal of Applied and Environmental Microbiology*
21. *Biomines*
22. *The Mother Earth News*
23. *Humanizing City Life*
24. *The Co-Evolutionary Quarterly*
25. *Alternative Sources of Energy*
26. *People and Energy*
27. *Self-Reliance*
28. *ACORN*
29. *New Roots*
30. *Dialogue*
31. *Tomorrow*
32. *Appropriate Technology*
33. *Compost Science*
34. *Journal of Environmental Science and Technology*
35. *Journal of Environmental Quality*
36. *Journal of the Water Pollution Control Federation* (WPCF)
37. *Journal of the American Water Works Association* (AWWA)
38. *Progress in Water Technology*
39. *Public Works*
40. *Water and Sewage Works*
41. *Water Pollution Control* (Britain)
42. *Water Resources Research*
43. *Journal of the American Society of Agricultural Engineers*
44. *American City and County*
45. *Municipal Wastewater Reuse News* (AWWA)

include patent listings, conference proceedings, symposia publications, monographs, technical reports and legal documents. Regular use is being made of a number of bibliographic tools, such as bibliographic indexes, separately published bibliographies, periodical indexes, publishers' booklists, computer data bases and government publications indexes.

Current research and demonstration projects in this field have been identified by examining current EPA grants and contracts and EPA in-house projects, and by performing a search of pertinent data bases that contain up-to-date listings of applicable projects.

The *Federal Register* and the *Code of Federal Regulations* were reviewed for federal regulations and guidelines pertaining to small wastewater systems. Data bases covering federal legislation, the *Congressional Record* and other congressional activities were searched. Sixteen foreign data bases were surveyed for applicable material.

Although the attempted coverage is extensive, it is recognized that it will be very difficult to identify and obtain copies of all pertinent documents and information sources. Therefore, the Clearinghouse solicits and welcomes any suggestions concerning additional materials that could be included in its information bank and made available to the system's users. (Manufacturers' advertising or promotional materials will not be included in the computer bank, but will be filed in the Clearinghouse library.)

OPERATION OF THE CLEARINGHOUSE

The Clearinghouse staff is currently abstracting all the information received and collected to date. For each entry selected, a legible hard copy (photocopy) is first secured for the Clearinghouse library. Each item is then catalogued and abstracted. These abstracts are then entered into a computerized information bank. Thus, the Clearinghouse possesses both an information bank of abstracts and a library containing all of the actual documents abstracted.

Specific descriptive keywords, selected from the Clearinghouse's thesaurus, are assigned to each abstract. Major category designations are also assigned to each abstract. The keywords are used primarily for literature searches, and the category designations are used for the preparation of tables of contents and as subject index headings for the abstract compendia to be published periodically by the Clearinghouse. All abstracts in the computerized information bank are retrievable through any of these descriptor elements.

Besides the creation of the computerized information bank and the library of documents, the Clearinghouse has also collected and plans to maintain an up-to-date list of contact people or offices with direct responsibility and/or knowledge in the development, review, design and management of small wastewater systems. This list of contact people is coded for each state and EPA region for each reference.

SERVICES PROVIDED BY THE CLEARINGHOUSE

The Clearinghouse eventually plans to provide a variety of services to its users. These services will include responding to individual mail and telephone requests for information; the annual preparation of a compendium of all available abstracts; conducting special literature searches on specific topics; preparing specialized bibliographies and technology updates; publishing a periodical abstract update bulletin; and participating in pertinent local, regional and national conferences, short courses and seminars.

As of September 14, 1979, there were 531 documents and abstracts available in the system, which have been published in the form of a compendium of abstracts and are for sale to the general public. The procedure for acquiring this document was described in the Clearinghouse bulletin mailed to all persons included in the Clearinghouse mailing list (presently about 20,000 names). Copies of this document are also available for public use at various libraries and EPA offices throughout the U.S.

Copies of any of the materials cited in the compendium of abstracts are generally available at government, university and public libraries. For out-of-print documents or articles from hard to obtain sources, the Clearinghouse will make single copies available for the cost of reproducing, handling and mailing the material when allowed by the current applicable copyright laws.

Persons seeking additional information and/or desiring to be included in the Clearinghouse's mailing list may mail their names and addresses to the EPA Small Wastewater Flows Clearinghouse, West Virginia University, Centennial House, Morgantown, West Virginia 26506, or call, toll-free, (800) 624-8301. Persons calling from within West Virginia may call 293-4191 collect.

REFERENCES

1. Senate Committee on Environment and Public Works. "The Clean Water Act Showing Changes Made by the 1977 Amendments," Serial No. 95-12, U.S. Government Printing Office, Washington, D.C. (1977).

35

VIRUS MOVEMENT IN GROUNDWATER

Flora Mae Wellings, Sc.D., Director
Epidemiology Research Center
Office of Laboratory Services
Central Operations Services
Department of Health and Rehabilitative Services
Tampa, Florida 33614

INTRODUCTION

Although this conference is addressing onsite sewage disposal systems, the problems associated with virus survival and movement in soils is a factor common to onsite as well as community systems. The major difference is the relative constancy of the presence of virus in sewerage as opposed to its sporadic presence in onsite systems. In urban areas particularly, enterovirus diseases that result in virus being discharged into wastewater systems occur year round, but are more frequent from May through September. Therefore, virus can be isolated from community wastewaters year round. Conversely, onsite systems would yield virus only when family members or visitors were experiencing an enterovirus infection.

No essentially definitive studies have been done to evaluate the effectiveness of onsite systems for inactivation of naturally occurring virus; i.e., excreted as an integral part of man's biological wastes. However, data are available indicating that enteroviruses enter the drainfields and eventually escape into lakes and streams [1]. This being the case, it is reasonable to assume that virus-containing leachate from septic tanks would eventually reach the groundwater, as has been shown for virus-containing wastewater at sewage effluent land disposal sites.

The importance of addressing the movement of virus in soil must be linked to the ultimate fate of the virus as related to man's well-being. A review of the waterborne disease literature over the past 25 years [2-4] shows that consumption of untreated or chlorinated groundwater was responsible for most waterborne disease outbreaks in the United States. These data also revealed that only a portion of waterborne disease outbreaks are reported to official agencies. When one adds to the number of reported and unreported outbreaks those that are never recognized because of the large numbers of subclinical infections caused by human enteroviruses, the relationship and importance of human enterovirus movement in soil is established.

VIRAL CHARACTERISTICS

The presence of virus in groundwater is thought to be facilitated by the innate characteristics of the virion per se. Unlike bacteria, viruses cannot multiply. They are replicated only within a living cell. Over a hundred different types of virus traverse the alimentary tract of man, are replicated within the cells of that system and discharged from the body as integral parts of the biological wastes of man.

Once viruses enter the environment, they can persist for relatively long periods of time [5,6] depending on the physiochemical conditions encountered. Unlike most bacteria found in sewage, viruses do not require nutrients for survival because they have no metabolism outside of a living cell. Virus survival depends primarily on the amount of protection from inactivating forces afforded the virion. Such protection can result from the virus being adsorbed to, or occluded within, a minute solid [7]. The propensity for virions to clump affords additional protection.

The size of a virus plays an important role, not only in virus survival, but in its entrainment by the percolating water. The size of the enterovirus ranges from 18 nm to 25 nm, as compared with a bacterium, which is on the order of 750 nm. It is evident that even if the viruses were encased in a solid resulting in a particle size ten times that of a single virion, the filtering capability of the soil would be much greater for a bacterium than for the occluded virion. Even a clump of virus composed of 100 enteroviruses would be small enough to escape entrapment in a medium that would trap a bacterium. It should be evident that the efficiency of the so-called "living filter" ascribed to soils based on bacterial studies cannot be assumed to apply to viruses because of the gross physiochemical differences between the two groups of organisms.

VIRUS REMOVAL BY SOILS

Although the efficiency of soils to remove virus from applied wastewater is much less than for bacteria, viruses are probably removed both by entrapment, if they are associated with large solids, and by adsorption onto soil particles, if they are present as free virions or adsorbed to a particulate that may facilitate adsorption onto soil. Unfortunately, adsorption is not an irreversible reaction. Because adsorption depends on many variables, such as pH, flowrate, the presence of cations, soluble organics and clay, as well as the soil composition, desorption may occur as these variables are altered. Therefore, the term "virus removal" may be inappropriate because of the adsorption reversibility phenomenon.

VIRUS MOVEMENT IN SOILS

Soil is dynamic. Its physiochemical status can be altered drastically by climatic changes and man's activities. As gross changes occur, the virus that had been concentrated by adsorption onto soil particles may be desorbed en masse and migrate through the soil in an ionic cloud or plume. Rainfall is particularly significant in this respect. The first indication of the importance of rainfall in virus migration through the soil matrix was obtained from the study reported at the first National Sanitation Foundation (NSF) conference in 1974 [8]. Following heavy summer rains, a burst of virus was demonstrated in groundwater obtained from both a 10- and a 20-foot-deep monitoring well at a wastewater land disposal site. Since that time, this field observation has been confirmed by laboratory experiments.

The effect of rainfall on virus desorption was simulated by the addition of distilled water to soil columns flooded with a wastewater–virus mixture. Columns 250 cm in length packed with loamy sand were subjected to flooding for two days, then dried for two hours [9]. A 10-cm amount of distilled water was added, followed immediately with wastewater. Considerably more virus desorption and vertical movement occurred, as shown by increased numbers of virions demonstrable at the 80- and 160-cm depths than when the wastewater–virus mixture was applied. However, the addition of wastewater immediately following the distilled water surge apparently encouraged readsorption at a deeper soil level. Only a few plaque-forming units (PFU) of virus were isolated from the outflow samples.

The effect of repeated cycles of rainfall on virus release from soil has been investigated [5]. Nonsterile cone samples of a sandy forest soil were used to determine virus migration and survival under simulated cycles of rainfall and effluent applications. A characteristic burst of virus, as noted in the earliest field study [8], was demonstrated in the soil columns. It was suggested that distilled water reduced the ionic strength within the column, facilitating virus desorption. During 84 days the capacity of the virus to migrate was unchanged. These data strongly support the contention that virus in groundwater is not a continuum but occurs in pulses, as dictated by the physiochemical changes taking place within the soil matrix.

The efficiency of soils for virus adsorption from wastewater is closely associated with the composition of the soil, as previously stated. Sandy soils that permit rapid percolation rates, ideal for land disposal of wastewater from the engineering standpoint, have the least capacity for virus adsorption. This was demonstrated at a U.S. Army installation where effluents from an Imhoff tank were distributed through a dosing tank to the rapid infiltration (RI) cells [10]. Each of the 22 RI cells had an average area of 0.8 acre (0.324 hectare) and fed into soils composed principally of unconsolidated silty sands and gravel of glacial origin atop bedrock.

Groundwater monitoring wells at depths ranging from 14.9 to 94.5 feet were installed immediately under the cells and at distances greater than 600 feet from the RI cells. Wastewater was applied to three RI cells for seven days and groundwater samples obtained before, during and at days 11 and 21 postdosing. Viruses were isolated from all wells on at least three of the nine sampling days and from one well located about 600 feet (183 meters) from the RI site on six of the nine sampling days. Virus isolations were not constant but were noted to present as bursts, which at times represented 10% of the composite average (276 PFU/l) of the virus present in the applied effluents.

This study confirmed lateral movement of viruses within the high water: soil ratio zone(s) of the soil, as noted in other field studies [11-13]. The actual lateral distance a virus might travel when entrained within an aquifer has not been established. The greatest lateral movement documented to date is the >600 feet obtained at the RI site. The reason that this great distance was demonstrable in only this study is probably attributable to the excellent placement of monitoring wells as related to groundwater flow and distance from the RI cell, and to the frequency of sampling. A tracer (f2 bacteriophage) was added continuously to the dosing tank at a level of 10^5 PFU/ml of wastewater applied to the RI cells. Groundwater samples were obtained three times daily. The f2 tracer was demonstrable in groundwater under the application site in a 94.5-foot-deep monitoring well 48 hours after application of wastewater began. Bursts of f2 appeared only in the first samples obtained on days 2, 3, 5 and 11 and in the third sample on day 4 drawn from the monitoring well located more than 600 feet lateral to the application site. The presence of the f2 tracer indicated that groundwater flow was in the direction of the well that yielded the indigenous enteric virus bursts. Thus, virus entrainment within the aquifer can result in significant lateral movement of virus.

The effect of recharge basins on groundwater quality was evaluated in studies conducted in Long Island [11]. Lateral movement of virus was demonstrated in a 20-foot-deep groundwater monitoring well 150 feet down gradient from the recharge site. Of the monthly samples, 30% were positive, yielding 3.7 PFU/gal in August 1976; 1.6 PFU/gal in December 1976; and 10.6 PFU/gal in February 1977. At a second site, 25% of the samples obtained from a 37-foot-deep monitoring well yielded 80 PFU/gal in June 1976; 6.4 PFU/gal in September 1976; and 100 PFU/gal in February 1977. At a third site, an 84-foot-deep monitoring well yielded no virus. Nevertheless, total and fecal coliform tests were positive at least 50% of the time in all wells. The absence of virus in samples was attributed to the depth of the well. This interpretation is moot because of the limited sampling schedule and the concentration technique employed. No rainfall data were given; however, the demonstration of 100 PFU/gal in a 37-foot-deep well using a virus concentration system having a 0–37% efficiency appears to indicate that significant amounts of viruses could reach the 37-foot level in soils comparable to those at the 80-foot-deep well site. The lower levels of virus anticipated to be present in the latter well may not have been demonstrable with the concentration system used, or virus present may have passed through the area prior to, or after, sampling.

VIRUS MOVEMENT IN LEACHATE FROM SEPTIC TANKS

Surface waters were tested in two areas where septic tank leachate was the only identifiable source of human enterovirus [1]. Virus was isolated from 28.8% (2:7) of specimens obtained from Lake Ronkonkoma. In September 1976, 2.3 PFU/gal were identified; and in March, 7.5 PFU/gal. At another site, Penataquit Creek, samples were positive for virus in June (25 PFU/gal) and July 1976 (8 PFU/gal) only, which corresponds well with the enterovirus season.

Shellfish-growing sites, including those approved for harvesting (open) and not approved (closed), were sampled in two bays. One, Great South Bay, received water from creeks carrying septic tank seepage; the other, Oyster Bay, received sewage effluent. The inflow site of the sewage effluents was located several miles from the shellfish-growing beds, whereas the creeks emptied into Great South Bay not too distant from the beds. Virus isolations were obtained from Great South Bay waters open for shellfish harvesting from three of the eight samples tested at levels of 8 PFU/gal in July 1976; 1.2 PFU/gal in August 1976; and 2.9 PFU/gal in

April 1977. Virus was also isolated from clams harvested at the site in April (0.3 PFU/gal) and June 1977 (0.1 PFU/gal). In the closed area of the bay, three of nine samples were positive at levels of 4.0 PFU/gal in July 1976; 4.4 PFU/gal in February; and 1.1 PFU/gal in June 1977. Isolates were obtained from clams at levels of 0.16 PFU/gal in July 1976 and 0.1 PFU/gal in June 1977. Tests done in five other months were negative. There was no major difference between the virological findings within the closed and open beds. However, total coliform counts between the two sites were remarkably different. Counts in the open beds ranged from 4 to 460 total coliforms/100 ml, with an average of 119.9 coliforms/100 ml and a median of 93. In the closed beds, total coliforms ranged from 23 to 2400 coliforms/100 ml, with an average of 693.9 coliforms/100 ml and a median of 130. This is additional evidence that bacterial counts are insufficient when determining the bacteriological safety of waters, whether for shellfish harvest control or drinking water protection.

At Oyster Bay, virus was isolated only once in eight samples of bay water over the open beds. In July 1976, 2.8 PFU/gal were obtained from the bay waters over the open beds. Oysters harvested from open beds over eight months yielded virus only once–0.48 PFU/gal in March 1977. Water over the closed beds yielded no isolates, but oysters harvested over the eight months yielded virus on three occasions: (1) 0.48 PFU/gal in July 1976; (2) 0.08 PFU/gal in November 1976; and (3) 0.2 PFU/gal in 1977. It would appear that virus monitoring of shellfish may provide a better basis for determining the microbiological status of waters for shellfish harvesting than do bacteriological counts.

CONCLUSIONS

This review of published data relating to virus survival and movement in soils indicates that human enteroviruses persist both in soil and water environments. At present, relatively little is known about the half-life of these organisms once they enter the environment. Nor are there sufficient data available to evaluate their true significance in terms of public health. Numerous cases of hepatitis have been associated with the consumption of groundwater and shellfish, but little is known about the number of enterovirus diseases that may have gone undetected or were not recognized as being waterborne. There appear to be no major differences in the survival and movement of human enteroviruses in soils between those discharged from septic tanks and those discharged in poorly treated sewage effluents. Once enteroviruses enter the soil system, their ultimate fate is dependent on countless variables, many of which cannot be controlled by man. Therefore, virus should be removed from sewage effluents before land disposal. More research should be devoted to onsite systems to determine whether virus contamination of groundwaters and surface waters through septic tank leachate results only from failed septic tank systems or from well-functioning systems as well, particularly during heavy rains or spring thaws. If it is determined that even functioning systems contribute to groundwater contamination, the use of new, innovative systems should be encouraged.

REFERENCES

1. Vaughn, J., and E. F. Landry. "Virus Study," Interim Report Series 6, Nassau-Suffolk Regional Planning Board, Hauppauge, NY (1977).
2. Craun, G. F., and L. J. McCabe. "Review of the Causes of Waterborne-Disease Outbreaks," *J. Am. Water Works Assoc.* 65:74 (1973).
3. Craun, G. F., L. J. McCabe and J. M. Hughes. "Waterborne Disease Outbreaks in the US," *J. Am. Water Works Assoc.* 68:420 (1976).
4. McCabe, L. J., and G. F. Craun. "Status of Waterborne Diseases in the US and Canada," *J. Am. Water Works Assoc.* 67:95 (1975).
5. Duboise, S. M., F. E. Moore and B. P. Sagik. "Poliovirus Survival and Movement in a Sandy Forest Soil," *Appl. Environ. Microbiol.* 31:536 (1976).
6. Lefler, E., and Y. Kott. "Virus Retention and Survival in Sand," in *Proceedings of Water Resources Symposium No. 7, Virus Survival in Water and Wastewater Systems,* J. F. Malina, Jr. and B. P. Sagik, Eds. (Austin, TX: Sweet Publishing Co., 1974), p. 84.
7. Hejkal, T. W., F. M. Wellings, P. A. LaRock and A. L. Lewis. "Survival of Poliovirus Within Organic Solids During Chlorination," *Appl. Environ. Microbiol.* 38:114 (1979).
8. Wellings, F. M., A. L. Lewis and C. W. Mountain. "The Fate of Virus in Florida Soils Following Secondary Effluent Spray Irrigation," in *Individual Onsite Wastewater Systems, Proceedings of the First National Conference* (Ann Arbor, MI: Ann Arbor Science Publishers, Inc., 1975).
9. Lance, J. C., C. P. Gerba and J. L. Melnick. "Virus Movement in Soil Columns Flooded with Secondary Sewage Effluent," *Appl. Environ. Microbiol.* 32:520 (1976).
10. Schaub, S. A., and C. A. Sorber. "Virus and Bacteria Removal from Wastewater by Rapid Infiltration Through Soil," *Appl. Environ. Microbiol.* 33:609 (1977).
11. Vaughn, J. M., E. F. Landry, L. J. Baranosky, C. A. Beckwith, M. C. Dahl and N. C. Delihas. "Survey of Human Virus Occurrence in Wastewater-Recharge Groundwater on Long Island, *Appl. Environ Microbiol.* 36:47 (1978).
12. Wellings, F. M., A. L. Lewis, C. W. Mountain and L. V. Pierce. "Demonstration of Virus in Groundwater after Effluent Discharge onto Soil," *Appl. Microbiol.* 29:751 (1975).

13. Wellings, F. M., A. L. Lewis and C. W. Mountain. "Assessment of Health Risks Associated with Land Disposal of Municipal Effluents and Sludge," in *Risk Assessment and Health Effects of Land Application of Municipal Wastewater and Sludges,* B. P. Sagik and C. A. Sorber, Eds., Proceedings of a conference sponsored by the Center for Applied Research and Technology, the University of Texas at San Antonio and the Applied Science and Research Applications Directorate, the National Science Foundation, December 12-14, 1977, San Antonio, TX (1978).

36

SEPTIC SYSTEM LEACHATE SURVEYS FOR RURAL LAKE COMMUNITIES: A WINTER SURVEY OF OTTER TAIL LAKE, MINNESOTA

William B. Kerfoot
K-V Associates, Inc.
Falmouth, Massachusetts 02540

INTRODUCTION

In porous soils, groundwater inflows frequently convey wastewaters from nearshore septic tanks through bottom sediments and into lakewaters, causing attached algae growth and algal blooms. The lake shoreline is a particularly sensitive area because (1) the groundwater depth is shallow, encouraging soil water saturation and anaerobic conditions; (2) septic tanks and leaching fields are frequently located close to the water's edge, allowing only a short distance for bacterial degradation and soil adsorption of potential contaminants; and (3) the recreational attractiveness of the lakeshore often induces temporary overcrowding of homes, which lead to hydraulically overloaded septic tanks. Rather than a passive release from lakeshore bottoms, groundwater plumes from nearby onsite treatment units actively emerge along shorelines, raising sediment nutrient levels and creating local elevated concentrations of nutrients [1]. The contribution of nutrients from subsurface discharges of shoreline septic tanks has been estimated at 30–60% of the total nutrient load in certain New Hampshire lakes [2].

Wastewater effluent contains a mixture of near ultraviolet (UV) fluorescent organics derived from whiteners, surfactants and natural degradation products, which persist under the combined conditions of low oxygen and limited microbial activity.

Figure 1 shows two samples of sand-filtered effluent from the Otis Air

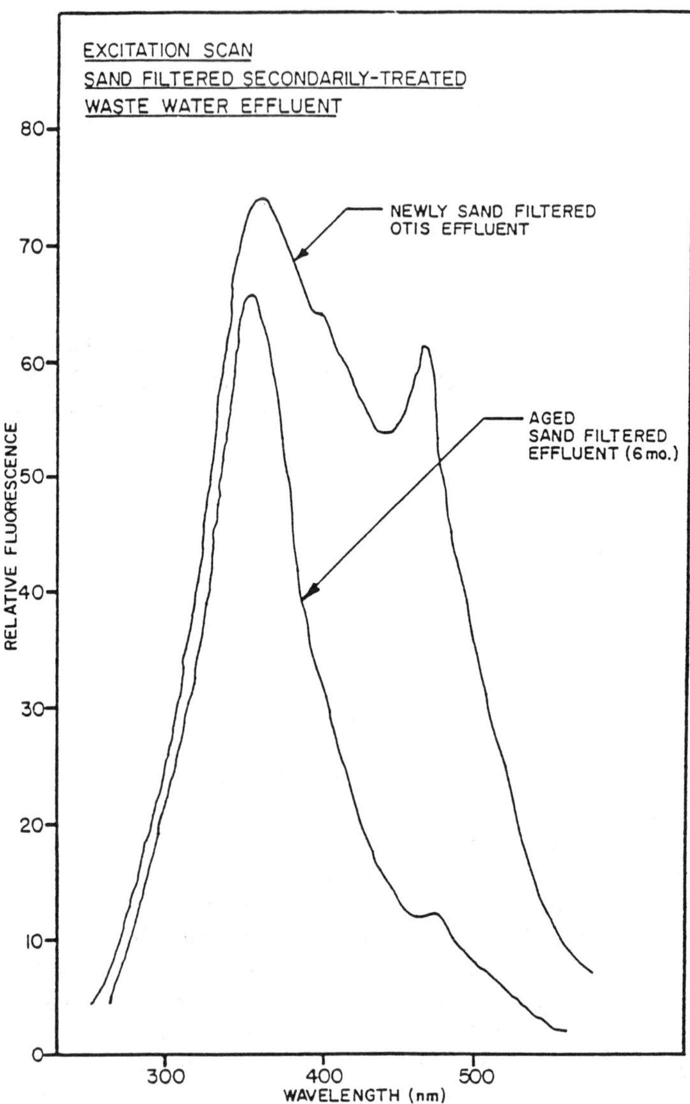

Figure 1. Sand-filtered effluent produces a stable fluorescent signature, shown here before and after aging.

Force Base sewage treatment plant. One was analyzed immediately and the other after it had remained in a darkened bottle for six months at 20°C. Note that little change in fluorescence was apparent, although during the aging process some narrowing of the fluorescent region did occur. The aged effluent percolating through sandy loam soil under anaerobic conditions reaches a stable ratio between the organic content and chlorides, which are highly mobile anions. The stable ratio (cojoint signal) between fluorescence and conductivity allows ready detection of leachate plumes by their conservative tracers as an early warning of potential nutrient breakthrough or public health problems.

Surveys for shoreline wastewater discharges were conducted with a modified "septic leachate detector" and the K-V Associates, Inc. Dowser® groundwater flowmeter. The septic leachate detector (ENDECO Type 2100 "Septic Snooper") consists of the subsurface probe, the water intake system, the analyzer control unit and a graphic recorder. Initially, the unit is calibrated against stepwise increases of wastewater effluent of the type to be detected, which are added to the background lakewater. The probe of the unit is then placed in the lakewater along the shoreline. Groundwater seeping through the shoreline bottom is drawn into the subsurface intake of the probe and travels upwards to the analyzer unit. As it passes through the analyzer, separate conductivity and specific fluorescence signals are generated and sent to a signal processor, which registers the separate signals on a strip chart recorder as the boat moves forward. The analyzed water is continuously discharged from the unit back into the receiving water. A portable unit obtained from ENDECO was used during the field studies, but was modified to operate under the conductance conditions encountered in the field.

PLUME TYPES

The capillary-like structure of sandy porous soils and horizontal groundwater movement induces a fairly narrow plume from malfunctioning septic tank systems. The point of discharge along the shoreline is often through a small area of lake bottom, commonly forming an oval-shaped area several meters wide when the septic tank is close to the shoreline. In denser subdivisions containing several overloaded units the discharges may overlap, forming a broader increase.

Groundwater Plumes

Three different types of groundwater-related wastewater plumes are commonly encountered during a septic tank system leachate survey: (1) erupting plumes, (2) passive plumes, and (3) stream source plumes. As the soil becomes saturated with dissolved solids and organics during the aging process of a leaching onlot septic tank system, a breakthrough of organics occurs first, followed by inorganic penetration (principally chlorides, sodium and other salts). The active emerging of the combined organic and inorganic residues into the shoreline lakewater describes an erupting plume. In seasonal dwellings, where wastewater loads vary in time, a plume may be apparent during late summer when shoreline cottages sustain heavy use, but retreat during winter during low flow conditions. Residual organics from the wastewater often still remain attached to soil particles in the vicinity of the previous erupting plume, slowly releasing into the shoreline waters. This dormant plume indicates a previous breakthrough, but sufficient treatment of the plume exists under current conditions so that no inorganic discharge is apparent. Stream source plumes refer to either groundwater leachings or nearstream septic leaching fields, which enter into streams that eventually empty into the lake.

Runoff Plumes

Traditional failures of septic tank systems occur in tight soil conditions when the rate of inflow into the unit is greater than the soil percolation can accommodate. Often leakage occurs around the septic tank or leaching unit covers, creating standing pools of poorly treated effluent (Figure 2). If sufficient drainage is present, the effluent may flow laterally across the surface into nearby waterways. In addition, rainfall or snow melt may also create an excess of surface water, which can wash the standing effluent into water courses. In either case, the poorly treated effluent frequently contains elevated fecal coliform bacteria, indicative of the presence of pathogenic bacteria and, if sufficiently high, must be considered a threat to public health.

METHODOLOGY–SAMPLING AND ANALYSIS

The septic tank system leachate survey covered two principal study areas in Otter Tail County, Minnesota. The first, and largest, water body area examined was Otter Tail Lake, an eight-mile-long glacial depression coursed from northeast to southwest by the south-flowing Otter Tail River. This lake shoreline is almost entirely ringed by seasonal cottages interspersed with year-round dwellings (10% of the total), a few cattle yards and cultivated croplands. The lake is very shallow along most of the shoreline, and the soils consist mainly of medium sand of high porosity. The second study area comprised the adjacent satellite lakes–Blanche, Deer, Round and

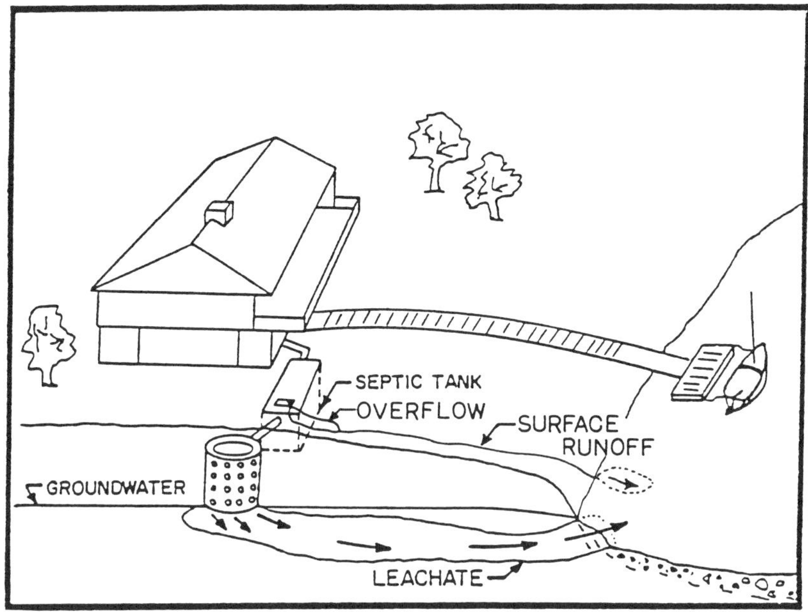

Figure 2. Excessive loading of septic tank systems causes the development of plumes of poorly treated effluent that may (1) enter nearby waterways through surface runoff, or (2) move laterally with groundwater flow and discharge near the shoreline of nearby lakes.

Walker. These lakes were much smaller than Otter Tail Lake and were slightly less populated. Again, soils were generally sandy and quite porous.

Objectives of this survey were as follows.

1. to perform a complete shoreline scan for evidence of septic tank system leachate (nutrient) intrusion using through-the-ice techniques for winter conditions, with forward progress related to prevailing weather conditions expected to be at least one shoreline mile per day;
2. to take discrete water samples for subsequent nutrient analysis only at those locations of alleged effluent plumes revealed by the leachate detector instrument;
3. to take samples for fecal coliform analysis from all moving surface tributaries or exceptionally high shoreline effluent plumes; and
4. to make visual observations relevant to sources of lakewater degradation.

This survey was executed from March 22–April 30, 1979. Daytime temperatures ranged from 5° to 45°F. Ice measured 3 feet in depth and was very solid. Snow cover rarely exceeded 2–10 inches.

Procedure

Otter Tail Lake was surveyed in a continuous clockwise direction starting and ending at the outlet of the Otter Tail River. The survey team consisted of two men and lightweight mobile survey gear. The basic equipment platform was a polyethylene sled 6 ft X 3 ft (actually a collapsed portable ice house by "Snoboat"). The septic leachate detector instrument was lashed securely with shock cords to a large plastic ice chest, which was lashed, in turn, to the sled. A 12-vdc snowmobile battery powered the instrument and small water pump. This centrifugal water pump lifted subice water from a drilled hole and discharged it through the instrument detector chamber and out a flexible plastic tube exhaust from which retained samples could be taken.

The large ice chest held chilled water samples as well as supplies and maintenance gear. Groundwater specimens were drawn through a rugged stainless steel well-point sampler developed by K-V Associates, Inc. This 7-foot-long, 3/8-inch bore tube could easily be driven by hand up to 18 inches into the porous bottom sediment. Groundwater samples were drawn from sandy sediments of those holes displaying a high relative fluorescence signal. Interstitial water was extracted via a simple hand vacuum pump and large plastic receiving chamber. All tubes were of large bore to minimize freezing obstructions. The captured groundwater could then be readily decanted apart from entrained sand and bottled for later analysis. Such bottom sample accompanied a surface sample for each significant plume discovery, and groundwater samples were withdrawn very easily through the loose sand bottom in nearly every case.

To gain access to the liquid water beneath the ice cover, a gasoline-powered "Jiffy" ice auger equipped with 5-inch-diameter, 3-foot-long drill bit on a 12-inch shaft extension was used.

In summary, the two-man team proceeded on foot in tandem around the lake perimeter with self-contained equipment in tow on lightweight plastic sleds. Skis or snowshoes were used as conditions required. The lead individual bored fresh holes on approximate 100-foot intervals, gauging the ice thickness as well as his freewater clearance to the sand bottom. He charted a path that would ensure 6–10 inches of freewater which, on Otter Tail Lake, frequently offset the team up to 100 yards from shore. The instrument operator, trailing closely behind, flushed his pump line in each new hole and processed a brief but steady stream of water through the detector. Relative fluorescence, conductivity and positional information were recorded in a bound log book. A U.S. Geological Survey (USGS) lakeshore map provided sufficient landmark detail for reasonable annotation of position versus hole number (Figure 3) [3].

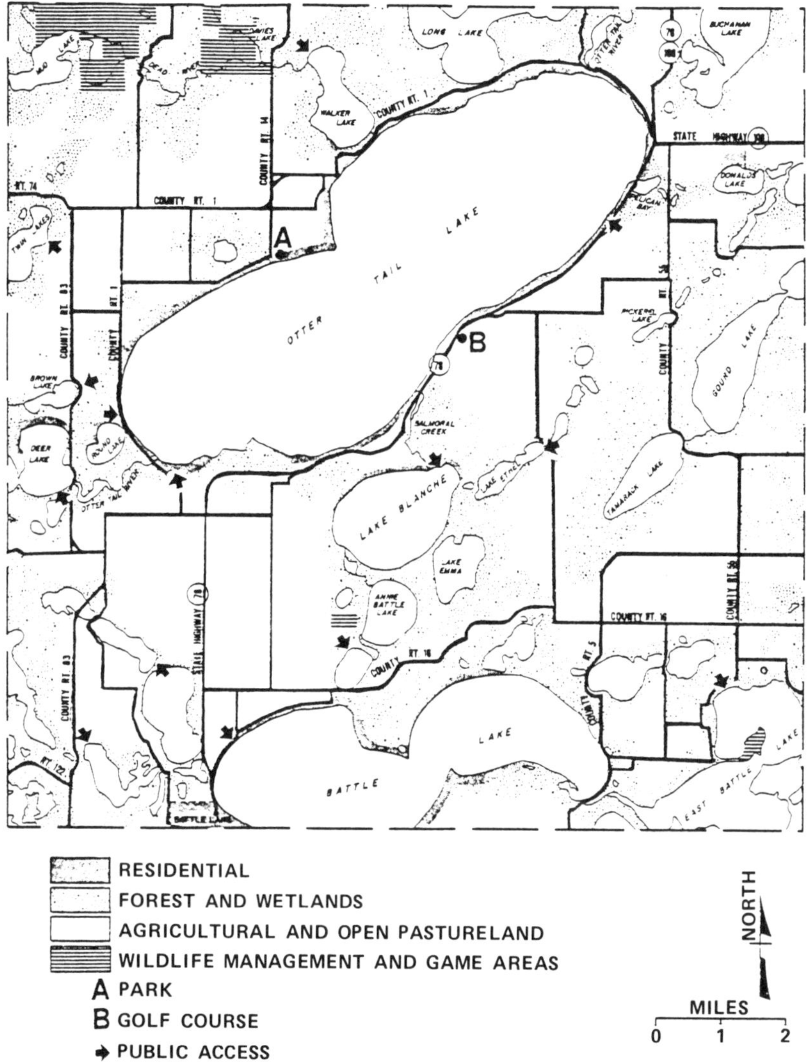

Figure 3. Existing land use in the Otter Tail study area (courtesy of the Otter Tail Lake Planning Advisory Commission and the U.S. Geological Survey [3].

Sample Handling

Both groundwater and surface water samples for nutrient analysis were retained in 250-ml clean plastic bottles, marked to correspond with hole numbers. The samples were preserved at 35°F or colder, pending laboratory analysis.

Bacteria samples were captured in sterilized 250-ml plastic bottles and shipped the same day to the Environmental Protection Laboratory in St. Cloud, Minnesota, for fecal coliform analysis.

Calibration

Each work day began with a calibration of the leachate detection. Two solutions were required: (1) a background sample drawn from an assumed unpolluted central portion of the lake; and (2) a 10% dilution in background water of local New York Mills treated effluent. An initial 20-liter volume of central lakewater lasted the entire survey as the background standard. A 1-liter bottle of lagoon effluent was taken from the treatment facility in the nearby town of New York Mills. This sample was filtered to remove suspended solids prior to use. Injection of these two solutions into the leachate detector instrument at ambient outdoor working temperature allowed us to set a reasonable ZERO and SPAN adjustment.

Satellite Lakes

Surveys of four smaller lakes followed the completion of Otter Tail Lake. The same procedure was used, fair weather allowing for conclusion of each lake within a day's time for the leachate scan with an additional day for bacterial sample retrieval. The north shore of Blanche Lake and Deer Lake, northern and eastern shores of Round Lake, and south shore of Walker Lake were surveyed. The shoreline areas represented the more populated shorefronts, which are candidates for sewerage collection facilities. Table I presents the results of bacterial analysis of all the lakes surveyed.

Groundwater Flow Determination

The direction and rate of inflow of groundwater was measured at eight locations around Otter Tail Lake and four locations at each of the satellite lakes surveyed (Table II). Snow cover and unsaturated sand cover were removed above beach regions and a Dowser groundwater flowmeter inserted into the saturated sand sediments. Conditions permitting, three separate flowrate determinations were made, often with small-scale dye tracings of interstitial flow for confirmation. The observed compass direction

Table I. Bacterial Content of Shoreline Samples

Station Number	Fecal Coliform No./100 ml	Location	Ice Hole Number
Otter Tail Lake			
1	0	Pelican Bay inlet	523
2	0	Balmoral Creek inlet	716
3	0	Melt spot–F.N. 521	642
4	0	Melt spot–F.N. 694	773
5	0	Big white barn	783
6	8	Spring near Rearing Pond	788
7	0	Soft snow–F.N. 747	810
8	0	Soft snow–F.N. 748	811
9	0	Otter Tail River outlet	915
10	0	Nursing home	79
11	0	House–F.N. 1060	201
12	0	Soft spot–F.N. 1063	203
13	0	Gas station–resort	333
14	0	Walker Lake outlet	343
15	2	Long Lake canal	450
16	0	Soft spot–F.N. 208	481
17	356	Otter Tail River–Rt. 1 bridge	–
17	0	Otter Tail River–2nd sampling	–
18	0	Inflow: first inlet	–
19	2	Inflow: second inlet	–
Blanche Lake			
1	0	Balmoral Creek outflow	20
2	0	House–F.N. 066	37
3	0	House–F.N. 010	71
4	0	Start of ice holes	1
Round Lake			
1	0	Snow melt–F.N. 34	34
2	0	Snow melt–F.N. 33	33
3	0	Snow melt–F.N. 27	29
4	16	Blue house–F.N. 7	10
Deer Lake			
1	0	House–F.N. 54	9
2	0	House–yellow ice	10
3	0	House–F.N. 28	29
4	0	House–clear ice	45
Walker Lake			
1	0	House–F.N. 79	5
2	0	House–F.N. 75	6
3	0	House–F.N. 59	19
4	0	House–F.N. 53	21
Well Water			
F.N. 67	0	Walker Lake well (Lien)	
F.N. 68	0	Walker Lake well (Whisher)	
F.N. 888	0	Round Lake well	

Table II. Observed Rates of Groundwater Flow

Station	Direction	Flowrate (fpd)	Comments
GW-1	300°	0.5–0.6	Covered with 5 feet of snow
GW-2	315°	10–12	Melted spot with vegetation
GW-3	330°	1–5	Covered with 3 feet of snow
GW-4	340°	0.6–0.9	Softer snow
GW-5	75°	11–13	Snow melt in broad area (nursing home)
GW-6	165°	15	Exposed beach sand off park
GW-7	150°	12–14	One foot of snow with exposed sand
GW-8	195°	17–19	Yellow snow around exposed area

and rate of flow were computed and compared with the rates anticipated by the Darcy equation from known groundwater heights.

Water Analysis

Water samples taken in the vicinity of the peak of plumes were analyzed by U.S. Environmental Protection Agency (EPA) Standard Methods for the following chemical constituents:

- conductivity (cond.)
- orthophosphate phosphorus (PO_4-P)
- total phosphorus (TP)

More than 200 small-volume (50 ml) water samples were obtained at locations of sample holes and 120 samples at selected plumes and background stations for analysis. The samples were placed in polyethylene containers, chilled and frozen for transport and storage. Conductivity was determined by a Beckman (Model RC-19) conductivity bridge; PO_4-P and TP by the single-reagent procedure following standard methods [4], and selected samples synchronous-scanned for fluorescence to confirm the organic source.

PLUME LOCATIONS

The Otter Tail Lakes study area included the shoreline of Otter Tail Lake and populated portions of the surrounding water bodies of Blanche, Deer,

Round and Walker Lakes. Based on the soil atlas of Otter Tail County, 90% of the study area contains sandy, highly permeable soils of glacial outwash deposits. The dominant soil types are (1) sand over sandy, well-drained soils (Salida, Sioux and Hubbard); (2) loamy over sandy, well-drained soils (Arvilla and Estherville); and sandy over sandy, poorly drained soils (Figure 4). The outwash deposits extend downwards to depths of 50–100 feet, below which is about a 200-foot thickness of undifferentiated glacial drift before bedrock (Precambrian crystalline rock) is intercepted, forming the "oasis," a large groundwater aquifer. Melting ice blocks caused the depressions, which, filled with groundwater, form Otter Tail and its satellite lakes.

On the basis of groundwater drainage, lakes fall into categories of "confined" or "withdrawal" lakes, or a combination of both. In confined lakes, the groundwater inflow along one side is offset by an equivalent exfiltration along opposing shorelines, resulting in little change in net groundwater contribution to the lake. In other cases, the lakewater body may behave as a withdrawal well, withdrawing groundwater from around most shorelines and discharging the net inflow of water as stream flow from the lake.

Otter tail is a withdrawal lake, the substantial drop in hydraulic head from the inlet to the outlet serving to withdraw groundwater into the lake along the entire length of shoreline. As described in more detail in the section entitled Groundwater Flow Characteristics and Nutrient Loading, the satellite lakes also induce even more rapid groundwater inflow along adjacent shorelines because of gravity leveling of water in the lakes, which create abnormally high hydraulic heads nearby the shoreline. On entering the groundwater, septic tank system discharges within the areas adjacent to the lake would be transported uncommonly fast towards the lake.

A total of 265 sample locations indicating plumes were observed along the surveyed shorelines (Figures 5-8). Of these, about 235 were found to be of groundwater origin; the others represented surface stream drainage inflows from lakes. Solid circles indicate locations of probable groundwater leachate sources, with plumes emerging from porous bottom sediments into the lake. Solid squares represent locations of observed surface discharges into lakewaters. These may result from overflowing septic tank systems or from leaching systems along the stream shoreline as sources. A line is drawn from each symbol to the location of the ice hole sampled where the plume was encountered. Fluorescent spectral analysis was used where necessary to separate the discharges from bogs from wastewater inflows. Almost a one-to-one relationship existed between the number of locations of groundwater plumes and the number of permanent dwellings (Table III).

Frequencies of groundwater plume locations above that expected based

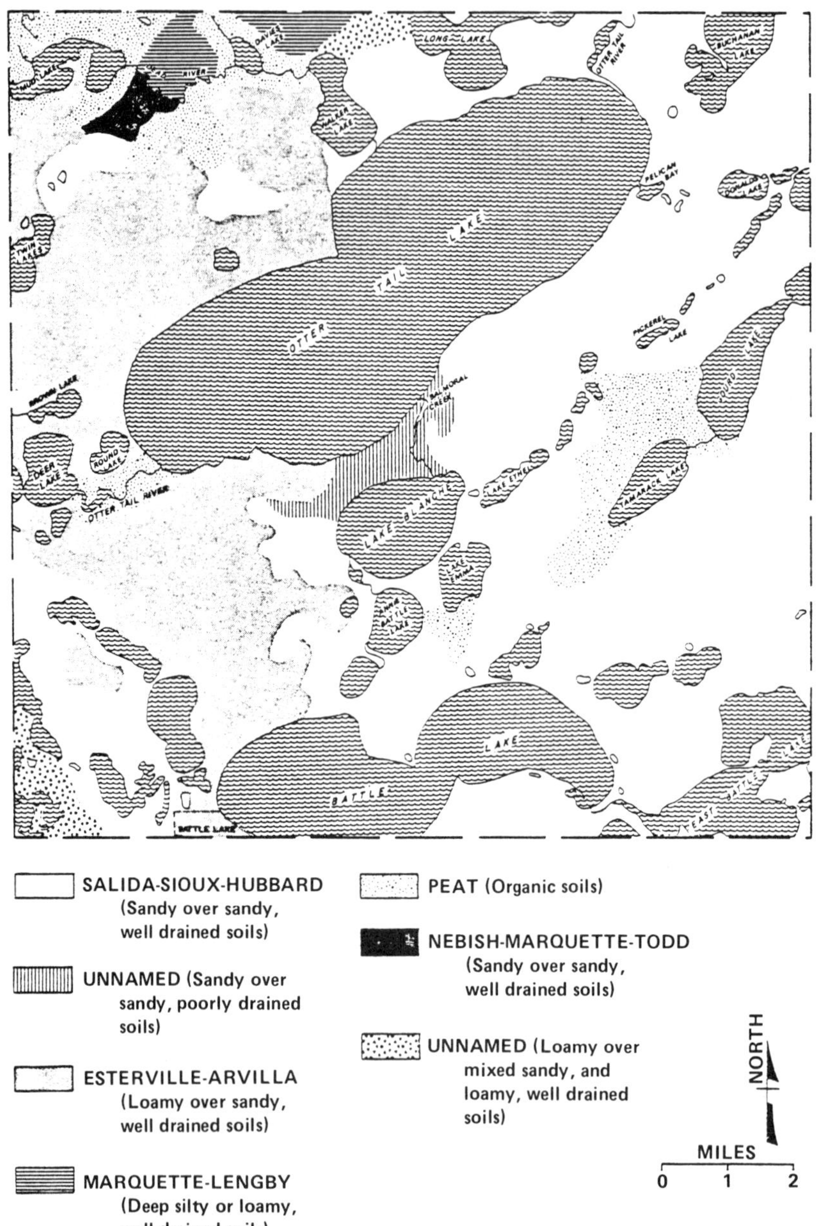

Figure 4. Soil landscapes in the Otter Tail Lake study area (courtesy of the University of Minnesota) [3].

Table III. Number of Groundwater Plumes Compared with Occupancy

Segment[a] Number	Residential Occupancy		Number of Groundwater Plume Locations
	Permanent	Seasonal	
1	7	23	5
2	21	64	21
3	14	45	21 (unnamed lake)
4	12	37	9
5	2	6	2
6	12	37	9 (Walker Lake)
7	14 (9)	40 (22)	14 (Walker Lake)
8	5	12	2
9	4 (1)	9 (7)	14 (Long Lake)
11	21 (?)	45 (?)	16 (Long Lake)
12	13	29	Inflow region
13	7	15	2
15	7	15	1
16	7	14	3
17	2	6	6
18	1	3	1
19	5	12	0
20	6	13	6
21	10 (8)	49 (31)	19 (Blanche Lake)
26	10 (8)	50 (29)	52 (Blanche Lake)
27	0	0	2
28	2	8	5
29	5	22	5
30+32	8	42	1 (exfiltration?)

[a]See Figure 11.

on permanent occupancy occurred along shoreline areas where adjacent lake areas induced rapid subsurface flows. The higher than expected frequency of plumes emerging along the Otter Tail shoreline may be attributable to the strong inflow of Otter Tail "capturing" plumes from the adjacent shorelines of the satellite lakes. Rather than intruding into Blanche Lake, septic tank system discharges from systems serving residences on the northern shore probably flow toward Otter Tail Lake. Few erupting plumes were found on Blanche Lake, although segments 19 and 26 along Otter Tail Lake downstream of their rapid groundwater flow show substantial areas affected by plumes. The same phenomenon appears to occur with an unnamed lake adjacent to segment 3 and Long Lake in segment 9.

An exceptionally low number of plume locations were observed in segment 30 + 32, which may indicate the most likely shoreline area where groundwater may come the closest to exfiltration rather than infiltration.

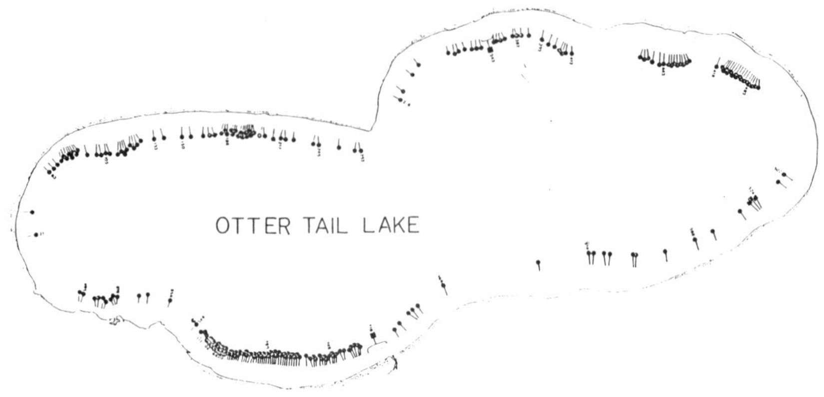

· ICE HOLE LOCATION

D1 BACTERIAL SAMPLE LOCATION

○ DORMANT GROUNDWATER PLUME

● ERUPTING GROUNDWATER PLUME

□ ORGANIC SURFACE WATER PLUME WITHOUT DISSOLVED SOLIDS LOAD

■ ORGANIC SURFACE WATER PLUME WITH DISSOLVED SOLIDS LOAD

Figure 5. Plume and bacterial sample locations on Otter Tail Lake.

The frequency of plume locations on Round Lake, in agreement with projected groundwater flow based on water height in the lakes, further supports the possibility of exfiltration.

The predominance of groundwater plumes corresponds to the observed soil conditions and conditions of septic tank–soil absorption systems. The study area contains highly permeable sandy soil and seasonally high water tables, where inadequately treated wastewater may be reaching the groundwater. In addition, a large number of septic leaching fields are submerged in groundwater, limiting aeration and treatment of the effluent. Coupled with the exceptionally rapid groundwater movement, the waste streams are entering the lake shoreline. The incidence of the high frequency of erupting plumes does not necessarily indicate a high transport of phosphorus to the lakewaters (see section entitled "Groundwater Flow Characteristics and Nutrient Loading"). High frequency of plumes and noticeable phosphorus loading from groundwater sources are apparent in shoreline segments of Otter Tail Lake near the satellite lakes of segments 3,6,6,21 and 26. The same is likely true for segments 9 and 11, but insufficient water quality information was available for confirmation.

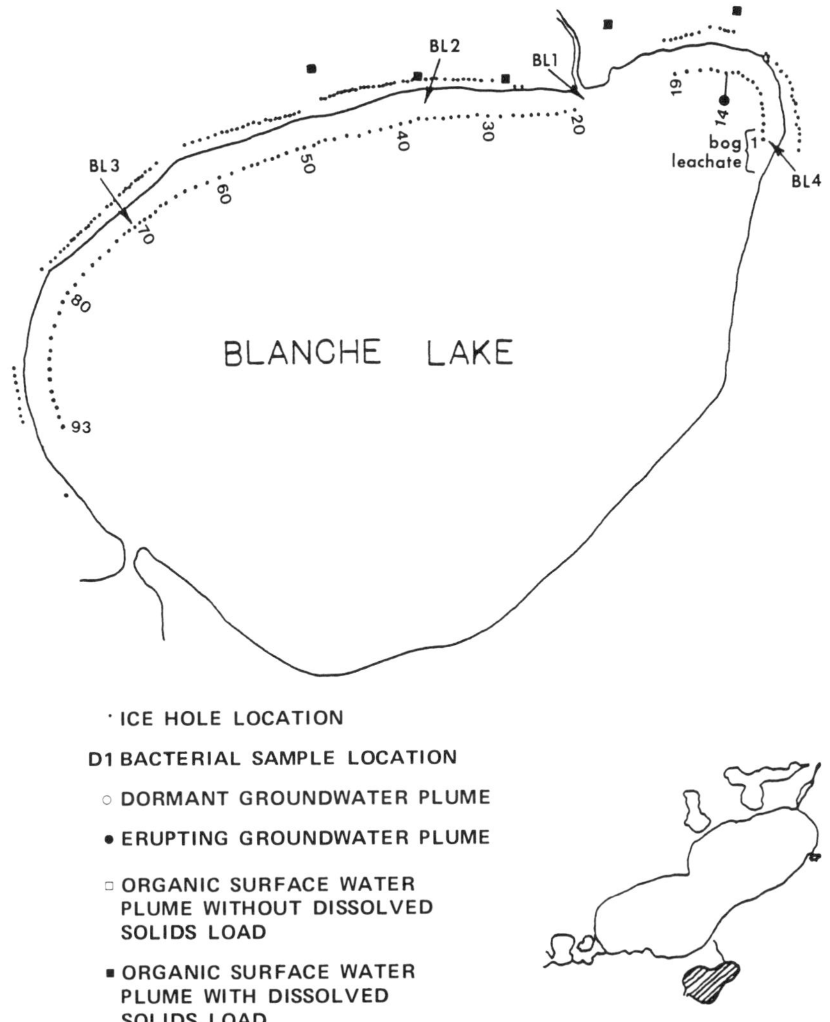

Figure 6. Sampling station, plume and bacterial sample locations on Blanche Lake.

NUTRIENT ANALYSES

Completed analyses of the chemical content of 130 samples taken along the shorelines of Otter Tail Lake and its tributaries are presented in Table IV. The sample letters refer to the locations given in Figures 5–8 and

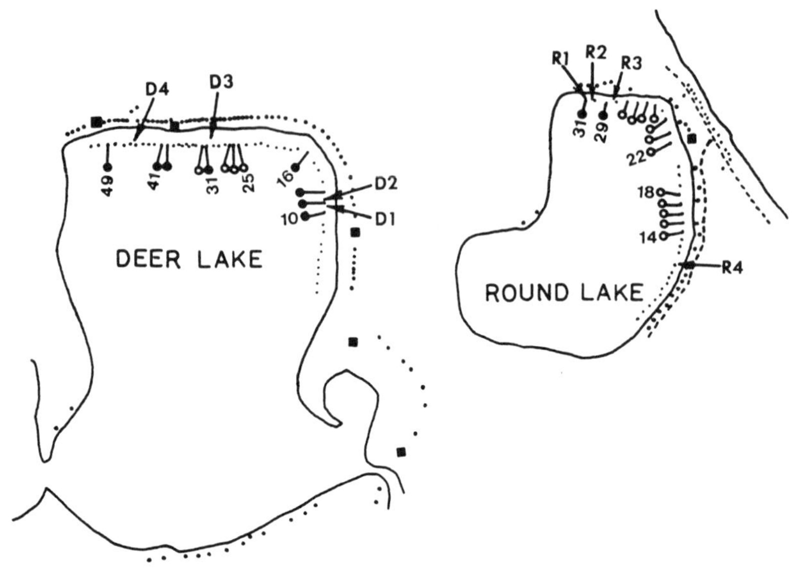

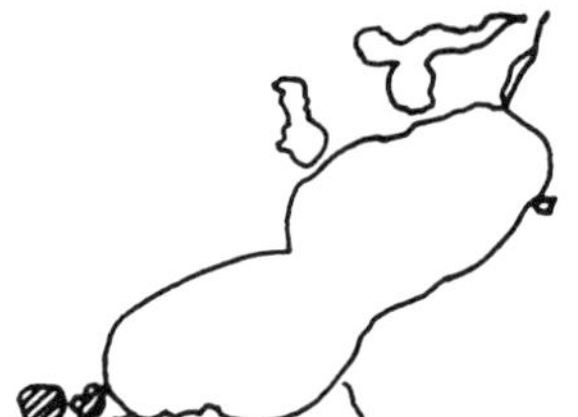

· ICE HOLE LOCATION

D1 BACTERIAL SAMPLE LOCATION

○ DORMANT GROUNDWATER PLUME

● ERUPTING GROUNDWATER PLUME

□ ORGANIC SURFACE WATER PLUME WITHOUT DISSOLVED SOLIDS LOAD

■ ORGANIC SURFACE WATER PLUME WITH DISSOLVED SOLIDS LOAD

Figure 7. Sampling station, plume and bacterial sample locations on Deer and Round Lakes.

the profiles of Figure 9. The symbol "S" refers to surface water sample and the symbol "G" to groundwater sample. Practically all groundwater samples represent easily flowing vacuum withdrawals from highly permeable sandy bottom sediments.

The conductivity of the water samples as conductance (μmhos/cm) is given in the second column. The nutrient analyses for PO_4-P and TP are presented in the next two columns in ppm–mg/1.

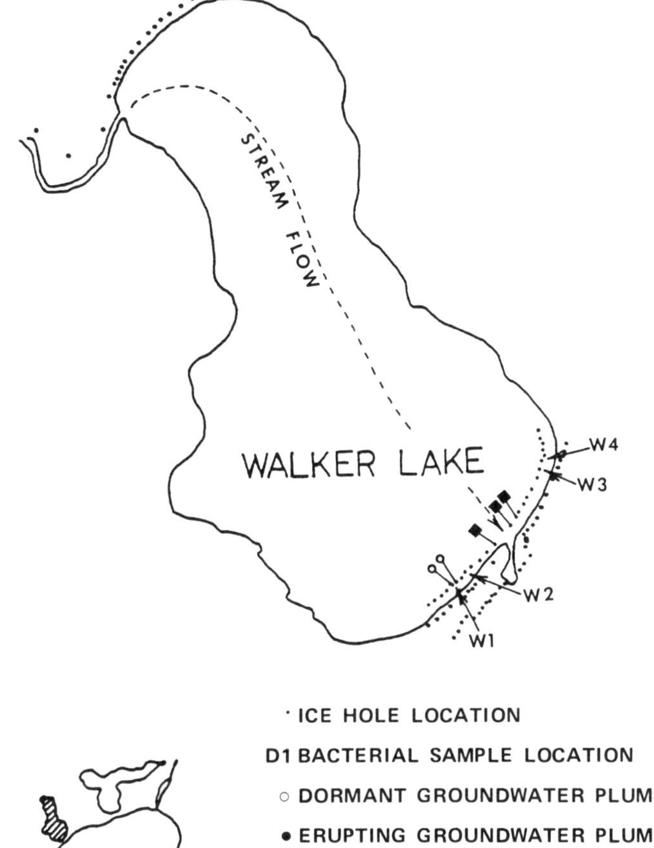

Figure 8. Sampling station, plume and bacterial sample locations on Walker Lake.

NUTRIENT RELATIONSHIPS

Two types of wastewater discharges were observed along the shoreline of the Salem Lakes: groundwater seepage and surface runoff. The two sources are treated differently in evaluating their loading contributions.

Table IV. Analysis of Surface Water (S) and Groundwater (G) Samples Taken in the Vicinity of Wastewater Plumes Observed on the Shorelines of Otter Tail Lake and its Satellites–Blanche, Deer, Round and Walker

Sample Number		Conductivity	PO_4-P (ppm)	Total P (ppm)	Ratio ΔC	Ratio ΔTP	Breakthrough P (%)
Otter Tail Lake							
Center 1	S	160	0.003	0.024			
Center 2	S	300	0.001	0.010			
1	S	250	0.001	0.049			
16	S	310	0.003	0.008			
54	S	250	0.002	0.008			
54	G	250	0.002	0.082			
71	S	310	0.001	0.006			
71	G	250	0.011	0.342			
79	S	365	0.000	0.006			
79	G	250	0.003	0.112			
81	S	380	0.001	0.007			
81	G	225	0.006	0.250			
83	S	235	0.002	0.011			
85	S	305	0.004	0.006			
85	G	300	0.008	0.221	50	0.21	78
87	S	260	0.001	0.007			
87	G	220	0.004	0.288			
105	S	300	0.001	0.005			
105	G	200	0.002	0.059			
106	S	340	0.004	0.007			
111	S	360	0.001	0.004			
111	G	245	0.001	0.038			
113	S	265	0.001	0.006			
113	G	140	0.001	0.004			
118	S	320	0.001	0.005			
118	G	245	0.001	0.015			
149	S	320	0.000	0.008			
149	G	240	0.003	0.034			
166	S	–	0.003	0.016			
186	S	275	0.003	0.007			
186	G	235	0.005	0.048			
190	S	265	0.001	0.010			
190	G	250	0.003	0.163			
194	S	320	0.004	0.004			
201	S	320	0.002	0.022			
207	S	350	0.001	0.008			
207	G	225	0.004	0.020			
309	S	325	0.004	0.009			
310	S	275	0.002	0.012			
310	G	200	0.002	0.082			

Table IV, continued

Sample Number		Conductivity	PO_4-P (ppm)	Total P (ppm)	Ratio ΔC	Ratio ΔTP	Breakthrough P (%)
Otter Tail Lake							
314	S	300	0.002	0.009			
314	G	175	0.001	0.053			
326	S	240	0.001	0.007	150	0.01	1
326	G	400	0.002	0.020			
333	S	265	0.004	0.017			
333	G	250	0.002	0.016			
340	S	320	0.001	0.007			
352	S	–	0.003	0.015			
352	G	250	0.006	0.050			
360	S	250	0.005	0.016			
360	G	175	0.003	0.006			
397	S	290	0.002	0.009			
407	S	280	0.003	0.012			
407	G	250	0.002	0.013			
432	S	370	0.003	0.013			
432	G	275	0.001	0.048	25	0.04	28
443	S	345	0.001	0.006			
443	G	345	0.001	0.073	95	0.06	11
448	S	415	0.010	0.050			
448	G	325	0.004	0.109	75	0.10	23
481	S	325	0.002	0.012			
486	S	320	0.004	0.008			
486	G	225	0.002	0.078			
500	S	270	0.001	0.020			
550	S	325	0.001	0.010			
550	G	375	0.009	0.074	125	0.06	8
584	S	335	0.001	0.007			
584	G	225	0.002	0.163			
608	S	300	0.002	0.015			
608	G	352	0.006	0.078	102	0.07	12
670	S	445	0.002	0.015			
670	G	280	0.007	0.508			
686	S	330	0.001	0.013			
686	G	215	0.007	0.047			
694	S	360	0.002	0.018			
694	G	550	0.002	0.140	300	0.13	8
696	S	415	0.001	0.022			
696	G	285	0.000	0.020			
718	S	250	0.004	0.021			
734	S	190	0.001	0.007			
734	G	310	0.001	0.010	60	0.00	<1
752	S	345	0.001	0.010			
752	G	390	0.001	0.029	140	0.02	3
760	S	250	0.006	0.009			
760	G	–	0.002	0.012			

Table IV, continued

Sample Number		Conductivity	PO_4-P (ppm)	Total P (ppm)	Ratio ΔC	Ratio ΔTP	Breakthrough P (%)
Otter Tail Lake							
773	S	330	0.002	0.010			
773	G	310	0.001	0.009	60	0.00	<1
777	S	400	0.001	0.007			
777	G	250	0.001	0.013			
786	S	310	0.001	0.016			
816A	S	485	0.002	0.078			
816A	G	275	0.005	0.151	25	0.14	98
822	S	415	0.002	0.019			
822	G	345	0.002	0.029	95	0.02	4
827	S	–	0.003	0.028			
827	G	275	0.001	0.028			
836	S	400	0.005	0.035			
836	G	275	0.002	0.063			
845	S	200	0.002	0.025			
845	G	345	0.003	0.206	95	0.20	37
854	S	200	0.001	0.010			
854	G	200	0.004	0.115			
869	S	300	0.003	0.031			
869	G	215	0.001	0.013			
877	S	390	0.002	0.011			
877	G	280	0.007	0.254			
888	S	215	0.002	0.012			
888	G	250	0.001	0.038			
Otter River Rt 1 Bridge Inlet	S	325	0.002	0.016			
Otter River 2nd Inlet	S	325	0.003	0.018			
Otter River Outlet	S	330	0.001	0.011			
Westig Canal	S	335	0.008	0.087			
Westig Canal	G	440	0.002	0.446	190	0.44	41
Balmoral Creek	S	380	0.002	0.018			
Walker L. Canal	S	410	0.002	0.016			
Pelican Bay	S	175	0.001	0.013			
Charney's Well	G	185	0.007	0.071			
Aerea Home & Well	G	275	0.025	0.065			
Well F.N. 1061	G	300	0.005	0.056			

Table IV, continued

Sample Number		Conductivity	PO_4-P (ppm)	Total P (ppm)
Round Lake				
1	S	215	0.001	0.017
1	G	260	0.001	0.096
14	S	250	0.001	0.018
14	G	415	0.001	0.106
15	S	325	0.011	0.115
15	G	200	0.012	0.260
30	S	200	0.001	0.011
30	G	400	0.001	0.042
34	S	250	0.005	0.026
34	G	310	0.003	0.102
Walker Lake				
1	S	400	0.001	0.012
1	G	450	0.000	0.031
6	S	275	0.001	0.017
6	G	150	0.001	0.038
22	S	300	0.001	0.031
22	G	540	0.001	0.043
24	S	300	0.001	0.024
24	G	350	0.003	0.130
Deer Lake				
1	S	300	0.001	0.012
1	G	350	0.002	0.446
10	S	250	0.001	0.009
10	G	430	0.001	0.037
16	S	300	0.002	0.014
16	G	250	0.001	0.068
29	S	100	0.001	0.016
29	G	250	0.005	0.267
46	S	350	0.003	0.024
46	G	380	0.002	0.192
Blanche Lake				
13	S	335	0.004	0.025
13	G	325	0.002	0.366
30	S	360	0.002	0.023
30	G	375	0.001	0.064
37	S	300	0.001	0.012
37	G	325	0.001	0.064
56	S	495	0.002	0.018
56	G	450	0.001	0.040
Background groundwater	G	250	0.002	0.010

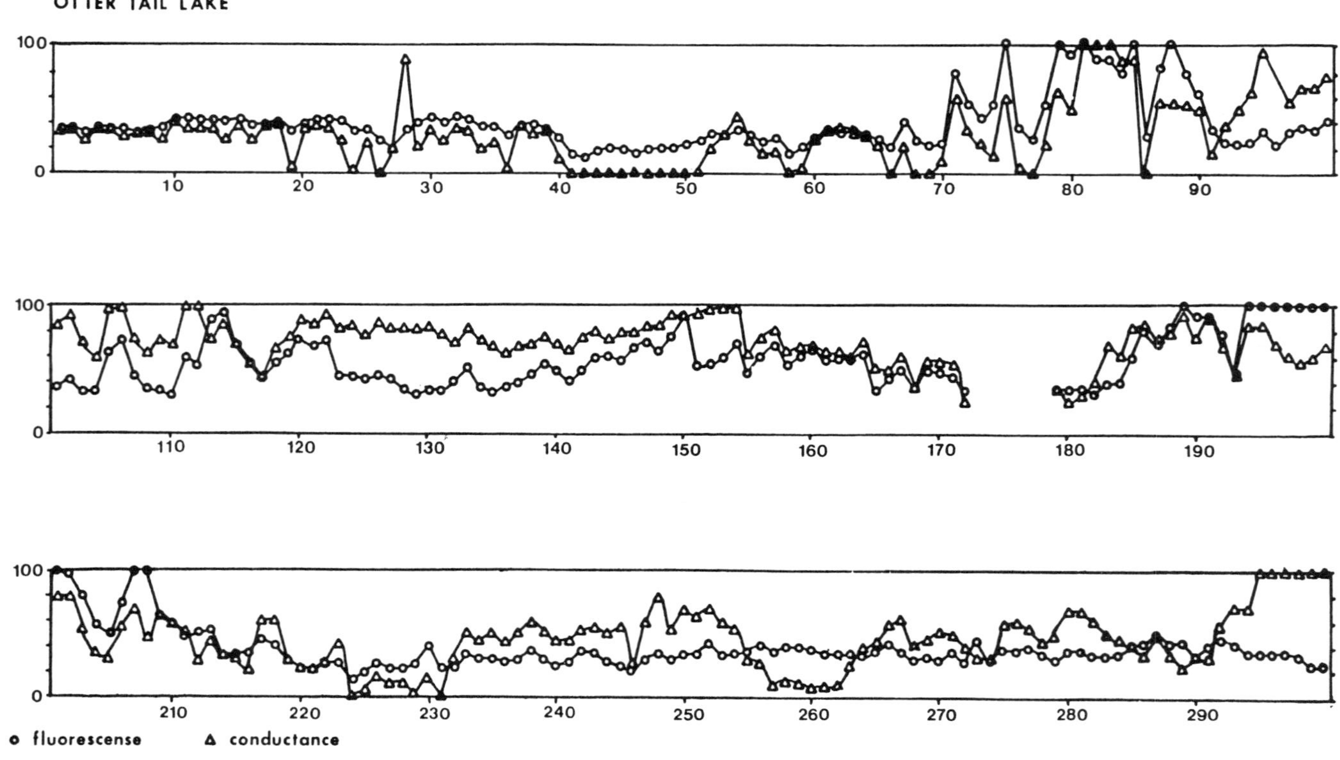

Figure 9. Shoreline leachate profiles for Otter Tail Lake and sections of its statellites: Blanche, Deer, Round and Walker Lakes (continued on next three pages).

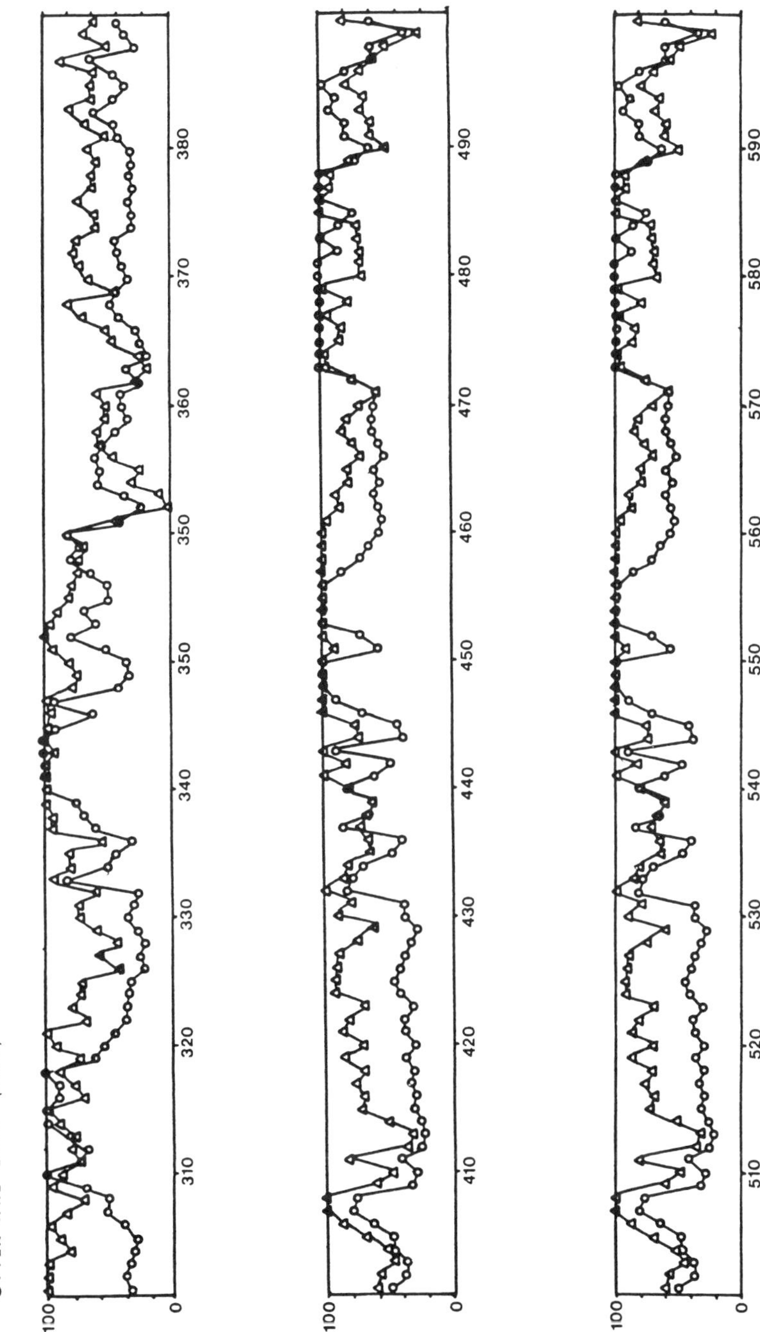
OTTER TAIL LAKE (cont.)
100
0
310
320
330
340
350
350
360
370
380
100
0
410
420
430
440
450
460
470
480
490
100
0
510
520
530
540
550
560
570
580
590

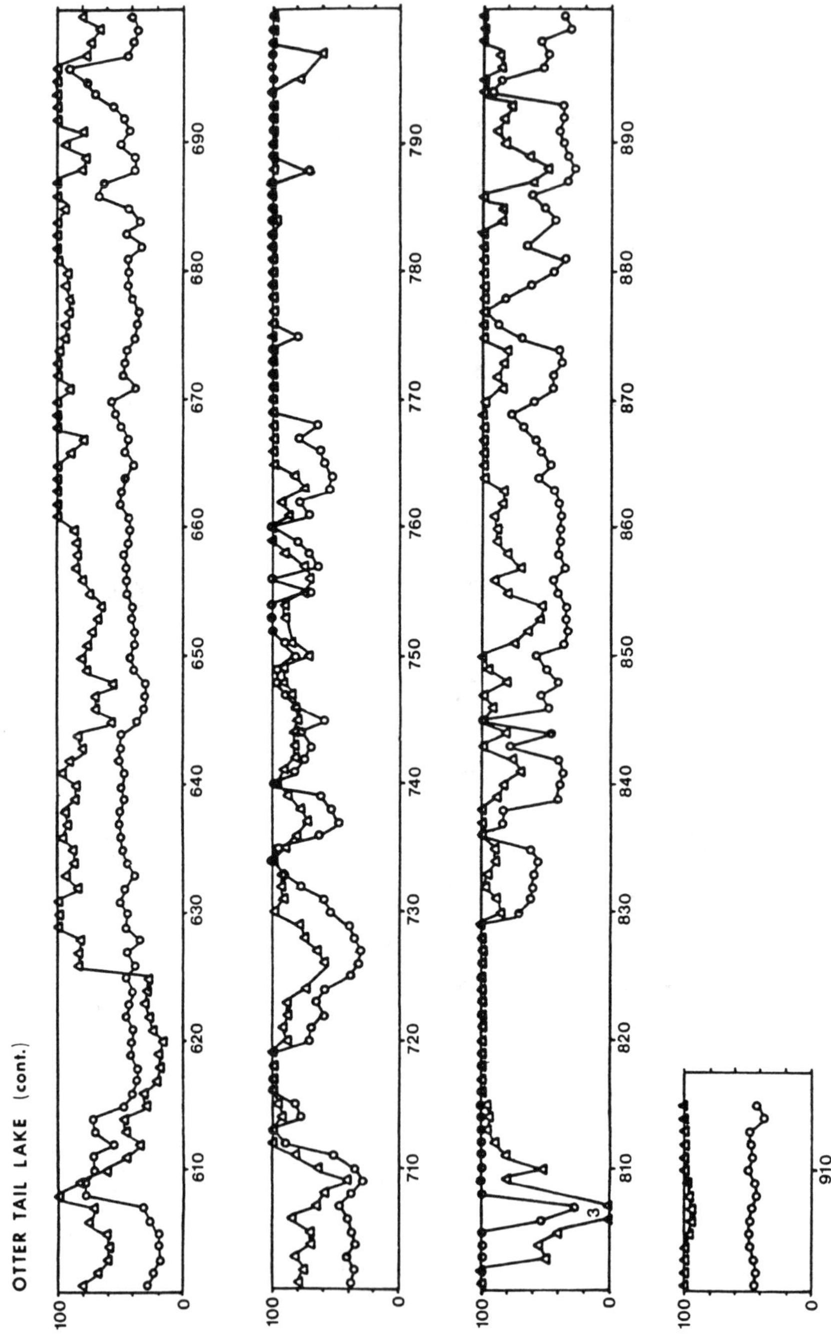

OTTER TAIL LAKE (cont.)
100
0
610
620
630
640
650
660
670
680
690
100
0
710
720
730
740
750
760
770
780
790
100
0
3
810
820
830
840
850
860
870
880
890
100
0
910

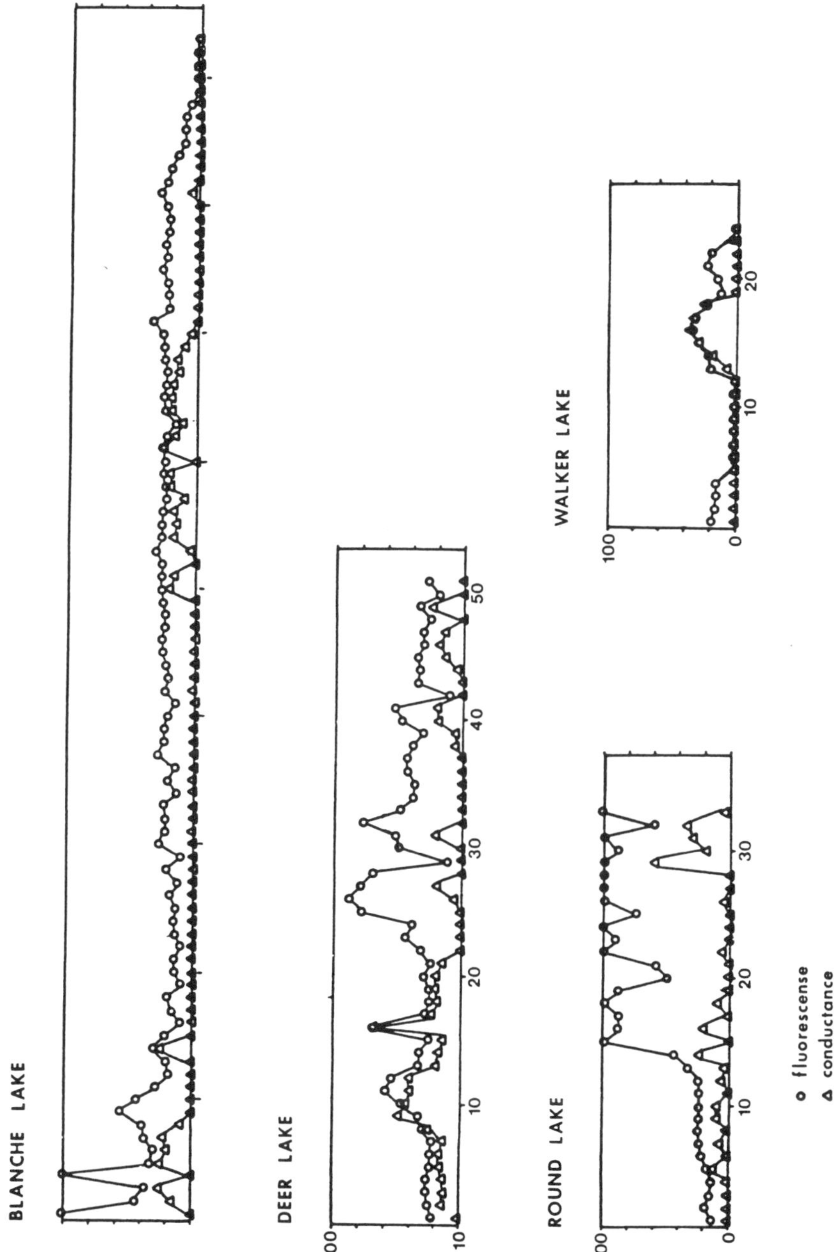
BLANCHE LAKE
DEER LAKE
100
10
10
20
30
40
50
ROUND LAKE
100
0
10
20
30
WALKER LAKE
100
0
10
20
o fluorescense
Δ conductance

Groundwater Plumes

By the use of a few calculations, the characteristics of the wastewater plumes can be described. First, general groundwater background concentration for conductance and nutrients is determined. The concentration of nutrients found in the plume is then compared with the background and with wastewater effluent from the lake region to determine the percentage breakthrough of phosphorus and nitrogen to the lakewater. Because the well-point sampler does not always intercept the center of the plume, the nutrient content of the plume is always partially diluted by surrounding ambient background groundwater or seeping lakewater concentrations. To correct for the uncertainty of withdrawal location of the groundwater plume sample, the nutrient concentrations above background values found with the groundwater plume are corrected to the assumed undiluted concentration anticipated in local standard sand-filtered effluent (assuming 100% of conductance should pass through). Then they are divided by the net nutrient content of raw effluent over municipal water. Computational formulae can be expressed as follows:

For the difference between background (C_0) and observed (C_i) values:

$$C_i - C_0 = \Delta C_i \quad \text{conductance}$$

$$TP_i - TP_0 = \Delta TP_i \quad \text{total phosphorus}$$

$$TN_i - TN_0 = \Delta TN_i \quad \text{total nitrogen (sum of } NO_3\text{-N and } NH_4\text{-N)}$$

For attenuation during soil passage,

$$100 \times \left(\frac{\Delta C_{ef}}{\Delta C_i}\right) \frac{\Delta TP}{TP_{ef}} = \text{breakthrough of phosphorus}$$

$$100 \times \left(\frac{\Delta C_{ef}}{\Delta C_i}\right) \frac{\Delta TN}{TN_{ef}} = \text{breakthrough of nitrogen}$$

where C_0 = conductance of background groundwater (μmhos/cm),
C_i = conductance of observed plume groundwater (μmhos/cm),
ΔC_{ef} = conductance of sand-filtered effluent minus the background conductance of municipal source water (μmhos/cm),
TP_0 = total phosphorus in background groundwater (ppm-mg/1),
TP_i = total phosphorus of observed plume groundwater (ppm-mg/1),
TP_{ef} = total phosphorus concentration of standard effluent,
TN_0 = total nitrogen content of background groundwater, calculated as NO_3-N + NH_4-N,
TN_i = total nitrogen content of observed plume groundwater, calculated as NO_3-N + NH_4-N (ppm-mg/1), and
TN_{ef} = total nitrogen content of standard effluent.

Surface Discharge Plumes

A number of locations were found where surface inflow under the ice entered the shoreline lakewaters. The inflow was analyzed as stream inflow carrying wastewater loads. Each inflow carries a certain dissolved solids load possessing its own peculiar nutrient concentration of TP and TN. The percentage of effluent was characterized in the surface water, based on a comparison with the New York Mills effluent standard. The fraction of TP and TN expected in a diluted sample of effluent with lakewater was then compared with the background-corrected solids load and observed nutrient concentrations. The fraction of phosphorus and nitrogen accounted for by the observed dilution wastewater load is given as percent nutrient residual. If the amount of effluent-related nutrients is only a small percentage of the observed loading, other sources must be contributing, presumably from road runoff, agricultural runoff or other nonpoint sources.

The computational formulae can be expressed as follows:

F_E = fluorescent units observed in water sample

F_B = fluorescent units corresponding with background lake surface water

F_S = fluorescent units corresponding with 100% standard effluent from nearby treatment plant

$$\Delta F = \frac{F_E - F_B}{F_S} = \text{fraction of effluent observed in shoreline water}$$

$$100 \times \Delta F = \%E_0 = \text{percentage of effluent observed in shoreline water}$$

for fraction of nutrients accounted for by effluent fraction,

$$100 \times \frac{\left(\frac{\Delta C_{ef}}{\Delta C_i}\right)\Delta TP}{\Delta F \cdot TP_{ef}} = \text{observed phosphorus as percentage of expected effluent fraction in shoreline water}$$

$$100 \times \frac{\left(\frac{\Delta C_{ef}}{\Delta C_i}\right)\Delta TN}{\Delta F \cdot TP_{ef}} = \text{observed nitrogen as percentage of expected effluent fraction in shoreline water}$$

Assumed Wastewater Characteristics

Local samples of effluent were obtained at the New York Mills sewage treatment plant near the study area. A conductance:total phosphorus ratio of 950:4.0 was obtained. Subtracting the background lakewater concentration of 300 μmhos/cm gives a $\Delta C{:}\Delta TP$ ratio of 750:4.0, representing the change in concentration to source water by household use in the Otter Tail Lake study region.

COLIFORM LEVELS IN SURFACE WATERS

A series of water samples were analyzed at each lake for fecal coliform content to confirm the presence of surface runoff or soil short-circuiting from malfunctioning systems. Previous field surveys of Otter Tail Lake have shown no indication of pollution of the lakewater by fecal matter [5]. Most previous values were at or below limits of detection (20 mpn/100 ml). With the exception of the inlet of the Otter Tail River, virtually all samples from Otter Tail Lake and the satellite lakes contained negligible bacterial concentrations. A resampling of the Otter Tail bridge at the river inlet showed no detectable fecal coliform bacteria seven days after the first sampling. Minnesota water quality standards specify that fecal coliform numbers not exceed a geometric mean of 200 organisms/100 ml of water based on five samples per month or 400 organisms/100 ml of water in more than 10% of all samples during any month of recreational use and aquatic life.

The results of the sampling confirmed that the sandy soils effectively filter out bacterial contamination even though certain chemical constituents penetrate readily with plume movement.

GROUNDWATER FLOW CHARACTERISTICS AND NUTRIENT LOADING

Otter Tail Lake is surrounded by very permeable surficial deposits of glacial outwash. The aquifer deposits consist of stratified sand and gravel with occasional lenses of silt. The sandy deposits vary in thickness from 50 feet in the eastern areas to about 100 feet in the western sections. The principal water source is precipitation, which falls directly onto its surface, then flows laterally to the central drainage canal of the Otter Tail River basin.

While silt and clay layers restrict flow in the far southeastern side near the town of Otter Tail, high rates of flow have been noticed for the sand and gravel sections of the northern shoreline and the southwestern segments. An estimated 5000 ac ft/yr of water (ca. 4.5 mgd) leave the aquifer as underflow in the vicinity of the Otter Tail River at the southwest end of Otter Tail Lake [5]. The transmissivity of the aquifer varies from 5000 to about 200,000 gpd/ft, with the highest values being found in the northeastern and southwestern sections of the study area.

Groundwater Flow Patterns

Because the mean elevation of nearby lakes represents the height of the groundwater levels, an approximation of inflow based on Darcy's equation can be constructed for Otter Tail Lake. The velocity of flow through porous media (V_S) is proportional to the first power of the hydraulic gradient $\frac{dH}{dL}$:

$$V_S = -P \frac{dH}{dL}$$

where P = intrinsic permeability of the aquifer. If an average aquifer thickness of 100 feet exists, the permeability for a 200,000 gpd/ft transmissivity is T/M, or 2000 gpd/ft^2 for a unit square area.

Using the observed hydraulic gradients for mean groundwater heights, the expected rates of flow were estimated for the Otter Tail shoreline (Figure 10). The direction of flow is indicated by the direction of the arrow and its rate of flow is proportional to length (units are in fpd). The flow net analysis indicated that groundwater inflows would be expected around the entire periphery of Otter Tail Lake, with the possible exception of the western shoreline near Round Lake. In general, the elevated hydraulic head differences caused by lakes or embayments would cause a probable doubling or tripling of groundwater inflow flowrates in segments adjacent to satellite lakes, particularly near the smaller sections of the segment 3 unnamed lake and Pelican Bay, plus the broader shorelines adjacent to Blanche Lake, Walker Lake and Long Lake (Figure 11) [3].

Field Investigations

Field observations of observed groundwater flow patterns added support to the assumed flow patterns. Groundwater flow was evaluated at eight discrete points around the Otter Tail Lake shoreline and at two locations on each satellite lake surveyed, using the Dowser groundwater flowmeter and the more conventional dye test.

Study sites were chosen along sandy beaches within a yard or two of the water's edge. Under winter conditions, visual observations of the extent

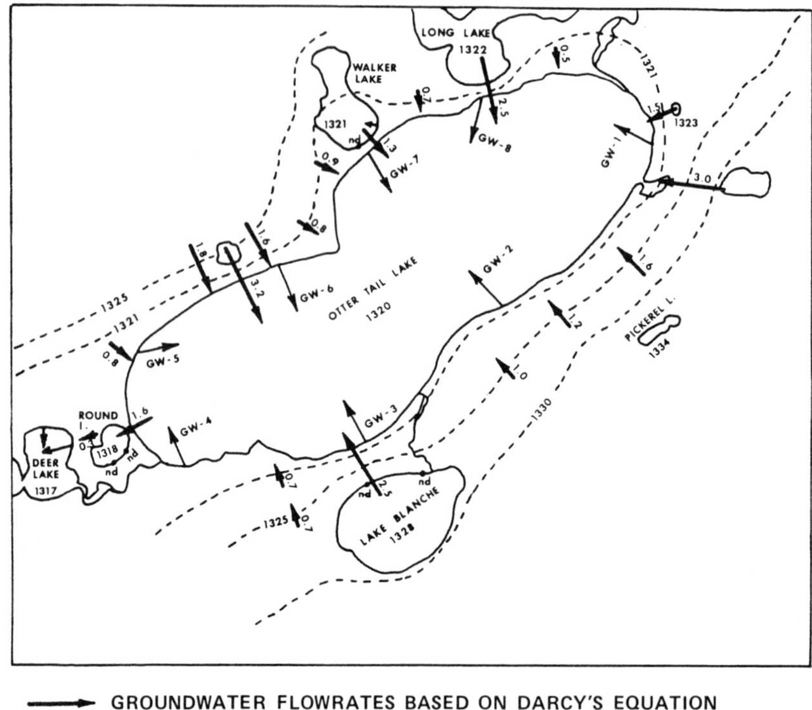

GROUNDWATER FLOWRATES BASED ON DARCY'S EQUATION

GROUNDWATER FLOW DIRECTION AND FLOWRATES MEASURED BY THE GROUNDWATER FLOWMETER

APPROXIMATE GROUNDWATER ELEVATION

nd NO DIRECTION

Figure 10. Groundwater flow patterns surrounding Otter Tail Lake.

of shoreline ice cover provided a noticeable clue to the locations of more rapid intrusion of warmer groundwater into the colder lakewaters. Heavy snow cover was correlated with limited groundwater flow, while exposed sandy beaches betrayed rapid groundwater movement.

To implant the sensitive probe, a shallow hole was dug in the loose sand to the depth of saturated soil. The instrument sensor was driven 3–5 inches into the sand (groundwater table) and the compass direction was set to due north (magnetic). Measurement of direction and flow was accomplished within 10 minutes and was usually repeated three times at each site. The direction of flow and approximate time of travel was noted for each individual measurement and the mean used (Figure 10).

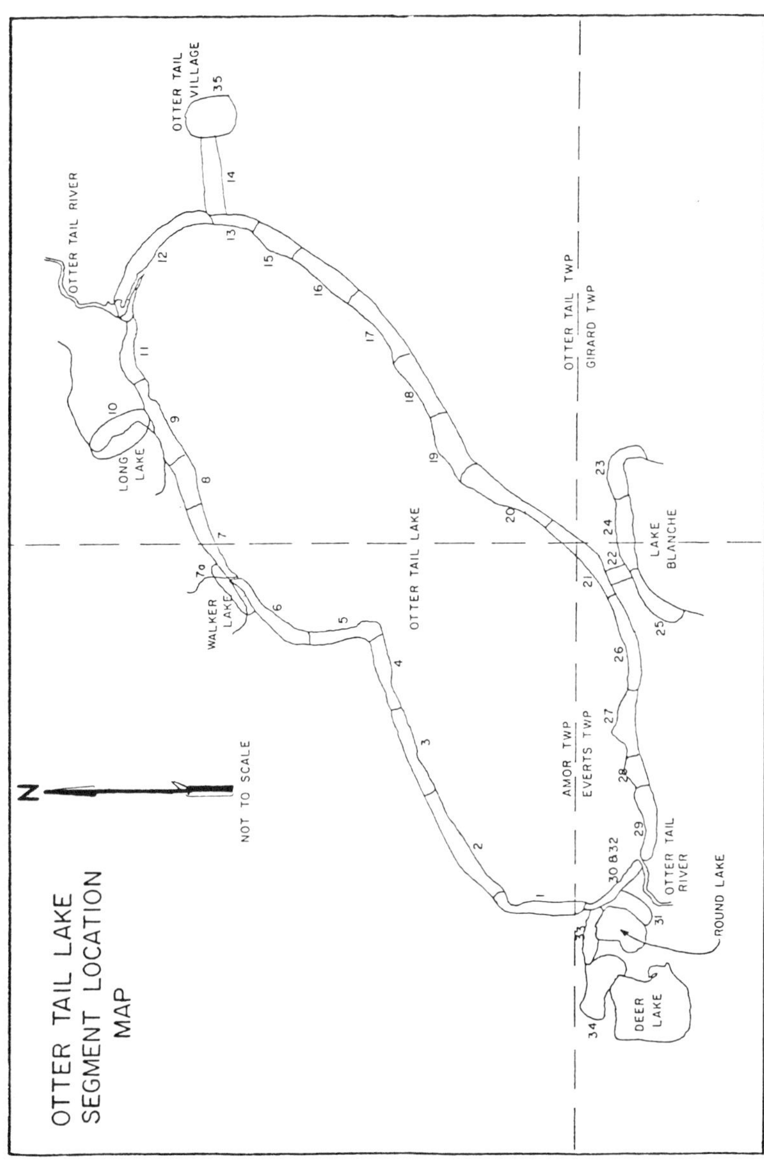

Figure 11. Segment locations within the Otter Tail Lake study area [3].

The observed directions of flow generally corresponded to that expected from the estimated groundwater gradients. The greatest difference was noted just north of a nursing home near the top of segment 1 (GW-5). A large discharge from the leaching field may have caused a local deflection of the flowrate, which would account for the observed discrepancy. Along northern regions of Blanche Lake, Walker Lake and the southern shoreline of Round Lake, no directional movement of the nearshore groundwater could be measured. These areas correspond to regions of anticipated exfiltration.

Shoreline areas had irregular rates of inflow, apparent through variations in snow thickness to even exposed snow melt areas of high flow. The naturally warmer groundwaters reduce snow cover by heat transfer, which is dependent on rate of movement. The shoreline north of Blanche Lake was laden with melt holes and depressions. Measurements of flow at exposed areas or melt holes revealed exceptional groundwater movement in excess of 10 fpd. Although melting snow along shoreline areas probably contributed to the high rates of flow, the permeability of deposits of sand and gravel is sufficient to accommodate such a rapid subsurface discharge.

Nutrient Relationships

Although previous investigations of groundwater-based lakes have verified a relationship between nutrient-leaching from nearshore septic tank systems and attached algae growth, especially *Cladophora sp.* [6], the interstitial phosphorus concentrations were rarely above 0.017 mg/l, or 2% breakthrough. Generally, phosphorus is not normally transported from septic tank disposal fields to surface waters by groundwater. However, under the high groundwater inflow rates and high water table levels surrounding Otter Tail Lake, which promote phosphorus mobility, substantial transport appears to occur. Frequencies of breakthrough of phosphorus from intercepter plumes average 26% with regions of substantial transport related to locations of exceptionally high groundwater flow.

The relationship of phosphorus loading to groundwater flow is emphasized by:

1. the occurrence of erupting groundwater plumes from nearshore septic tank systems around almost the entire periphery of Otter Tail Lake, consistent with a "withdrawal" lake;
2. a statistically significant correlation between (a) density of permanent residences and number of erupting plumes, (b) groundwater phosphorus concentrations and surface water concentrations, and (c) frequency of plumes and estimated groundwater flowrates; and

3. an exceptionally high groundwater flowrate sufficient to "flush out" seasonal septic tank systems located within 100 feet of the shoreline in at least a five-month period.

Groundwater nutrient loadings from septic tank systems become significant for certain segments of Otter Tail Lake. An estimate of their impact can be seen from Table V. The method used to estimate phosphorus loadings from the National Eutrophication Survey [7] assumes 7% (0.25 lb/capita/yr) of a 3.5 lb/capita/yr of total phosphorus found in raw wastewater will reach the lake. Sampling of groundwaters where plumes were present indicated a mean of 26% penetration of phosphorus, with high groundwater flow areas showing substantially higher leaching. With ice holes drilled at 100-foot intervals, similar to the average distance between house lots, each plume intersected should be indicative of leaching from that lot. Because of the high groundwater flow, the number of plumes was compared with only the permanent residences. A high correlation existed between the two columns, with a mean frequency of 78% incidence of plumes from the number of projected permanent residences per segment. The per capita loading for Otter Tail Lake is 2.8 times the presumed national mean phosphorus loading of 0.25 lb/capita/yr, or 0.7 lb/capita/yr.

The highest shoreline phosphorus loadings from groundwater sources are expected for segments 26, 3 and 0. Attached algal growth may be anticipated for these areas. The extent of any algal growth could not be determined during this study because of ice cover. However, total phosphorus contents of water samples from the different segments showed the highest mean levels in segments 26 and 9. The lowest was observed for segment 30 + 32, the only segment where exfiltration was considered likely.

CONCLUSIONS

A through-the-ice septic leachate survey was conducted along the shoreline of Otter Tail Lake, Minnesota during April of 1979. The following observations were obtained from the shoreline profiles, analyses of groundwater and surface water samples, and evaluation of groundwater flowrates and patterns:

1. More than 200 of the 975 ice holes drilled at house lot intervals along the shoreline showed evidence of erupting groundwater plumes of septic leachate origin.
2. Erupting plumes occurred around the entire periphery of the lakeshore front, significantly correlated with the number of permanent residences.
3. The highest frequency of plumes was found in shorelines of lakes exhibiting induced high groundwater inflow due to adjacent satellite lakes.

Table V. Calculated Winter Phosphorus Loading per Shoreline Length Based on Observed Frequency of Intercepted Plumes and Percent Breakthrough of Nutrients with Expected Relative Groundwater Flow and Observed Winter Surface Total Phosphorus Content Compared to the Phosphorus Loadings in the Last Two Columns

Segment	Existing Houses (R)	No. of Major Plumes (P)	Estimated Frequency (%)	Nutrient Loading (kg/yr)	Approx. Shoreline Length (mi)	Loading per Shoreline Length (kgP/mi)	Mean Surface Phosphorus Content	Groundwater Flowrate (ft/day)
1	7	5	71	5	0.92	5.4	0.007(3)	0.8
2	21	21	100	22	1.29	17	0.006(10)	1.8
3	14	21	100[a]	22	1.15	19	0.011(6)	2.2[b]
4	12	9	58	9	0.99	9	–	0.8
5	2	2	100	2	0.79	2.5	–	0.9
6	12	9	75	9	1.11	8	0.009(4)	1.3
7	14	14	100	14	1.03	14	0.014(4)	1.0
8	5	2	40	2	0.64	3.1	0.012(1)	0.7

9	4	14	100[b]	14	0.83	17	0.023(3)	2.5
11	21	16	76	16	1.19	13	0.010(2)	0.5
12	13	Inflow			1.01	–	0.016	–
13	7	2	29	2	0.53	3.8	0.020(1)	1.5
15	7	1	14	1	0.48	2.1	0.013(3)	3.0
16	7	3	43	3	0.84	3.6	0.010(1)	1.6
17	2	6	100[a]	6	1.04	5.8	0.011(2)	1.2
18	1	1	100	1	0.69	1.5	–	1.0
19	5	0	0	0	0.55	0	–	1.0
20	6	6	100	6	0.99	6.1	0.016(4)	1.0
21	10	19	100[a]	19	1.10	17	0.018(4)	2.0
26	10	52	100[a]	52	1.31	40	0.022(5)	2.5
27	0	2	100[a]	2	0.63	3.2	0.016(2)	0.7
28	2	5	100[a]	5	0.38	13	0.011(1)	0.5
29	5	5	100	5	0.79	6.3	0.012(1)	0.5
30+32	8	1	13	1	0.76	1.3	0.008(1)	-1.6

[a] Based on mean house loading (2.5 persons × 3.5 lb/capita/yr) × % breakthrough (0.26) × no. of plume locations.
[b] Average across segment since small lake area.

4. In general, the attenuation of phosphorus from nearshore septic tank systems was not high, with a mean breakthrough of 26% found for intercepted erupting plumes. The per capita loading for Otter Tail Lake has been estimated as 2.8 times the presumed national mean phosphorus loading of 0.25 lb/capita/yr, or 0.7 lb/capita/yr.

5. During winter, the mean concentration of total phosphorus in the surface waters of nearshore lake segments was generally lower ($\bar{x}$ = 0.013) than that of the inflow of the Otter Tail River (0.016 mg/l). However, the segments adjacent to Blanche Lake (0.022 mg/l) and Long Lake (0.023 mg/l) showed elevated levels in regions of high anticipated groundwater phosphorus loadings.

6. No evidence of fecal bacterial contamination of surface waters was found, despite the high incidence of erupting plumes.

REFERENCES

1. Kerfoot, W. B., and E. C. Brainard. "Septic Leachate Detection–A Technological Breakthrough for Shoreline On-Lot System Performance Evaluation," in *State of Knowledge in Land Treatment of Wastewater,* H. L. McKin, Ed., (Hanover, NH: Cold Regions Research and Engineering Laboratory, 1977).
2. Lakes Region Planning Commission Discussion of Natural Retention Coefficients Graphed Report gF2 From Phase II, Non-Point Source Pollution Control Program, Lakes Region Planning Commission, Meredith, NH (1977).
3. Water Pollution Research Associates. Draft Environmental Impact Statement, Ottertail Lake, Ottertail County, MN, prepared by U.S. EPA, Region V, Chicago, IL (1978).
4. U.S. Environmental Protection Agency. "Methods for Chemical Analysis of Water and Wastes," U.S. EPA, NERC, Analytical Control Laboratory, Cincinnati, OH (1975).
5. Water Pollution Research Associates. Draft Environmental Impact Statement, Alternative Wastewater Systems for Rural Lake Projects, Case Study No. 5, Ottertail County Board of Commissioners, Ottertail County, MN, prepared by U.S. EPA, Region V, Chicago, IL, and WAPORA, Washington, DC (1979).
6. K-V Associates. "Investigation of Septic Leachate Discharges Into Crystal Lake Michigan; Interpretive Report," prepared for WAPORA, Inc., Washington, DC (1978).
7. "USEPA National Eutrophication Survey: National Eutrophication Survey Methods for Lakes Sampled in 1972," Working Paper No. 1, Corvallis Environmental Research Laboratory, Corvallis, OR (1972).

37

AERIAL SANITARY SURVEYS IN RURAL WASTEWATER PLANNING

Barry M. Evans
Remote Sensing Specialist
Development Sciences, Inc.
Sagamore, Massachusetts 02561

INTRODUCTION

Historically, information on failing septic systems has been obtained solely via discussions with local sanitarians, questionnaires mailed to community residents, house-by-house investigations, examination of soil maps and/or "windshield" surveys. Because of the great deal of time, money and labor involved in these conventional procedures, however, other methods are being sought by the U.S. Environmental Protection Agency (EPA) and state and local government bodies to efficiently, economically and quickly assess septic system problems in a given area. A recently developed aerial photographic survey method that has been utilized successfully in rural wastewater facilities planning studies in Ohio, Michigan, Wisconsin, Minnesota, Indiana, Pennsylvania, South Dakota, Virginia and Massachusetts to identify and locate malfunctioning septic systems appears to more than meet these requirements.

There are three basic types of failures that can occur with septic tank or cesspool systems:

1. The wastewater contained in the system can back up into the home.
2. The wastewater can "short-circuit" to underlying groundwater before it is adequately filtered and purified.
3. The wastewater can make its way to the surface in the form of a "surface breakout."

It is this last type of failure that is detectable using this aerial photographic technique.

SEPTIC SYSTEM TYPES AND ASSOCIATED PROBLEMS

There are several types of onsite sewage disposal systems currently being used in this country. However, most can be categorized as either a septic tank–absorption field or leach pit septic system. The leach pit or cesspool system is usually found with older homes, whereas the septic tank–absorption field system is almost always found with homes built within the last 15-20 years.

A cesspool system usually is a covered pit with an open-jointed lining in its bottom portions into which raw sewage is discharged. The liquid portion is disposed of by seeping or leaching into the surrounding soil, while the solids or sludge are retained in the pit to undergo partial decomposition before occasional or intermittent removal. It is sometimes filled with rock, brick, cinder block or similar material that functions as an absorption/filtration medium.

Septic tank–absorption field systems are regarded as conventional septic systems and are interchangeably called septic field, filter field, leach field or drainfield systems. These usually consist of at least a septic tank and a subsurface disposal area, and sometimes have a distribution or "drop box" unit as well. The trench disposal system is the most common absorption field design, and the seepage bed method is a frequently used variation.

As mentioned earlier, only those malfunctions that are noticeable on the surface can be detected with aerial imagery. Those failures related to sewage backing up into the home or too rapid transport of wastewater effluent through the soil into the groundwater cannot be detected via remote sensing. In instances involving the latter, the use of a soil lysimeter or similar apparatus and water quality data collection may be necessary to determine the existence and extent of a problem.

Surface failures of septic systems can usually be attributed to one or more of the following causes:

1. The soil used in the absorption field has too slow a percolation rate to allow for adequate assimilation, filtration and biodegradation of sewage effluent flowing into it.
2. The septic system is installed too close to an underlying impervious layer.
3. The septic system is installed in an area where the seasonal water table is too high for its designed use.
4. The system is built on too steep a slope for proper drainage.

5. The system is overloaded because either too many people are using it or it is not being maintained properly.
6. Mechanical malfunctions or breakage in the septic tank, distribution box and/or drainpipes have occurred.
7. Caustic, toxic or otherwise harmful substances that could kill bacteria (which break down organic matter in the septic tank and leach field) have been flushed into the system and solids have passed into the leach field, resulting in clogging of the leach field and subsequent surfacing of wastewater.
8. All or part of the system has been improperly installed.

Based on work undertaken to date, it has been determined that the primary surface manifestations associated with this type of failure are:

1. conspicuously lush vegetation;
2. dead vegetation (specifically grass);
3. standing wastewater or seepage; and
4. dark soil where excess organic matter has accumulated.

All of the above are results of the upward movement of partially treated or untreated wastewater to the soil surface, and usually appear directly above, or adjacent to, one or more components of the septic system. Often, two or more of these manifestations will occur simultaneously at a homesite experiencing a septic system failure. In some cases, depending on the soils makeup of the particular area, the outline of the drainage line(s) of a properly functioning septic system can be distinguished with aerial photography. This peculiarity points up the need for tailoring photo interpretation keys to specific geographic areas.

IMAGE ANALYSIS METHODOLOGY AND CASE APPLICATIONS

The three types of film used in most of the aerial surveys are (1) normal color (Ektachrome 2448), (2) color infrared (Ektachrome 2443), and (3) thermal infrared imagery exposed at scales ranging from 1:4000 to 1:12,000. In the photo interpretation procedure, these aerial films were viewed simultaneously in a "multispectral" approach to identify those manifestations mentioned above that might be associated with malfunctioning septic systems and distinguish them from unrelated surface phenomena. These "signatures," in conjunction with a knowledge of what type of system might be used with homes having various ages and styles, and where they should be situated in relation to the house, were used to devise a photo interpretation key for detecting and locating failing septic systems. After the photo analyses were completed for each area, field checks were made of the suspect sites to verify actual failures and discriminate them from "false" signatures. Figure 1 illustrates a typical "surface breakout" in the Massachusetts study area and how it appeared on color infrared film (note the dark spot indicated by the arrow).

Using the image interpretation key, potentially failing septic systems were successfully identified in all study areas. As mentioned earlier, some degree of variability in photo signatures was expressed in different geographic areas. Two study areas—Steuben Lakes (Indiana) and three adjacent townships northwest of Philadelphia in particular—demonstrated this point.

In Warminster, Warrington and Horsham Townships in Pennsylvania, approximately 120 potentially failing systems were located and chosen for subsequent ground inspection. Of these, 68 were determined to have failing septic tanks and/or absorption fields at the time of the inspection. An additional 25 systems exhibited signs of having failed in the past or having the potential to malfunction during periods of excessive use or moderate-to-heavy rainfall. In the Steuben Lakes area, approximately 45 suspect homesites were located and chosen for subsequent ground inspection. Of these, only four were determined to have failing absorption fields or drainage pipes.

The disparity in the number of suspect versus confirmed failures in the two areas can be partially explained by the variability of signatures in those areas. In the study area northwest of Philadelphia, for example, excessively lush grass directly above the absorption field (as viewed on the aerial imagery) indicated almost certain system failure. In the Steuben Lakes area, however, many of the absorption fields exhibiting this particular signature did not necessarily have a significant problem. Because of poor water-holding capacity of the sandy soils in this area, any yard that exhibited conspicuously lush growth and/or excess soil moisture tended to be greatly enhanced with respect to their surroundings. These characteristics (i.e., "signatures") are very closely correlated with surface failures or septic systems and, consequently, any homesite exhibiting these characteristics was suspected of having a potentially failing system and was checked in the subsequent field inspection.

Despite the large number of suspect homesites located initially, however, most (if not all) of the major surface-related failures in both areas were believed to have been identified and located. In both instances, the use of the aerial survey techniques described greatly reduced the number of sites requiring ground inspection (e.g., in the case of the three townships in Pennsylvania, only 120 homes had to be ground-checked versus 2000–3000 possible homes). Again, these results imply the need to adapt the general image interpretation key outlined above to specific geographic areas for the most effective results.

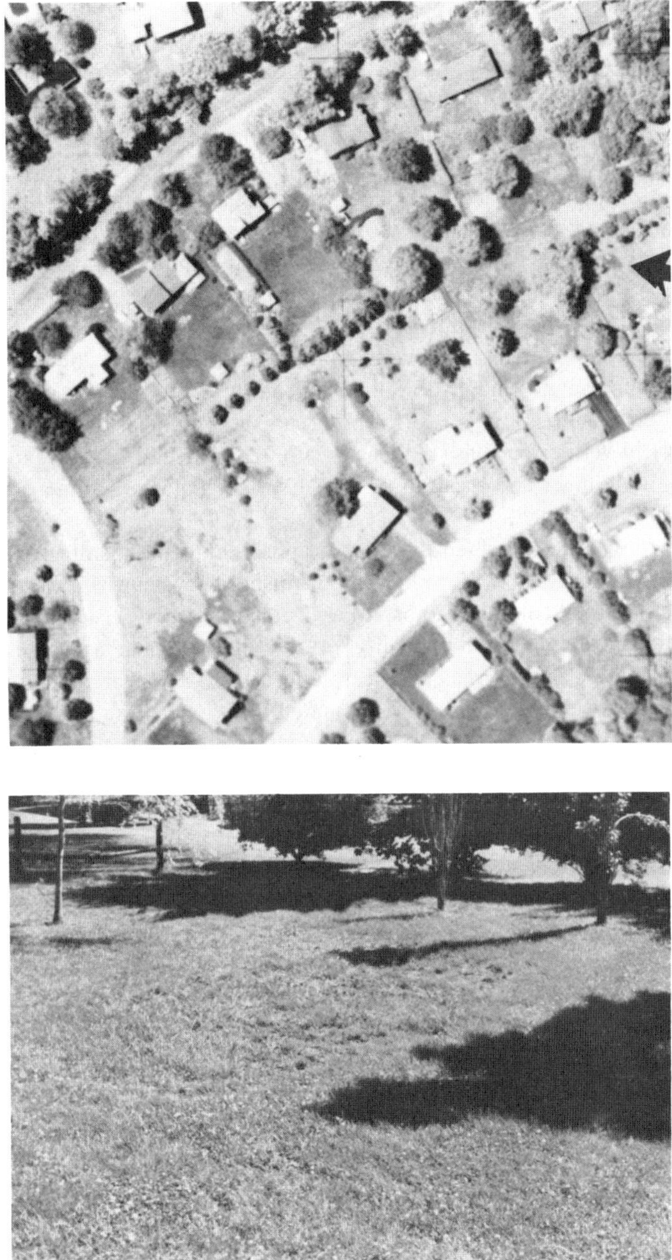

Figure 1. Enlargement of aerial color infrared photo (top) and photograph taken on the ground (bottom) of typical surface breakout in Holliston, Massachusetts.

CONCLUSIONS

As implied earlier, one of the greatest assets of this technique is the realization of savings in time, money and labor with respect to conventional sanitary survey methods in addition to securing objective, hard-copy data. This savings is derived from the fact that those homes that do not have septic systems with surface breakouts are "screened out" in the photo interpretation procedure. Thus, only those systems exhibiting "failing" signatures (i.e., suspect sites) need to be field-checked. What is important here is not the percentage of probable failures actually confirmed, but whether most of the significant failures have been located.

For example, if there are 25 actual failures in an area with 2500 homes, it is more important to find all 25 failures in a group of 90 suspect sites than to find only 16 failures out of 20. In both cases, the number of homesites requiring field verification has still been greatly reduced, and objective information on the number and location of actual surface failures within a specified area has been obtained.

Based on results obtained thus far, it appears that the manifestations, or signatures, associated with failing onlot disposal systems are best distinguished on normal color and color infrared film exposed at scales of 1:10,000 or larger, depending on the quality of the film or camera system used. Thermal infrared imagery has not been judged to be as valuable in discerning failing septic systems and has been eliminated for use in future projects.

Some limitations in the use of remote sensing for septic tank system failure analysis have been encountered. Two of the most significant limitations are related to soil/vegetation homogeneity and tree cover. Failing systems situated in soils that exhibit a wide range of photo signatures, such as varying soil color/tone and patchy vegetative cover (e.g., some sandy soils around lakes), are sometimes difficult to distinguish from naturally occurring phenomena. In areas in which a large percentage of tree cover is present, failing septic systems may be cured by foliage and/or shadows cast by trees and large shrubs.

Additional limitations and/or advancements in this aerial survey technique may be discovered as ongoing projects are completed, and future studies are undertaken in different geographic locations under varying climatic and seasonal conditions. In areas where there are few or no limitations, however, the use of remote sensing techniques can be, and have been, applied successfully in the detection of malfunctioning onlot sewage disposal systems.

38

ELECTRO-OSMOSIS: A REVIEW OF RECENT FIELD EXPERIENCE

James Peterson, President
Electro-Osmosis Western
Santa Barbara, California 93101

INTRODUCTION

Sanitary disposal of human sewage and liquid waste becomes more difficult as world population increases. Sanitary waste disposal problems have been compounded by both urban flight and the inability of cities to enlarge their sewage systems to meet environmental standards. The attempt is being made to install and/or improve sanitary waste disposal systems through the use of septic tanks and leaching fields.

The septic tank system has been in use for many years and, for the most part, is generally satisfactory; however, disposal of septic tank effluent was, is and probably will continue to be a problem [1]. When introduced to some soils, principally the fine-grained, tightly bonded clays, septic tank effluent will not migrate rapidly enough to be economically practical for sanitary disposal.

Earl Peterson of Minneapolis, Minnesota was acutely aware of these problems and made an exhaustive study to find a solution. His studies included a review of the literature. In the exchange of letters between William Whewell and Michael Farady in April and May of 1834 [2], they indicated a need to give names to cathodes and anodes. Further, they determined that in a decomposable body (water), hydrogen will travel in one direction and oxygen in the opposite when the body is exposed to a specific electrical system.

Further studies in a similar vein have indicated the following:

> "When silt or clay particles are immersed in water, they develop a negative charge around their outer edge. The negative electrical charge attracts and holds positive charged water to the clay particles. When an electrical field develops, the anode repulses the positive charge of the outer water layer and attracts oxygen ions and other negative charge ions. The cathode affects the positive charge of the outer water layer. As the outer water layer is displaced, or drawn away, it is replaced by free water, producing the movement toward the cathode" [3].

This statement was confirmed in the ASAE Proceedings of 1977 [4]. "Water may be moved through a porous media, such as soil under the application of an electrical potential because of the phenomenon of Electro-Osmosis." The basis for this phenomenon is the existence of a positively charged double layer about the surface of the solid material. Application of an electrical field draws the outer layer towards the cathode, drawing with it a quantity of water [5].

To obtain a system for electrically assisted subterranean moisture migration, a source of electricity was required. To be ideal, this system should be relatively free of maintenance, economical, dependable and relatively easy to install. All this could be accomplished using "made in the ground" cathodes and anodes.

Cathodes are approximately 6 ft X 6 ft X 2 ft dug into the ground. The cavity is filled with carbon and contains graphite piles for the full depth. Normally, an inspection station and vent line are installed. The anode is generally 5 ft X 5 ft X 2 ft and filled with high-metallic-content rock, such as trap rock or dolomite. With the addition of an electrolite (water), a complete system has been established.

Earl Peterson, who designed this system, made his first installation in 1970 [6], in Dakota County, Minnesota. Peterson says that the systems installed have been in continuous use since that time and exhibit no sign of open discharge. One lift pump had to be replaced on the original system. Further, Peterson stated that an electro-osmosis system installed near Watertown, Minnesota in 1972 is not only still functioning satisfactorily, but that it also has dried up a spring that was in the leach field.

Peterson claims that the most serious problem is to find conscientious installers.

The state-of-the-art, research and development are continuing. In San Bernardino County, near Fullerton, California, Charles L. Senn [7] has designed and supervised the installation of a small-scale system for two lots on a 42-lot subdivision for Covington Brothers of Fullerton, California.

Percolation tests on two sites by H. V. Lawmister and Co. of Stanton, California, indicate rates of 500 minutes on one lot (No. 3) with sections of that same lot indicating infinity, and the other lot (No. 25) indicating 240 min/in. Soils at the test sites had the following general characteristics.

Depth (ft)	% Sand	% Silt	% Clay	% Moisture	% Saturation	Resistivity (ohms/cm^3)
3	66	24	10	4.6	20.9	390
5	78	12	10	6.4	24.5	390
15	64	24	12	3.3	22.1	1000

In his test design, Senn elected to use short sections of actual leach lines and trenches. Water was clear and metered into the trenches.

Each test section consisted of a trench 20 inches in length, 2 feet wide, and 3 feet deep. A 4-inch perforated pipe was placed on 2 feet of rockfill. The system was then connected to a metered clear water supply designed to maintain the water level slightly above the invert of the 4-inch perforated distribution line.

Percolation test sites were established to act as referees for the liquid transmissibility of the leach trenches (Figure 1). On Lot 25, both percolation rates and metered rates were determined to be 240 min/in. On Lot 3, the ratios were determined infinite. A cathode (6 ft X 2 ft X 4 ft) filled with carbon and 4-inch graphite piles was constructed approximately 30 feet from, and parallel to, the leach line trench; an anode (4 ft X 2 ft X 3 ft) was constructed adjacent to the trenches.

In his report, Senn says, "At Lot 25, the Electro-Osmosis system almost immediately produces a dramatic improvement in soil permeability. The percolation test rate jumped from 240 min. to 13 min. per inch and remained between 13 and 14 min. per inch for 30 hours. The trench rate was 9 cubic feet per hour. In a minimum trench length of 75 ft., this translates into approximately 6075 gallons per day."

Coolbroth-Sitton Septic Tanks, Inc. of Minneapolis, Minnesota has been an Electro-Osmosis licensee for some time. In a letter to Jim Peterson, Coolbroth [8] indicates that he has made 137 installations using the Electro-Osmosis concept. The first was in October of 1972. Of the 137, only two systems required any modification. Nix Anderson, a Registered Sanitarian, has only recently submitted copies of his findings on 25 installations near Casper, Wyoming. Some are used here and are included in Figures 2–4.

Studies of the Electro-Osmosis concept have not been limited to "in house." In his Master of Science thesis, David Effert [9] compares four different types of sewage disposal systems. He reports that:

> The Sewage-Osmosis system is designed and constructed for the purpose of increasing the infiltration rate of septic tank effluent into soils which would not normally accept the liquid. The system appears to accomplish this because

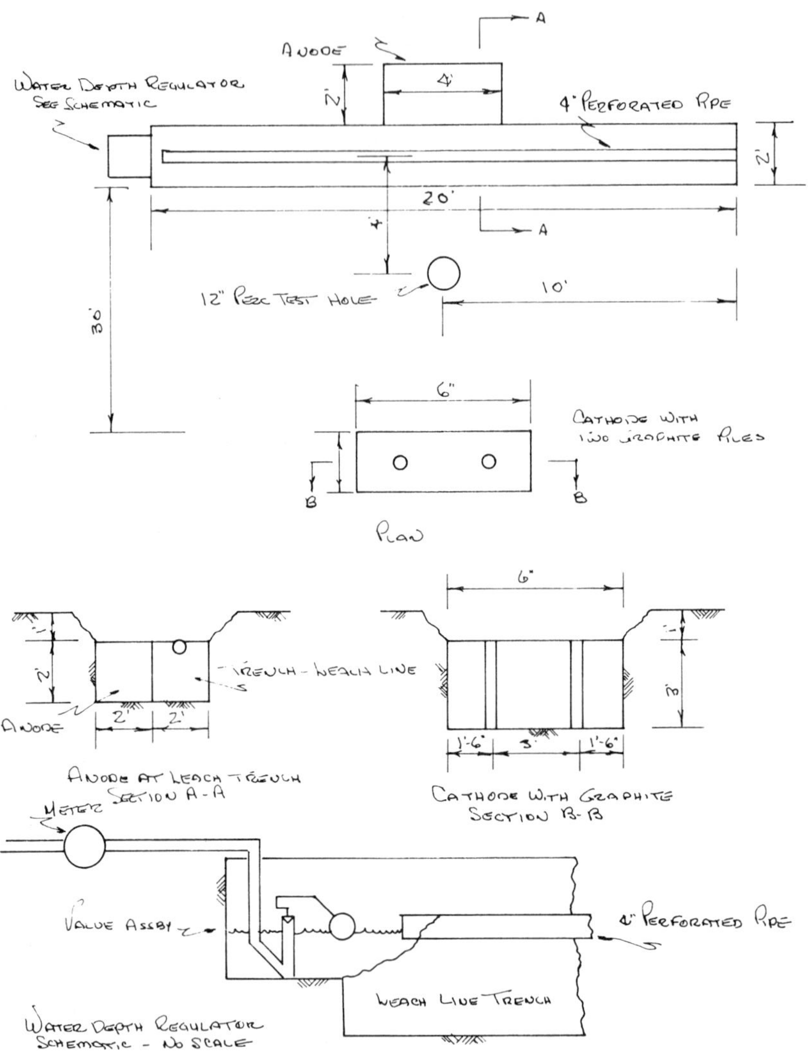

Figure 1. Electro-Osmosis Western demonstration site, San Bernadino County, California (after C. L. Senn RCE 6018).

over 114,533 gallons of liquid has been applied to the first section (10 feet) of absorption trench with only 9% passing through the second section and none passing into the third section in a seventeen-month study.

An important feature of the sewage osmosis system is the fact that it interferes very little with the normal operation of a home. The system

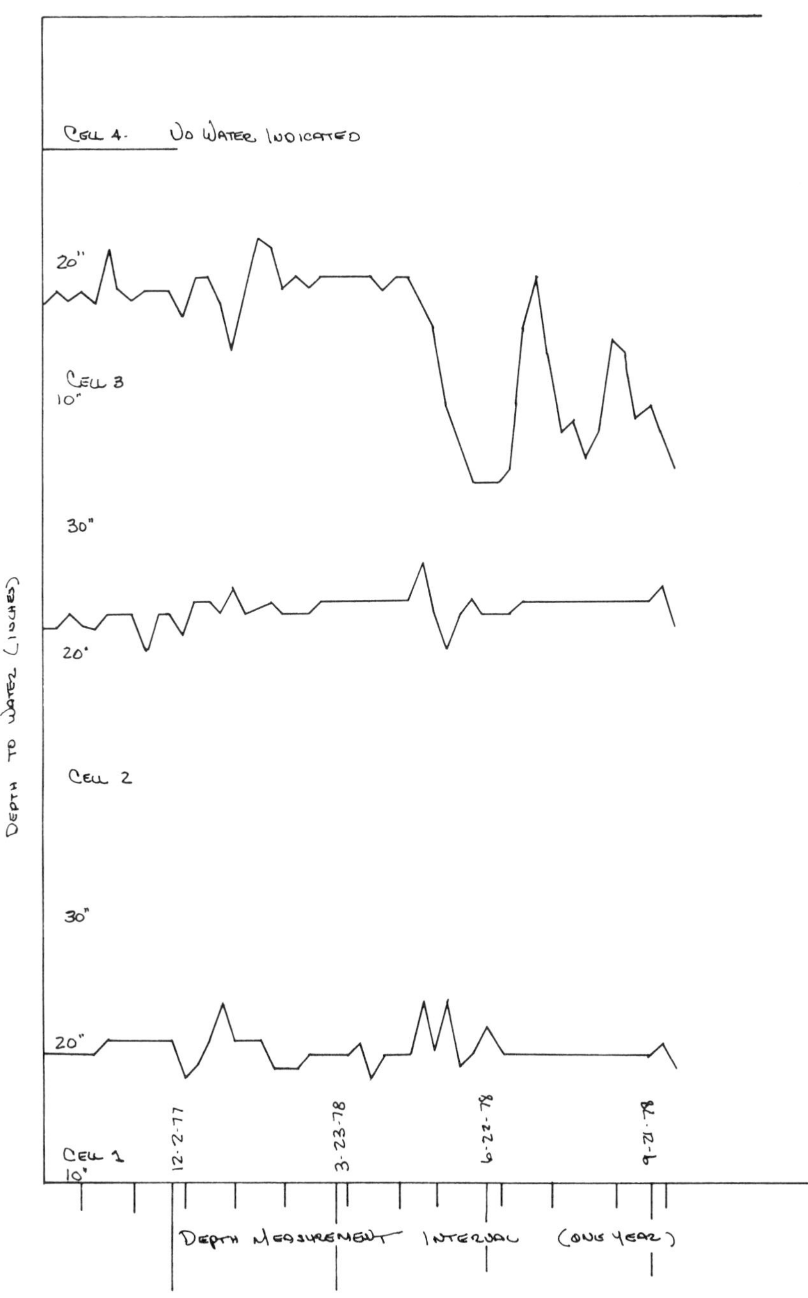

Figure 2. Electro-Osmosis System No. 1, Casper-Natrona County District, Wyoming.

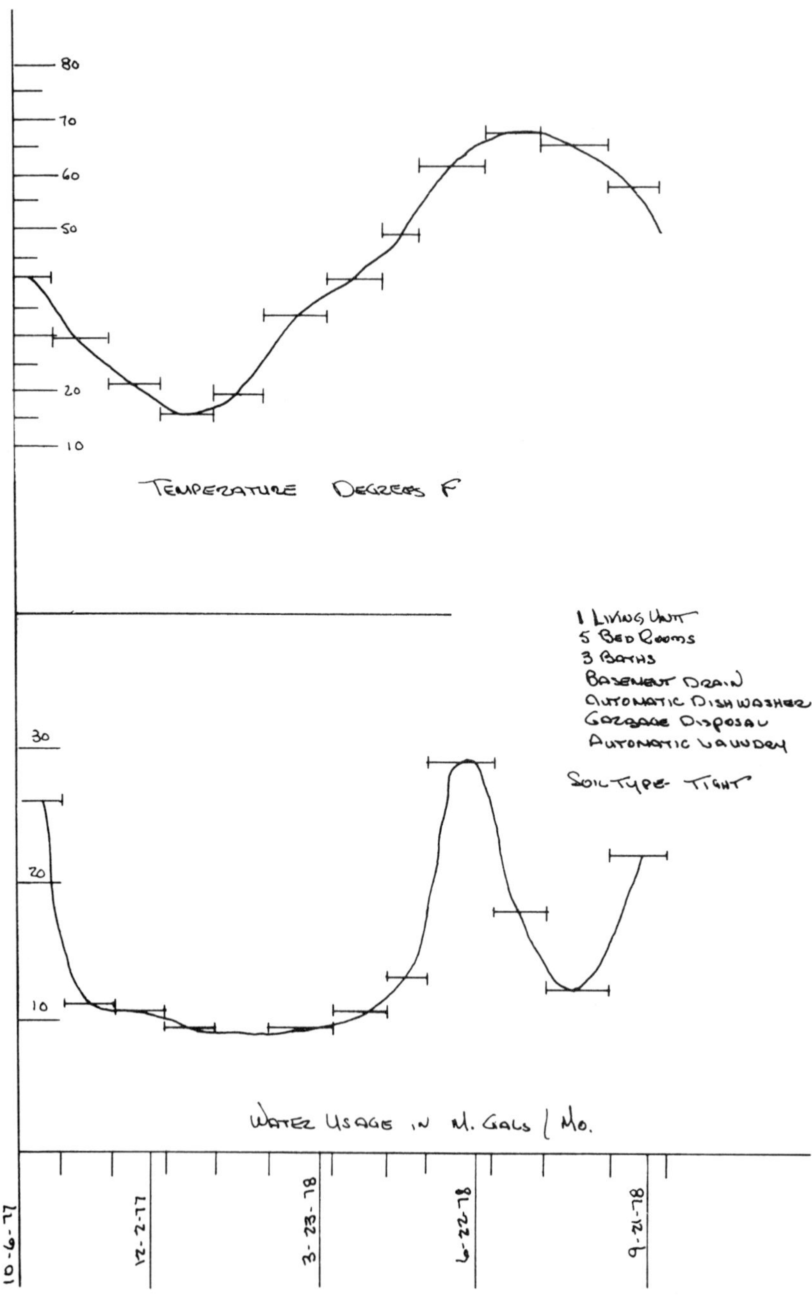

Figure 3. Electro-Osmosis System No. 1, Casper-Natrona County, Wyoming.

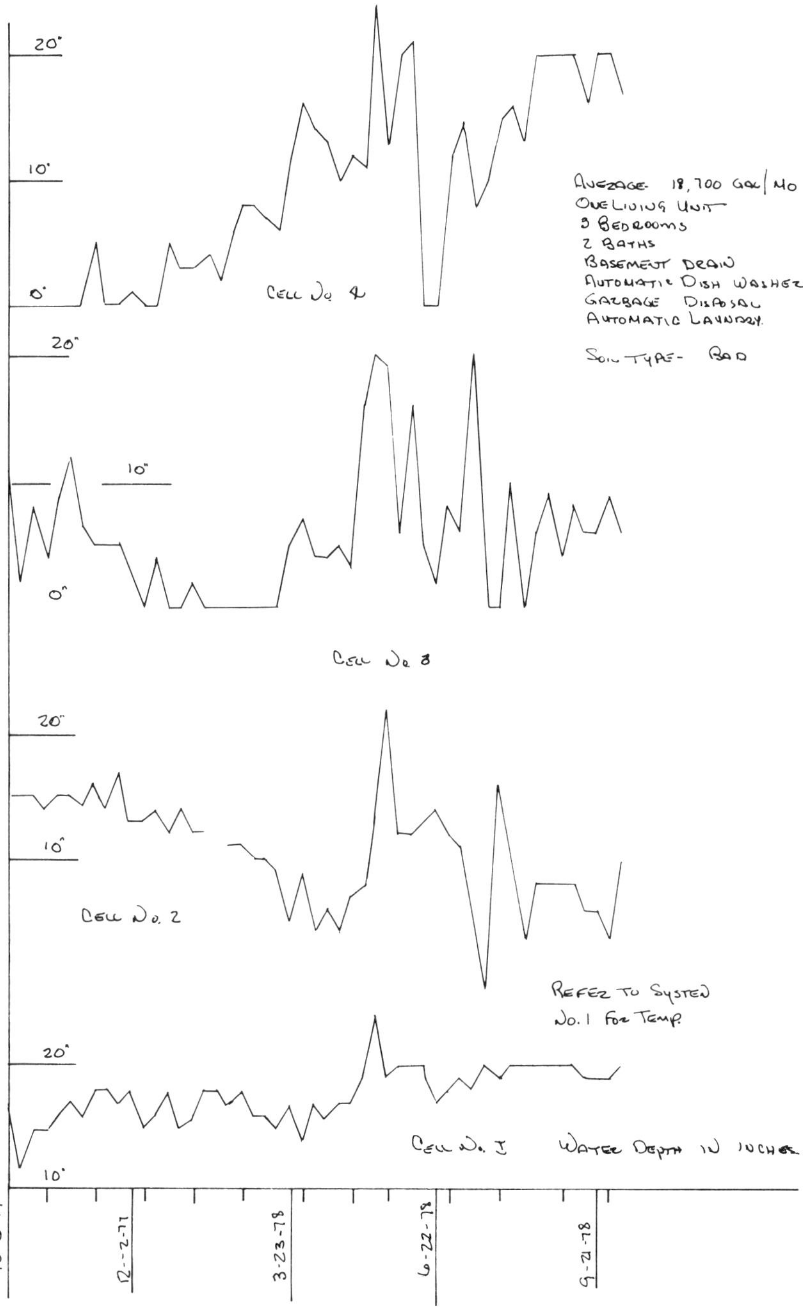

Figure 4. Electro-Osmosis System No. 6, Casper-Natrona County, Wyoming.

requires very little maintenance and it does not interfere with the home-owner's use of the land. It has no visual effect on the environment because all the equipment is located below the surface of the ground. The system is also reasonably priced. Annual costs are based almost exclusively on initial purchase and installation costs. The experimental system studied used only 22% of the available absorption trench which implies that the size of the system may be decreased with no harmful effects, thereby reducing installation costs.

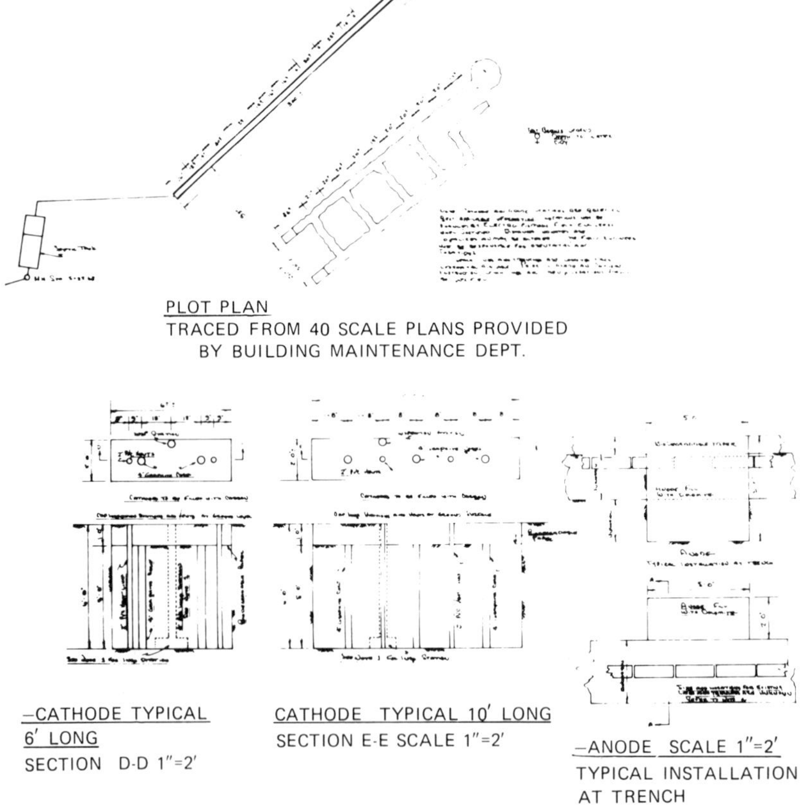

Figure 5. Use of the Electro-Osmosis System to rejuvenate

There are presently 14 systems installed and in operation in California, not all of which are new construction. Several systems have been used to rejuvenate existing systems.

In its evaluation of the Sewage Osmosis System, the Cornell Consulting Company [10] states in part, referring to the absorption rate of leach line trench sidewalls:

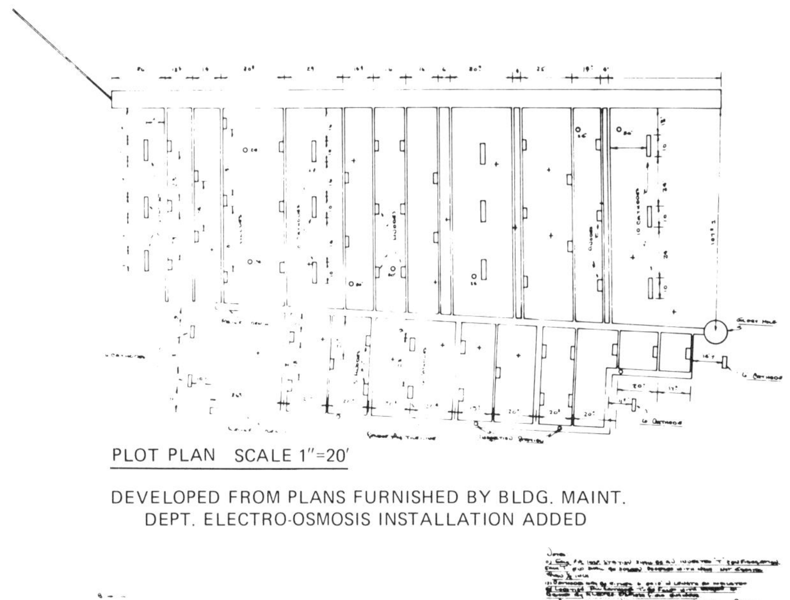

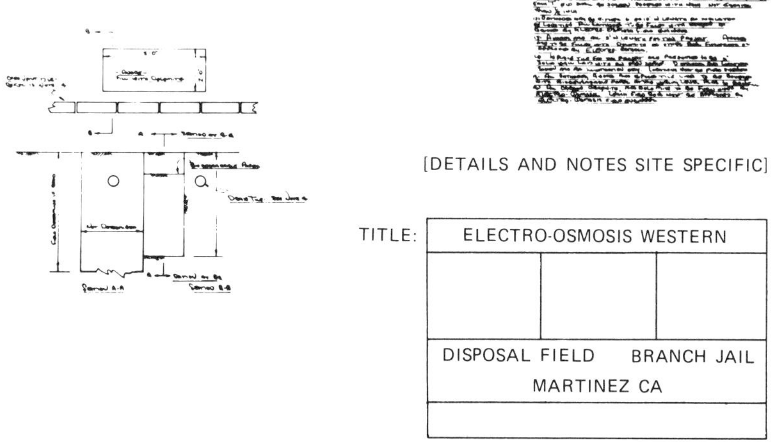

the disposal field of the Branch Jail in Martinez, California.

> ". . . but by far the greatest decrease is due to the soil pores clogging with a biological sludge. This blocking in the tight soils is by the lack of oxygen and the relative lack of micro-organisms. With small pore openings and a continuous influx of oxygen demanding sewage, it is all but impossible for the required oxygen to be supplied from the ground surface. Also the larger, more effective organisms such as Amoebas, and free swimming Protozoa cannot survive in the small openings so only Stalked Ciliate remain to complete digestion.
>
> ". . . the design of the system in effect creates an electric field to include electrolysis. As a brief review, electrolysis is the disassociation into the elements of hydrogen and oxygen. The oxygen is then drawn to the positively charged anode and the hydrogen is drawn to the negatively charged cathode. The sewage osmosis system does not attempt to create a field strong enough to break down all the water into hydrogen and oxygen. Rather the field is created to supply oxygen for aerobic digestion and to create a water flow in the soil down and away from the trench.
>
> "Because of the arrangements of the anodes, all of the oxygen produced by electrolysis is drawn through the absorption trench. To this extra oxygen is added oxygen received from the atmosphere since the disposal lines are only six inches underground. In addition to supplying oxygen in quantity, the system supplies a 2.5 foot depth of washed rock to provide an area for active biological contact and digestion. Thus the system creates an environment that prevents an anaerobic sludge from forming in the soil."

This concept is being proposed to rejuvenate the disposal field of the Branch Jail in Martinez, California (Figure 5).

New construction can also be associated with rejuvenation. At the Refugio Beach State Park, near Santa Barbara, California, Electro-Osmosis Western installed an Electro-Osmosis system to replace a failing system serving one comfort station (Figure 6). The system works so well that two additional comfort stations were added. However, the safety factor apparently was not great enough and sewage began to surface. Four additional cathodes were added to the system and it is now functioning satisfactorily. Further studies were to be made at this site during the winter rainy season.

As Peterson mentioned in his earlier statement, "The most serious problem is to find conscientious installers." So as to preclude the installation of systems that fail to function as designed, Electro-Osmosis has prepared technical memos and letters for the use of all licensees. These include, but are not limited to, "Percolation Tests and Transmissibility Determination," "Shipping Soil Samples" and "Site Report for Electro-Osmosis Installation" (see Appendixes A, B and C).

Much remains to be learned about electrically assisted subterranean moisture migration. It is the intent of Electro-Osmosis to maintain a research section and to work as closely as possible with its licensees. Information and knowledge properly distributed can provide for happy homeowners.

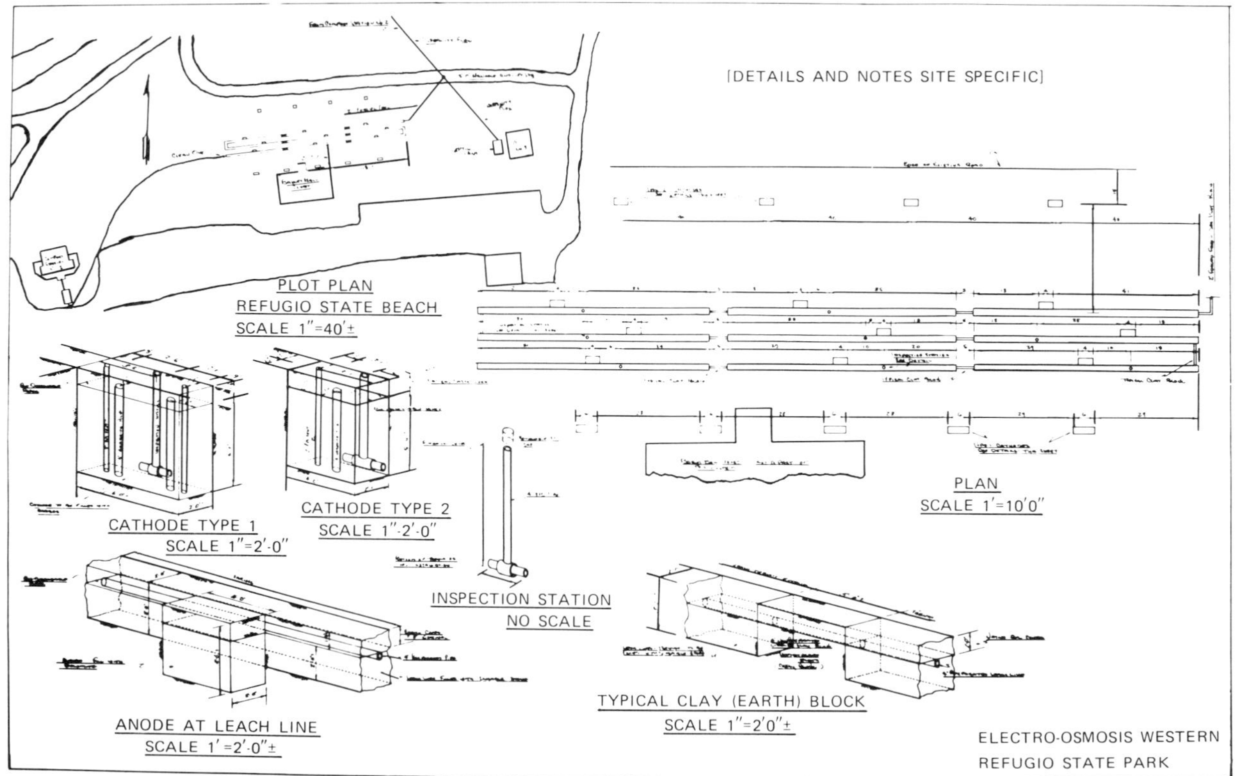

Figure 6. Electro-Osmosis System installed to replace a failing system serving comfort stations at Refugio Beach State Park, California.

APPENDIX A

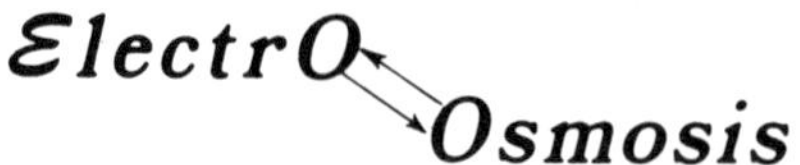

ELECTRO OSMOSIS WESTERN • 800 Garden St., Suite A • Santa Barbara, CA 93101 • 805/966-2027

M E M O

TO: All ELECTRO-OSMOSIS Licensees DATE: March 9, 1979

FROM: ELECTRO-OSMOSIS Western
Mr. Jim Peterson

SUBJECT: Percolation Tests and Transmissibility Determination

In order to present sufficient documentation to satisfy the "Administrative Authority" as defined in the current Uniform Plumbing Code, a percolation rate or rate of hydraulic transmissability must be prepared.

Unless local specifications conflict, the following methods should be used:

Percolation Test:

The percolation rate test hole shall be approximately 12" in diameter, and to a depth presumed to be the depth of the leaching field trench. All loose soil shall be removed from the bottom of the hole.

A screen sleeve approximately 36 inches in length and 8 to 10 inches in diameter, with not greater than ¼" mesh wrapped with one layer of burlap or muslin shall be placed in the approximate center of the test hole and rested on the bottom. Pervious material similar to pea gravel shall be placed on the outside and inside bottom of the sleeve. Not more than 3 inches of pervious material shall be placed on the inside bottom of the sleeve.

Clear water shall be introduced into the test hole at a volume and velocity not great enough to erode the sidewalls and bottom of the test hole to a depth not to exceed the 10 inches until the surrounding soil becomes saturated, or 24 hours, whichever is greater, and a transmissiblity or percolation rate becomes constant.

As soon as the percolation rate becomes constant, a falling head rate may be determined. The falling head rate shall be determined for a minimum of 8 inches inside the screen sleeve and a minimum of two trials.

The report shall include the following:

1. Test Hole diameter and depth
2. Size of screen sleeve including mesh size
3. Times of readings
4. Distance of head drop per reading
5. Percolation rate in minutes per inch

In some cases, hydraulic transmissibility may be determined by a short leaching field system. In this event, the leaching trench should be constructed the same as proposed for the finished product and oriented so that it will become a part of the finished leaching field system.

A device, attached to a water meter and set to control the water depth of approximately 1 to 1½ inches inside the perforated leach line pipe should be installed. There are no known vendors of such a device. ELECTRO-OSMOSIS is presently designing a control valve. It will be made available to Licensee holders.

Whether the percolation test or the transmissibility system is installed, tests should be run both before and after the ELECTRO-OSMOSIS system is installed.

Cathodes and anodes should be full size. Pits may be dug for both cathodes and anodes and the anode constructed as the leach line is constructed. For preliminary percolation or transmissiblity tests, carbon and graphite should not be installed in cathode.

Questions relating to this or any other ELECTRO-OSMOSIS problem should be directed, in writing, to the Santa Barbara office. As information is gathered and compiled, each licensee holder will be kept apprised of developments.

APPENDIX B

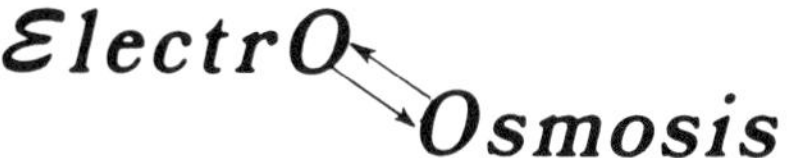

ELECTRO OSMOSIS WESTERN • 800 Garden St., Suite A • Santa Barbara, CA 93101 • 805/966-2027

M E M O

TO: ELECTRO-OSMOSIS Licensee DATE: March 9, 1979

FROM: ELECTRO-OSMOSIS Western
Mr. Jim Peterson

SUBJECT: Shipping Soil Samples
Please refer to Memo - Site Report for ELECTRO-OSMOSIS Installations

In the event that testing facilities are not available, or the franchise holder elects to send samples directly to ELECTRO-OSMOSIS Western, the following guidelines are offered for your consideration.

For all soil tests, except unit weight of undisturbed soil, five to ten pounds of native soil from the trench excavation should be placed in a plastic bag before any appreciable moisture change has occurred. The bag should be tied securely so as to preclude moisture loss.

Considerable care should be exercised to be sure that each soil sample is identified.

Identification should include job name and location, location of soil sample, and name of licensee. Typical identification would be:

Jones Residence, 2730 Foothill Road, Santa Barbara, CA.
Sample from bottom of center trench
Sample 1 of 1
Able Digger - Licensee

For in-place density samples, leave in the sampling ring, identify, and place in a plastic bag tied securely.

All samples should be placed in a suitable shipping container and shipped as soon as possible.

United Parcel Service and Greyhound Bus both have fairly inexpensive rates.

Samples may be sent to:

ELECTRO-OSMOSIS Western
800 Garden Street, Suite A
Santa Barbara, California 93101

APPENDIX C

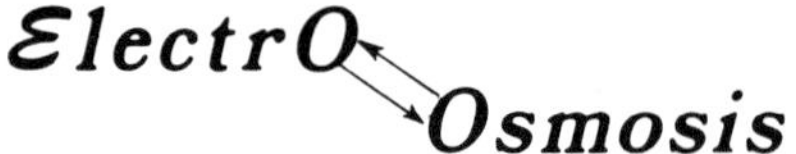

ELECTRO OSMOSIS WESTERN • 800 Garden St., Suite A • Santa Barbara, CA 93101 • 805/966-2027

M E M O

TO: All ELECTRO-OSMOSIS Licensees DATE: March 9, 1979

FROM: ELECTRO-OSMOSIS Western
Mr. Jim Peterson

SUBJECT: Site Report for ELECTRO-OSMOSIS Installations

In order to gather engineering information and data, and to provide licensee holders with engineering information, all franchise holders are requested to submit information from each site.

In order to maintain uniformity and information correlation, the following are submitted as guidelines:

1. Information should be submitted to ELECTRO-OSMOSIS Western, 800 Garden Street, Suite A, Santa Barbara, California, 93101. If facilities are not available for testing, such as a reputable laboratory, soil samples may be submitted to ELECTRO-OSMOSIS Western. Please refer to the soil shipping memorandum. Licensee holders who submit soil samples will be billed at actual cost plus 10% for handling. Estimated costs are $150.00.

2. In many respects, until more information can be gathered, a percolation or fluid transmissibility rate is the determining factor for ELECTRO-OSMOSIS installations. Please refer to the percolation or transmissibility

memo for methods and times. Any conflict with this memo and local custom should be brought to the attention of ELECTRO-OSMOSIS.

3. The report should contain a visual examination of the site. Included should be: (a) slope of the ground, (b) vegetation, (c) previous use of the site, (d) approximate depth of cut or fill at the site, and (e) estimated soil type.

4. Mechanical analysis of soil, including hydrometer analysis for each site. If radical soil changes are encountered, each should be sampled and a sketch made of the change limits. Soils should be graded from top size to two (2) microns. Screens should include U.S. Standard #4, #8, #16, #30, #50, #100 and #200.. Refer to Test Method No. ASTM #422.

5. Specific Gravity of Soil (True).
Refer to Test Method No. ASTM* D-854.

6. Moisture Content of Soil

The moisture content should be obtained from a soil sample at or near the bottom of the leaching trench. The sample should be not less than 100 g. and dried to a constant weight in a thermostatically controlled oven at 110° C ± 5° C (230° F ± 9° F). Normally, 24 hours in the oven is acceptable.

A microwave (radar) oven should not be used unless the submitting laboratory can provide suitable justification for its use.

Refer to Test Method ASTM* No. D-2216.

7. Unit Weight of undisturbed soil at or near the anticipated bottom of the leach line trench or percolation test hole.

The unit weight may be obtained using a thin wall sampler (4" seamless Shelby tubing), a standard penetration spoon, or an undisturbed soil sample treated the same as an asphalt concrete sample coated with paraffin. In all cases, the moisture content and test method shall be indicated.

Refer to Test Method ASTM* D-1188.

8. Soil pH

Refer to meter manufacturer's instruction manual.

9. Methods to determine electrical transmissibility are presently under study. Methods cited by this memo are tentative and subject to change.

(a) Resistivity-Conductivity of site soil.
Refer to Test Method California 643 (Service Life of Culverts) or to U.S. Department of Agriculture Hand Book No. 60. Test Method No. 5 for determination of resistance. At the date of this memo, Test Method California 643 is preferred and may be found at most California Department of Transportation offices, and all Caltrans Laboratories.

(b) In situ (in place) conductivity-resistivity readings should be obtained by driving $\frac{1}{4}$" threaded mild steel rod probes into the ground at or near the proposed leaching field area. Probes may be connected to a multimeter (Radio Shack Micronta Cat. 22-208 or equivalent) and the ohms resistance read directly. Unless

*ASTM - American Society for Testing Materials
Current publication

otherwise reported, all readings should be transverse to the leach lines and near the anode-cathode locations.

Questions relating to this or any other ELECTRO-OSMOSIS problem should be directed, in writing, to the Santa Barbara office. As information is gathered and compiled, each licensee holder will be kept apprised of developments.

REFERENCES

1. Otis, R. J., et al. "Effluent Distribution," *Proc. ASAE* (1977).
2. "Making the Language of Science," *Corrosion/73* (October 1972).
3. Cloud, J. J. "Electroosmosis–A Solution to Frost Heaving," Minneapolis Division FHWA (1971).
4. Beer, C. E., et al. "Analysis and Performance of a Sewage Osmosis System" (1977).
5. Shaw, D. J. *Electrophoresis* (New York: Academic Press, Inc., 1969).
6. Peterson, E. C. Personal communication (1976).
7. Environmental Consulting Associates. "Report on use of Electro-Osmosis Western System for Tract 9679," Los Angeles, CA (April 1978).
8. Coolbroth, F. Personal communication (October 8, 1979).
9. Effert, D. D. MS Thesis, Iowa State University, Ames, IA (1977).
10. Cornell Consulting Co. "Evaluation of the Sewage Osmosis System," Fort Collins, CO (1977).

39

STATUS REPORT ON THE POROX® (HYDROGEN PEROXIDE) PROCESS

John M. Harkin
Department of Soil Science
University of Wisconsin
Madison, Wisconsin 53706

INTRODUCTION

The following is a brief account of how the POROX process was devised and developed to repair septic tank systems that have failed because of soil clogging below the drainfield. Further, it shows how applications of this treatment led to the recognition of other causes of serious failures in septic tank systems, which can be conveniently avoided by minor modifications in installation practice.

Sanitary surveys of 613 homes around 8 recreational lakes in Wisconsin conducted in August 1967 indicated that approximately 22% of the septic tank systems then in use were failing by surface discharge of untreated effluent [1]. Reasons for system failure were ascribed to high groundwater (26.2%), steep slopes (20.5%) and poor soil permeability (11.2% of the systems examined). Recognizing the severity of environmental damage and public health hazard created by this situation, the Natural Resources Council of Wisconsin State Agencies recommended that a research project be created to investigate problems with septic tank systems and develop low-cost alternatives for onsite disposal of household sewage at problem sites. In 1971 the Wisconsin Legislature passed a bill providing funding for the University of Wisconsin to investigate the cause of failures and to devise methods or technologies to help avoid or remedy them.

DEVELOPMENT OF THE POROX PROCESS

One major development of this program, the so-called Small-Scale Waste Management Project (SSWMP, or "swamp") was a modified mound system for use at sites with problem soils. This design was intended to forestall failures of systems attributable to installation at inappropriate sites [2]. Recent studies of typical mounds installed by commercial contractors in Wisconsin have revealed that these modified systems perform as well as, or better than, conventional septic tank–absorption systems with respect to both wastewater acceptance and purification, despite the deficiencies in the soils at the installation sites [3]. Another development was a method to rehabilitate systems that had been properly installed at acceptable sites but which had failed naturally through prolonged use [4]. Such systems fail simply because the soil underneath their absorption areas gradually loses its initial permeability because the soil pores become clogged with a black, slimy deposit composed of organic wastes, bacteria, inorganic precipitates and other debris. These are then removed from septic tank effluent as it percolates through the soil. Rehabilitation is accomplished by removing any stagnant water from the system and treating the soil with strong solutions of hydrogen peroxide. This treatment removes the bulk of the organic and some of the inorganic materials and essentially restores the soil to its initial permeability [4].

Prior to this discovery, clogging of soil by these black, slimy deposits or "biological crusts" following applications of septic tank effluent had been studied repeatedly in the laboratory using columns of sand or lysimeters [5-7]. Partial restoration of soil permeability had been observed when effluent applications were discontinued for several days or weeks and the soil was "rested" [5]. However, the recovery of soil permeability on resting was usually partial and short-lived [5]. On the other hand, clogged columns treated with small amounts of hydrogen peroxide were restored to essentially their initial permeability within minutes to hours [4].

Following the successful unclogging of crusted sand columns in the laboratory in November 1973, in May 1974 the silt loam soil under two trenches of a failed household septic system at the University of Wisconsin Experimental Dairy Farm near Arlington, Wisconsin was unclogged by peroxide treatment. A soil tensiometer—a simple device used to measure the moisture content of soils by observing the height to which a column of mercury is raised against gravity by the surface tension in the soil capillaries [8]—indicated that the soil below the crusted trenches was much drier before the crusting material was destroyed by peroxide. The higher soil moisture indicated by the tensiometer after peroxide treatment revealed that water started to percolate easily into the soil again because the clogging layer had been destroyed

(Figure 1). These experiences were reported at the Second National Symposium on Individual Onsite Wastewater Systems [4]. This system is still working satisfactorily; tensiometer readings taken for three years following treatment showed that water continued to percolate readily from the gravel leach field into the soil below, but a small gradual increase in the soil moisture tension or "dryness" suggested that the system was slowly beginning to clog again.

Three other systems in sandy soils in a mobile home park at Rhinelander, Wisconsin, a second system at the University Dairy Farm, and a fifth system in a clayey soil just north of Madison's Lake Mendota were also treated in the summer and fall of 1974. Again, tensiometer readings indicated that the soil

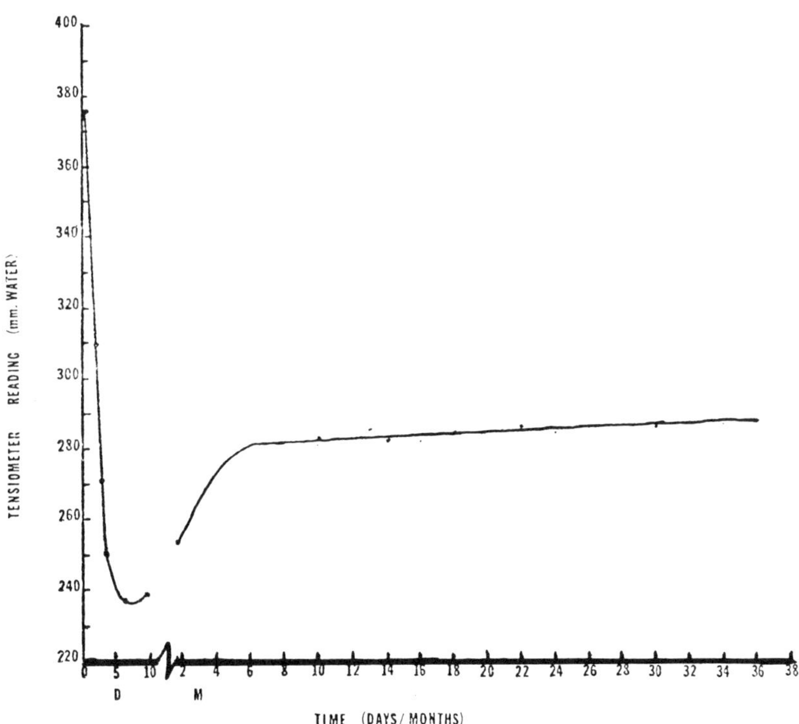

Figure 1. Changes in subcrust moisture tension following a POROX treatment in a field system. The initial steep drop indicates wetting of the soil as the crust is dissolved. The rise in tension during the first few days probably reflects resorting of soil agitated by decomposing peroxide. The slow rise over several months suggests gradual reformation of a biological clogging layer.

below these ponded, clogged systems became wetter after treatment, indicating that the clogging layer that had been inhibiting percolation of septic tank effluent into the soil had been destroyed by peroxide. These systems were also monitored by tensiometry. One of the systems in the sandy soil failed again soon after treatment, but was properly rehabilitated by a second treatment. Insufficient chemical had been added during the first treatment to dissolve the crust satisfactorily. Similar observations had been made previously with clogged soil columns in the laboratory; unless enough peroxide was added, the crust was not completely dissolved and permeability not adequately restored. In the laboratory, too, a second treatment invariably destroyed the residual crust left after the first inadequate treatment and returned the column to its initial permeability.

The advantage of this chemical method of system repair is that it restores soil permeability without creating major disturbances at the site or inconveniencing the users of the system by restricting water use [4].

Following the success of these laboratory and field experiments, an application was submitted for a patent covering chemical rehabilitation of septic tank systems, sand filters, etc., which had become clogged by biological crusts following applications of wastewater. This patent was issued in May 1977 and was assigned to the Wisconsin Alumni Research Foundation (WARF), the organization that handles patents for the University of Wisconsin [9]. WARF also coined the name POROX to designate the process and received a registered trademark for this name. Anyone practicing chemical treatments of such systems as failed septic tanks using hydrogen peroxide must be licensed by WARF. Further, in Wisconsin, anyone performing chemical treatments of failed septic tank systems must be licensed by the State Division of Health [10].

Since 1974 several hundred failed systems have been treated using the POROX process, either by licensees of WARF or by the author and his associates, who continued to experiment to determine the limitations of the process and improve ways to simplify and ensure uniform treatment of the clogged soil. A variety of system sizes, types and configurations have been treated: absorption trenches, beds and seepage pits (drywells) in a variety of soil types serving single-family dwellings, multiple housing units (mobile homes, small apartment buildings, etc.); retirement homes; restaurants; and even industrial plants. Modifications of the treatment solution have been developed to improve the treatment. For example, special stabilizers are sometimes added to inhibit enzymatic breakdown of the peroxide by catalases in the soil bacteria, and special equipment has been developed to facilitate the peroxide additions and ensure its thorough dispersal throughout the system. Details of the exact procedures for performing POROX treatments cannot be revealed because this is information supplied only to licensees by WARF.

Although a large measure of success was registered in these treatments, not all were successful. Paradoxically, many systems, (especially in sandy soils) that were expected to work well after treatment did not respond, while others performed amazingly well, even though treatment seemed unlikely to help because the systems were undersized, poorly constructed, etc. Closer inspection of systems where POROX treatments were ineffective generally revealed peculiarities with the system, which explained the lack of success. Recognition of these problems revealed patterns of shortcomings in system installation. Some interesting case histories are described in the following so that these inadequacies can be recognized and avoided in future.

CASE HISTORIES

Inappropriate Use of an Aerobic Unit

While a treatment was being performed at an industrial plant in upstate New York it was discovered that the system was not clogged in the customary fashion. Instead, in addition to the soil clogging, it was found that the distribution lines were half-filled with a black, greasy material, so that water could not drain out through most of the holes in the pipes. A small distribution box at the head of the system was also half-filled with the same material. The system was being served by an aerobic unit, which had been installed to replace a 5000-gallon septic tank used initially. The aerobic unit had been purchased because of an increase in the number of employees. It was expected that the aerobic unit would more effectively treat the wastewater and forestall any problems with the system. In fact, the aerobic unit was the real cause of the problem.

Workers in the plant used large amounts of barrier creams or hand cleaners containing lots of lanolin; the lanolin was not being degraded in the aerobic unit and was held in suspension as a fine dispersion by the agitation caused by the aeration device. Most of the lanolin passed out of the unit with the effluent. As soon as the effluent passed beyond the aeration unit, it became anaerobic. The lanolin settled out as a sludge in the pipes and in the soil of the absorption area, which was colored black by precipitates of metal sulfides formed under the anaerobic conditions. This system was rehabilitated by cleaning out the lines, regenerating the field permeability with a POROX treatment and reinstalling the septic tank in series in front of the aerobic unit. The quiescent flow conditions in the septic tank allowed the lanolin to separate before the septic tank effluent entered the aerobic unit, where further biological treatment was continued before the water passed into the absorption field, which now functions properly.

Improper Septic Tank Baffles

In several systems that were examined to determine whether they should be given a POROX treatment, problems with the outlet baffles were observed that had led or contributed to failure of the system. In some tanks the outlet baffles or sanitary tees were too long, so that the septic tank effluent flowing into the field was coming from a layer in the tank just above the sludge layer. Incompletely settled solids were forced into the absorption area, increasing the clogging in the soil and sometimes blocking the pipes in the distribution system. It has been shown that the amount of suspended solids in septic tank effluent is a major contributor to clogging and failure of soils [11]. In these systems, shorter baffles had to be installed and the pipes cleaned in addition to POROX treatment of the field to rehabilitate each system.

In several other systems, the outlet baffles were found to be so badly damaged or corroded that they were ineffective in retaining the scum layer in the tank. In some cases the baffles were missing altogether. Here, the load of solids from the scum layer was helping to clog the soils and sometimes completely blocking the outlet pipe from the septic tank, so that cleaning of the pipes and unusually large amounts of peroxide were required to rehabilitate these systems.

Problems were encountered with both metal and concrete baffles. Some metal baffles were so pitted and corroded that they were totally ineffective at retaining scum. No scum layer was observed in these tanks. The hydrogen sulfide and organic acids produced in septic tanks by bacterial action on the sulfates and putrescible organics in the wastewater are probably responsible for the dissolution of the iron in the baffles. In several other cases, metal baffles had fallen into the bottom of the tank because they had been inadequately anchored into the walls; either the bolts securing the baffles or metal anchors embedded in the concrete to hold the fastening bolts had corroded away. Some anchors had been set too shallow to begin with. Presumably galvanic cells are set up when baffles and bolts and metal anchors of different materials are exposed to the aggressive atmosphere in a septic tank and accelerate corrosion of the metals. Lightweight fiberglass baffles secured with plastic anchors or polyvinylchloride (PVC) sanitary tees were used to replace metal baffles in these systems.

Many concrete baffles were found to be damaged or missing. These were usually half-round baffles in monolithic concrete tanks. Where baffles were missing, the original baffles had not been reinforced with wire mesh. In some reinforced baffles the concrete had eroded away and the residues adhering to the wire were weak and of powdery, sandy consistency. Apparently, a weaker concrete mix had been used to facilitate slumping in the formation of the thin baffle walls because the tank walls were strong and undamaged. In the alkaline environment of septage, the poorer quality concrete had evidently deteriorated rapidly, leading to failure of the baffle and subsequent failure of the system by accelerated clogging.

Systems Installed in Sloping Sites

A variety of problems were encountered with systems installed on sloping sites. In at least four different systems examined, which had been installed parallel to the slope, the elevation of the normal water level in the septic tank was higher than that of the soil surface at the end of the seepage beds or trenches. Here soil clogging created a type of artesian well that regurgitated untreated effluent to the surface almost as rapidly as wastewater entered the systems. POROX treatments provided temporary relief for these systems, but they soon clogged and failed again at the bottom end because the bulk of the water entering the system was running down to the end of the system, overloading it in a localized area. Holes augered into the upper part of one of these systems revealed that the upper part of the bed was dry and unclogged, although water was surfacing at the low end.

Most sanitary codes and installation guidelines recommend that beds or trenches should be laid across slope at sloping sites. However, here too problems were encountered. In at least four systems, water was observed in the seepage trenches or beds soon after they had been unclogged by POROX treatments. Samples of water taken from the distal end of one of these systems were examined for fecal indicator organisms (total coliforms, fecal coliforms and fecal streptococci) and found to be nonseptic. The water levels in the trenches of two systems that were monitored varied according to the patterns of precipitation. Measurement of the water levels in shallow groundwater wells placed upslope from the systems frequently revealed that the water table came close to, or rose above, the level of the trench bottoms. The trenches actually were acting as interceptor drains and occasionally collecting groundwater moving down the slope at a high level in the soil horizon following heavy rains. Such systems could have been easily protected by drainage lines (curtain drains) installed upslope from the seepage trenches.

Similar problems were observed with some deep systems at the downslope end of long slopes; the homeowners had installed deep systems to accommodate toilets and showers in the basement level of their houses while avoiding the extra expense of a grinder pump to elevate the waste to a higher level in a shallow system. These deep systems also intercepted groundwater moving downslope through the soil; homeowners with shallow systems upslope from these sites experienced no such problems. Cross-slope systems are apparently particularly vulnerable to unusual groundwater flows. Therefore, careful soil inspection for signs of mottling (or preferably monitoring of the site) seems advisable before any system is installed at sloping sites. In any case, shielding of the system by a curtain drain is recommended before the site is landscaped.

Intrusion of Soil into Gravel Beds

The most frequently observed reason for lack of success of POROX treatments, especially in sandy soils, which are very easily unclogged in the laboratory, was intrusion of soil into the gravel within the absorption field.

When a soil absorption field is being installed, after gravel has been placed in the trenches or bed, and the septic tank effluent distribution system (perforated pipes or drainage tile) has been installed and embedded or covered over with a further thin layer of gravel, normally some barrier material is placed above the gravel before the system is backfilled with the soil removed during excavation. Typical materials used to cover the gravel are untreated building paper, straw or marsh hay, or pea gravel, which often are prescribed in state sanitary codes.

These materials are supposed to prevent soil from falling down into the gravel during backfilling. Untreated building paper is recommended for two reasons: (1) it is easy to apply, and (2) it is intended to be only a temporary barrier, remaining in position only until the soil has become consolidated above the gravel. In time, untreated paper rots away so that no barrier is left between the gravel and the soil. This is supposed to be beneficial because nothing is left to prevent movement of water vapor up through the soil or of air down into the soil. This situation is supposed to enhance both loss of moisture from the system by evapotranspiration and biological treatment of the wastewater by admission of oxygen to the soil bacteria. On the basis of such reasoning, use of impermeable barriers (plastic sheet, treated paper or roofing felt) is not permitted in many states.

The benefits of this theory are not realized in practice for unforeseen reasons. At fault is again the clogging of the system by biological crusts. As the system clogs and begins to pond, water becomes deeper and deeper within the gravel bed. Some ponded water seeps laterally into the soil, clogging the side walls of the trenches or bed as well (Figure 2). In time, the ponded water becomes so deep that it fills the whole absorption area, thus impinging on the soil overlying the gravel. Although this soil may have remained in place until that time, it is easily dislodged when wetted and can trickle down into the gravel.

The forces normally holding soil particles together in a consolidated mass above the gravel are the cohesive forces (mainly hydrogen bonding) of the

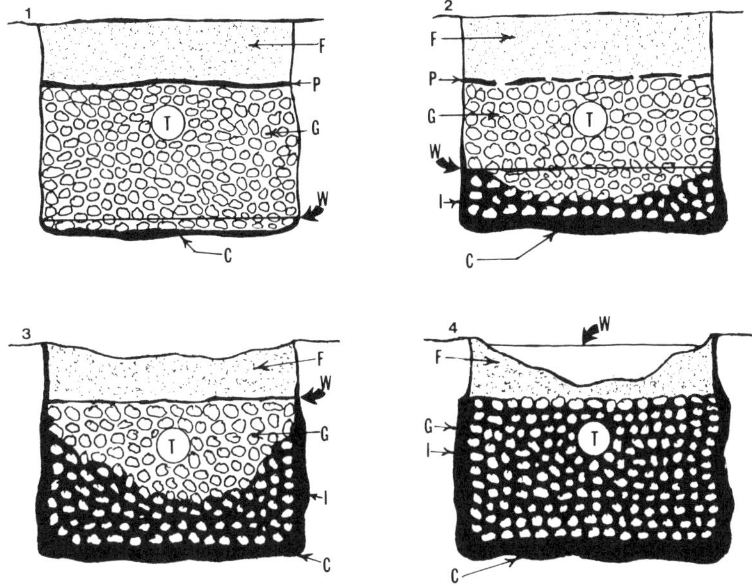

Figure 2. Schematic representation of the progressive stages in failure of a field system installed in sandy soil with untreated building paper as barrier material (C = biological clogging material, W = level of ponded water, P = paper in barrier layer, G = gravel, F = backfilled soil, T = drain tile or distribution pipe, I = infiltrated soil in gravel):

1. A thin biological clogging mat is forming under the gravel, causing water to begin to pond; paper is still undecomposed and retains backfilled soil.
2. Sidewalls are beginning to clog, ponded water is becoming deeper, paper is beginning to rot, some soil (probably mainly from sidewalls) is invading lower gravel.
3. Paper is totally decomposed, water level is now at top of gravel, sidewalls and bottom are more heavily clogged, soil from the fill is beginning to wash into the gravel.
4. The gravel is almost totally filled with soil, the backfill is slumping, and ponded water is surfacing.

extremely thin films of moisture surrounding the individual grains in the soil. Because these moisture films are so thin, the cohesive forces are strong when the soil is relatively dry; however, when the soil becomes waterlogged (saturated) as the effluent rises in a clogged and ponded system, the moisture between the soil particles is abundant and the cohesive forces become weak or are totally overcome. Thus, the soil particles are loosened and can trickle down into the gravel, filling up all the spaces between the stones. Some soil from the sidewalls of trenches or beds may invade the gravel in the same way while the water depth is increasing in the system. The soil that intrudes into the system fills up the pore space between the gravel and rapidly reduces the seepage area available for septic tank effluent infiltration (Figure 2).

This phenomenon was readily demonstrated using a laboratory model of a clogged drainfield (Figure 3). A Plexiglas® cylinder 12 inches in diameter and 4 feet high was sealed with a Plexiglas base and filled with gravel (1- to

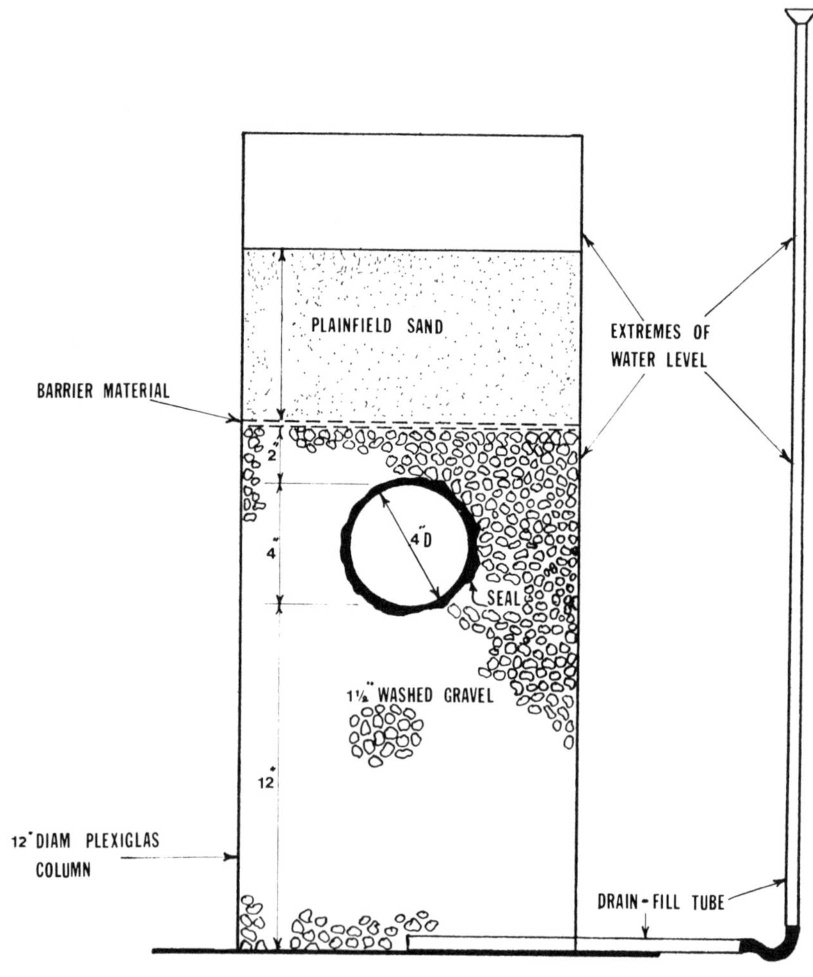

Figure 3. Laboratory model for testing barrier materials. Water levels were raised from the gravel–sand interface into the sand or the surface of the sand (ponding) and vice versa by adding or draining water from the tube.

1.5-inch diameter) to a depth of 12 inches. A section of 4-inch perforated pipe was puttied onto the sides. The pipe was surrounded with gravel and covered to a 2-inch depth with gravel. One of a variety of barrier materials was then placed above the gravel, being taped to the Plexiglas sidewalls if needed to provide an adequate seal, and 1-2 feet of Plainfield sand (C horizon) was placed above the barrier material and compacted by tamping. Plainfield sand was the soil chosen because (1) it is a common soil in the central sand plains of Wisconsin; (2) it has a fast percolation rate and is therefore considered ideal for installation of conventional septic tank–absorption systems; (3) it has the texture recommended for fill material for Wisconsin mound systems [2]; and (4) it is the soil that had invaded the gravel in several septic tank systems that did not respond well to POROX treatments.

Using this model, the efficacy of different barrier materials in preventing invasion of soil into the gravel in the unponded and ponded conditions was easily measured. To simulate ponding of a system, water was filled into the gravel using a tube sealed into the bottom of the plexiglass cylinder. When the water level was close to the barrier material and just above or below it, the water level was raised and lowered at different rates to simulate two different conditions: first, the slow minor fluctuations that result in a ponded system from normal patterns of household water use (increased water level during the day corresponding to peaks of water use in the house, drop in water level overnight) [12]; second, a sudden drop in water level that would occur if the septic tank were pumped in a system that was ponded and overfilled.

The barrier materials tested were: untreated building paper ("Red Rosin" paper); a 2-inch uncompressed layer of marsh hay; an 8- to 10-inch layer of marsh hay compressed to a thickness of 1–2 inches; a 2-inch unbacked fiberglass (building insulation); and a spunbonded polypropylene filter fabric.

Fresh undamaged building paper was an effective barrier that prevented both dry and wet sand from falling into the gravel and allowed both air and water to pass through the barrier. However, torn paper did not retain the dry sand, and even pinholes in the paper allowed wet sand to trickle into the system, especially when the water level was fluctuating in the vicinity of the barrier. Dry sand fell easily through holes in torn paper during "backfilling" and tamping. Wet sand cascaded through holes or tears in the paper when the system was flooded, regardless whether the water level was rising or falling and whether the rate of change of water level was fast or slow.

To examine how paper used as a barrier material in a real system might behave after it was weakened or rotted by biological action in the soil, undamaged paper was taped onto the sidewalls of the cylinder above the gravel and covered with tamped sand in the usual manner. The paper was then attacked chemically with strong acid or alkali. Paper weakened in this way was not an effective barrier to prevent wet Plainfield sand from invading the gravel when the water level fluctuated near the paper.

A loose layer of marsh hay was also not an effective barrier to either dry or wet sand. Some sand fell into the gravel immediately during "backfilling" and tamping of the sand layer. More sand trickled in when "ponded" water reached and fluctuated around the gravel/hay/sand interfaces. On the other hand, the 2-inch layer of compressed hay was quite an effective barrier. Dry sand did not flow easily through the compressed hay layer, and very little wet sand passed through this barrier. The practical disadvantages of using such a barrier are the expense of a sufficient amount of hay and the amount of labor needed to spread and compress it uniformly. Hay does not rot as easily in the soil as paper because hay contains some lignin [13]. Most of the lignin in paper is removed by Kraft pulping [14]. Consequently, hay will remain in position and prevent soil from entering the gravel for a longer time than paper, although eventually it may not, especially in well-drained, aerobic soils.

Pea gravel obviously will not rot in the soil, but is not a good barrier material. Some dry sand and more wet sand pass through a 2-inch layer of pea gravel. Experiments with soil drainage, graded sand filters, etc. have shown that particles pass easily through the interstices between particles that are more than seven times larger in diameter.

Unbacked fiberglass also does not rot in the soil and forms an excellent barrier to movement of both dry and wet soil. The only problems with fiberglass are its relatively high cost and occasional scarcity, because of the competing market for building insulation and difficulty in its application. A large amount of material would be needed to cover a field absorption area, and normally only batts or rolls of the relatively narrow standard widths used for building insulation are available. Fibers that penetrate the skin or are inhaled cause itching or throat irritation.

These problems are not shared by a large number of synthetic filter fabrics presently available on the market (Table I). These are also excellent barrier materials, as indicated by tests in the model system. They are applied in long rolls of varying widths and are also easy to cut, either with a saw while still rolled up, or with scissors when unrolled. The advantage of these materials over all others is that they can be used to prevent soil intrusion from trench or bed sidewalls as well. A layer of filter fabric can be placed around, or tacked into, excavation sidewalls before spreading the gravel during installation of field systems.

The choice of material used should be determined by cost, performance, strength and ease of application. Production costs are largely determined by the nature of both the synthetic fiber used and the fabric. Polyolefins are cheaper to manufacture than polyesters or nylon; nonwoven felts are cheaper to make than spunbonded (compressed felts whose individual strands are

Table I. Synthetic Filter Fabrics (Suggested for Use as Barrier Materials in Septic Systems)

Name	Fiber	Weave	Producer	U.S. Distributor	Efficiency[a]	Type	Approx. Cost ($\$/yd^2$)	Weight (oz/yd^2)
Typar	Polypropylene	Spunbonded	DuPont	DuPont	120	3201	0.38	2
						3301	0.55	3
						3401	0.75	4
						3601	1.00	6
Bidim	Polyester	Nonwoven	Rhone-Poulenc (France)	Monsanto	60	C-22	0.75	4.5
						C-28	0.95	6
						C-34	1.25	8
						C-38	1.55	10
						C-42	2.40	17
Mirafi	Nylon-polypropylene	Nonwoven	ICI (Britain)	Celanese	140	140	0.90	5
Supac	Polypropylene	Nonwoven	Phillips Petroleum	Phillips Fibers	120	4P	0.75	4.1
Stabilenka	Polyester	Nonwoven	Dutch ENKA (Holland)	American ENKA	40		0.68	2.5
							0.73	3.2
							1.05	4.4
Cerex	Nylon	Spunbonded	Monsanto	Monsanto	50	–	–	2
Polyfilter X	Polypropylene	Woven	Carthage Mills	Carthage Mills	210	PFX	1.75	7.2
						FX	2.55	6.6
						PFGB	2.80	12

[a] 100% retention of particles greater than given diameter (μ).

bonded by melting) or woven fabrics. The strength and performance of the materials are determined by their weight (thickness), weave and pore size. Thick felts are relatively impermeable to soils but of lower tensile and tear strength; woven materials are expensive and relatively porous; spunbonded materials are strong and relatively impermeable. Considering all factors, spunbonded polyolefins seem best suited. Unlike building paper, when spread over gravel in field systems they do not tear or rupture when walked on or when backfill soil is dumped on them. Although more expensive than the paper, they supply lasting protection to soil intrusion while allowing unhampered passage of liquids or gases through the soil. Field systems installed on sloping sites using these materials are currently being monitored and performing well, even though one trench was intentionally allowed to pond completely.

DISCUSSION AND CONCLUSIONS

The POROX process is an effective method for rehabilitating septic tank systems that have failed because of soil clogging. The process is much less expensive and far less upsetting to the users of the system and their property than replacement of the failed system. However, complicating factors such as those described above can thwart the effectiveness of the chemical treatment or expedite recurrence of failure. The process should be applied only by properly trained and licensed practitioners who have been taught safe handling of the chemicals involved, appropriate techniques for their application, proper methods of diagnosing causes of failure, and proper techniques concerning how to decide whether a treatment should be performed and how much chemical should be used. Inappropriate application of the procedure can only result in failure and disappointment and bring the process into disrepute.

In time, as the design and quality of septic tank system installations improve, the natural process of biological clogging caused by aging of systems should become the only reason for system failure, so that the applicability of the POROX process should increase. Research is continuing to determine whether there are yet other factors that complicate or frustrate application of the process and to improve diagnosis of system problems and the quality of POROX treatments.

ACKNOWLEDGMENTS

The following students and technicians assisted the author in performing many POROX treatments in field installations—the work that led to improvements in the treatment and recognition of problems with septic systems: Richard J. Apfel, Peter Glassen, David G. Kroll, Charles J. Fitzgerald and Colin P. Duffy.

REFERENCES

1. Miller, R. "Preliminary Environmental Impact Statement for Three Alternate Systems (Mounds) for Onsite Individual Wastewater Disposal in Wisconsin," Department of Health & Social Services, Madison, WI (1978).
2. Converse, J. C. "Design and Construction Manual for Wisconsin Mounds," Small Scale Waste Management Project, University of Wisconsin, Madison, WI (1978).
3. Harkin, J. M., C. J. Fitzgerald, C. P. Duffy and D. G. Kroll. "Evaluation of Mound Systems for Purification of Septic Tank Effluent," Tech. Rept. WIS WRC 79-05, Water Resources Center, University of Wisconsin, Madison, WI (1979).
4. Harkin, J. M., M. D. Jawson and F. G. Baker. "Causes and Remedy of Failure of Septic Tank Seepage Systems," in *Individual Onsite Wastewater Systems, Proceedings of the Second National Conference,* (Ann Arbor, MI: Ann Arbor Science Publishers, Inc., 1976), pp. 119-124.
5. McGauhey, P. H., and J. T. Winneberger. "A Study of Methods of Preventing Failure of Septic Tank Percolation Systems," SERL Rept. No. 67-17, Sanitary Engineering Research Laboratory, University of California, Berkeley, CA (1967).
6. Jones, J. H., and G. S. Taylor. "Septic Tank Effluent Percolation Through Sands Under Laboratory Conditions,' *Soil Sci.* 99:301-309 (1965).
7. De Vries, J. "Soil Filtration of Wastewater Effluent and the Mechanism of Pore Clogging," *J. Water Poll. Control Fed.* 44:565-573 (1972).
8. Richards, S. J. "Soil Suction Measurements with Tensiometers," in *Methods of Soil Analysis,* Vol. 1, C. A. Black, Ed., American Society of Agronomy, Madison, WI (1965), pp. 153-163.
9. Harkin, J. M. "Method for Treating Septic Tank Effluent Seepage Beds and the Like," U.S. Pat. 4,021,338, assigned to the Wisconsin Alumni Research Foundation, Madison, WI (May 1977).
10. Wisconsin State Board of Health. "Wisconsin Administrative Code H62.20," Madison, WI (1976).
11. Laak, R. "Pollutant Loads from Plumbing Fixtures and Pretreatment to Control Soil Clogging," *J. Environ. Health* 39(1):48-51 (1976).
12. Siegrist, R., M. W. Witt and W. C. Boyle. "The Characteristics of Rural Household Wastewater," *J. Environ. Eng. Div., ASCE* 102:533-548 (1976).
13. Harkin, J. M. "Lignins," in *Chemistry and Biochemistry of Herbage,* Vol. 1, R. W. Bailey and G. W. Butler, Eds. (New York: Academic Press, Inc.), pp. 323-373.
14. Wenzl, H. F. J. *Kraft Pulping Theory and Practice* (New York: Lockwood Publishing Co., 1967).

40

ONSITE SYSTEMS MANAGEMENT

Thomas E. Shannon
Executive Vice President
Thetford Corporation
Ann Arbor, Michigan 48106

INTRODUCTION

This chapter focuses on suggestions for improving communications among the manufacturers and developers of alternative systems, the respective regulatory bodies and the buying public, which includes the engineering professions, construction industry, architects, developers, financial communities, and the ultimate customer for products and systems that are innovative in the sanitation industry.

First it will be helpful to review the current situation—the problems confronting the manufacturer, the position of the regulatory bodies and the disposition of the purchaser. Perhaps the best way to approach this task is simply to relate some experiences, to indicate what has and has not worked, and why it did or did not.

THE NEED

Utmost in the minds of the manufacturer or developer of onsite products must be his vision of what the conditions and situations can be. He must be able to "look over the wall."

In the United States in 1979 $5,500,000,000 was spent in public and private funds for devices to accept and dispose of sanitary wastes. In addition,

$26 million will be spent on alternative onsite treatment systems. Somewhere between 60 and 70% of this nation's land mass is unpercable. This is especially true of the more attractive land sites in mountainous areas, adjacent to lakes and streams, and along our beautiful shorelines. Urban sprawl has reached proportions that have caused state governments to discontinue the use of funds set aside by the Department of Agriculture for subsidizing housing. Too much farm land was being usurped for residential developments. In addition to the 1,700,000 homes built in 1979, commercial, industrial and institutional building starts were up 12% over 1978. Prices for percable land or land serviced by sanitary sewers soared to prices 30% above 1978 prices.

Moritoria for both freshwater service and sewer service reached all-time highs during this period. These statistics indicate a burgeoning demand. Evidence of the strength of this demand was experienced recently. A single release in a popular science magazine elicited 30,000 inquiries from the readers who were promised an onsite waste treatment system that would allow them to build anywhere in a safe, reliable and ecological manner.

TAKING ADVANTAGE OF THE SITUATION

Where there is an exceptional need for a solution, there is also a business opportunity; and, like any business opportunity, the same criteria for success are applicable. The product must fill the need for those persons who will buy it. It must be reliable, with the quality characteristics expected by our technical society. It must meet the requirements proscribed by our regulatory agencies and be economically feasible to operate and maintain. Society has always set up a review to control the introduction of new products and developments. Unfortunately, this review seems both circuitous and redundant. Too often we condemn our regulatory and professional groups as being too conservative and bureaucratic. Innovative, onsite alternative sanitation systems must be classed as business development ventures.

Throughout history such enterprises have experienced the same resistance or hesitancy. For example, in Charles Dickens' *A Little Dorrit*, the author conjured a department in London referred to as the Office of Circumlocution. The Office of Circumlocution's purpose was to consider matters in such a way that they would become lost in endless circles. All matters that came up for consideration were destined never to come out, but to be captured in the never-ending rounds of review. It has already been mentioned that to be successful in this innovative industry one must take the longer view. In addition to this broader perspective, a realistic and scientific approach is required. In an attempt to develop this approach, an analysis of the buying process might help.

CONSENSUS PURCHASE

Every sale involves a multiple-purchase decision and a multiple-sale decision. In each case there is a chain of customers to convince, beginning with a consulting engineer, then the regulatory body (usually a sanitarian), the architect, the contractor, the developer, the lending source, and finally the owner or purchaser of the property or building. It is a multiple-sale situation because the seller is dependent not only on his own selling efforts to influence the positive decision, but also on each participant in the selling chain to sell each of the other participants. This is true of most every new product and is not exclusive to the innovator of a sanitation system.

Too often it is forgotten that as much time and resources of the marketing sales variety are required as the technical expenditures. The manufacturer is frustrated when the prospective participants in the acceptance chain are not readily convinced of the "magnificent" benefits of his product. Anxiety reaches high proportions and sometimes is converted to anger and hostility because of the slow acceptance, which then may create doubt and negative response on the part of the potential consumer. How many times is a manufacturer or developer told by an important decision-maker that he has seen many such "paper toilets," that they simply do not work and that he is not going to be the guinea pig? The manufacturer then is convinced that the consumer's mind is closed and the manufacturer becomes the victim of a modern-day Office of Circumlocution.

These negative responses and feelings are not peculiar to the alternative sanitation industry. The July 1979 issue of *Chemical and Engineering News* contained a reference to a recent meeting of the Club of Rome. In the Club's most recent proceedings, a paper was presented indicating that society's acceptance lagged almost twelve years behind innovation. This is only the sixth conference of *this* type. It is only realistic to approach the marketplace and the regulatory environment knowing that a period of time must pass before the technology will be given equal treatment to traditional sewerage.

Ralph Biggadike [1] has pointed out that a positive return on investment usually does not occur until the eighth year after the product is introduced. He also suggests that an equivalent amount of money is required for marketing as for the technical development. In addition to the quantity of resources required to launch a unique product, the quality of the introduction is just as important. Innovation and creativity in addressing the sales, distribution, pricing and promotion of a new product are equally as perplexing as the technical considerations. Everyone realizes that society does not beat an eager path to the new improved mousetrap, regardless how useful or unique it might be; the societal acceptance model slows down the rate of return.

Since its beginning in 1965, the Thetford Corporation has been introducing new and innovative products. At no time has a product been instantly successful; rather, it normally takes at least three years before there seems to be a modicum of acceptance. The more complex the product, the longer the time before it receives recognition and the more delicate the introductory approach should be, especially for technological products. There is definitely an etiquette and a discretion required in the introduction of a product of the variety discussed at this conference. Without careful documentation and sensitivity to the scientific community and regulatory bodies, a marketing venture is doomed, especially if a product is developed *before* looking for a market. Even if the product fits precisely the needs of a marketplace, a lengthy period of trial and error is necessary to find the formula of words and presentations that will cause the marketplace to recognize its benefits.

Sanitary Products

The above applies particularly to sanitary devices and systems. There are inhibitions in society regarding discussing, buying or selling products related to human elimination and disposal. To discover what the customer really wants and needs in a sanitary system and what society will accept and buy is a very perplexing problem. Years of advance market research and prototype testing are required. Many anxieties and fears are associated with products relating to public health. Although these are easily overlooked, nevertheless they are essential to adaptation. It is important that the proposition of the product be put into words, pictures and presentations that are crystal clear and simple enough to the purchaser to stimulate the need. Much scientific investigation is necessary to develop clean, clear and simple messages that convince the person who will expend the resources for the innovation. To introduce a product that involves educating the public for acceptance entails even greater difficulty. Today, no one questions that a refrigerator satisfies a specific need, nor is there any special education required on the part of the buyer to purchase a refrigerator. It was twelve years before electric refrigerators began to sell in a large enough quantity to encourage large investments for mass distribution. The same period of time was required for the acceptance of the telephone, and the light bulb was accepted only after many years of promotion and education. Oddly enough, these products are now manufactured and distributed by industrial giants. They were introduced, developed and pioneered by companies no larger than those represented at this conference. This is true of many innovations.

Dr. Frank Press, advisor to the President of the United States on scientific matters, recently made this point and indicated that the patent law was being amended to encourage the small company. In a recent monograph published by the Chase Manhattan Bank, the same point was made that innovation was truly the product of the smaller company. Xerox and Polaroid originally were struggling ventures led by entrepreneurial manager–scientists with visions. Even the fast-food industry struggled for years before the "Big Mac" reached the million plateau or Colonel Sanders became a household name.

STEREOTYPE SELLING

The Thetford Corporation has discovered that it takes almost eleven sales calls to the prospective customer before he is convinced enough to sign a purchase order. This is four times as much effort as is required for the sale of a more traditional product such as the Porta Potti®. The stereotype approach will not sell a Cycle-Let®.

First, a problem-solving environment must be established. The relationship with the prospective buyer or regulatory person can proceed only after a relationship of mutual participation and trust has been established. The salesperson involved needs special skills—only about one out of twenty seems to fit the mold. In addition to problem-solving skills, this individual must have patience, special talents in empathy, and a definite and credible technical approach.

Few discussions of value are less than two and a half hours long. Presenting the product proposition too soon will foreclose the opportunity. The sanitarian or consulting engineer will not be overpowered by facts, figures and testimonials. His interest and acceptance attitudes will not be triggered until he is convinced that the product solves a problem he is faced with and that the manufacturer is genuinely interested in helping him solve it.

Problems cannot be solved when feelings are very strong. Therefore, a certain behavior is necessary to show that the manufacturer is interested in obtaining the customer's ideas and opinions and wants to incorporate them in the decision-making process. Allowing input and recognizing the productive ideas on the part of the decision-maker is extremely important. New product marketing is characterized by this problem-solving climate, as opposed to the traditional or "systems" selling effort. Cutting off the prospect's ideas or objections, discarding his ideas, nonlistening attitudes, and an appearance of being too interested in getting a sale to worry about his feelings forever damage the relationship. Unfortunately, this has been true of too many charlatans and fast-buck operators who merely have pretended to have onsite solutions. All too many of us have had to listen to lengthy horror stories of systems that were abandoned by the manufacturer. If the presentation of the product could be characterized in two words it would be *helpful listening*.

Helpful Listening

Among others, helpful listening includes the following traits:

1. Invites theories, ideas and questions on the part of the prospect.
2. Organizes the information in a most courteous and logical manner.
3. Allows for an explanation of all the objections.
4. Reviews the details of the discussion.
5. Refocuses the discussion by persistently tracking the key issues as indicated by the customer.
6. Develops a congenial environment that allows for sharing of the true and deep-felt objections, fears and needs on the part of the participants, which is the essence of the meeting.

This is true not only of selling innovative sanitation products and systems, but of all business development ventures. Business development is characterized by the problem-solving and information-exchanging strategies. To ignore this fact is to invite failure. To accept this proposition and to adhere to these suggestions might be fruitful. A careful look at the statistics presented briefly at the beginning of this presentation reveals the great opportunity for those who have the perseverance and imagination to pursue the onsite endeavor.

CONCLUSIONS

Manufacturers of alternative and innovative systems are on the first wave of a new technology, participating in an industry that is alive and well and will become more healthy. Even in its infancy, it is populated by such exceptional professionals as inventors, scientists, business people and educators. These professionals need to adhere to the ethics and etiquette that have been portrayed in many other successful new ventures. This report has attempted to present the obligations and situations confronting the manufacturer of alternative and innovative waste treatment products. There is also an equal obligation on the part of the decision-makers to consider these products according to the same etiquette and ethics. Together they can participate in solving the major health problem facing society with fresh technology that promises the most ecological and economical resolution.

REFERENCES

1. Biggadike, R. "The Risky Business of Diversification," *Harvard Bus. Rev.* (May-June 1979).

INDEX